Mentorship in Veterinary Medicine

Mentorship in Veterinary Medicine

Edited by

Dani Rabwin, DVM
Ready, Vet, Go
Benicia, CA, USA

WILEY

Published by John Wiley & Sons, Inc., Hoboken, New Jersey.

Library of Congress Cataloging-in-Publication Data
Names: Rabwin, Dani, 1977- editor
Title: Mentorship in veterinary medicine / edited by Dani Rabwin, DVM.
Description: Hoboken, New Jersey : Wiley, [2027] | Includes index.
Identifiers: LCCN 2026022424 (print) | LCCN 2026022425 (ebook) | ISBN 9781394335381 Paperback | ISBN 9781394335404 adobe pdf | ISBN 9781394335398 epub
Subjects: LCSH: Veterinary medicine–Vocational guidance | Mentoring in medicine
Classification: LCC SF756.28 .M46 2027 (print) | LCC SF756.28 (ebook)
LC record available at https://lccn.loc.gov/2026022424
LC ebook record available at https://lccn.loc.gov/2026022425

Cover Design: Wiley
Cover Images: VTT Studio/Shutterstock, The Good Brigade/Getty Images

Set in 9.5/12pt STIXTwoText by Straive, Pondicherry, India

Printed and bound by CPI Group (UK) Ltd, Croydon, CR0 4YY

C978139433581_250826

For Buff and for the Ready, Vet, Go mentors, mentees, and community.

Contents

List of Contributors

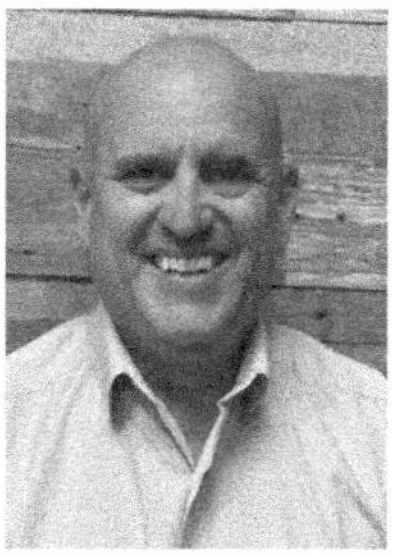

Gershon L. Alaluf DVM MBA DBA
Canyon Animal Management, Laguna Beach, CA, USA

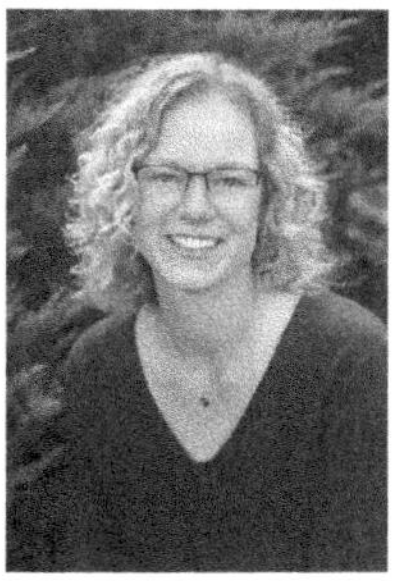

Kelly C. Cooper DVM
Reality Vet Coaching & Consulting, Oregon City, OR, USA

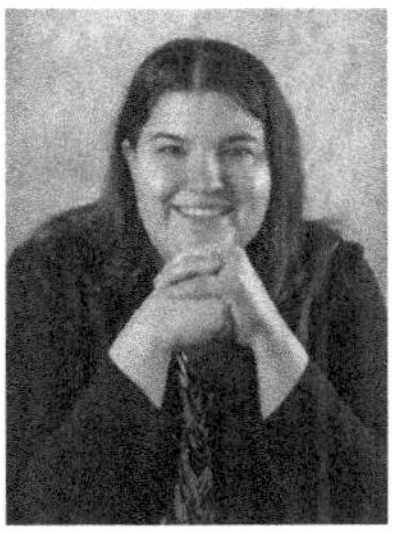

Kate Boatright VMD
KMB Veterinary Media LLC, Grove City, PA, USA

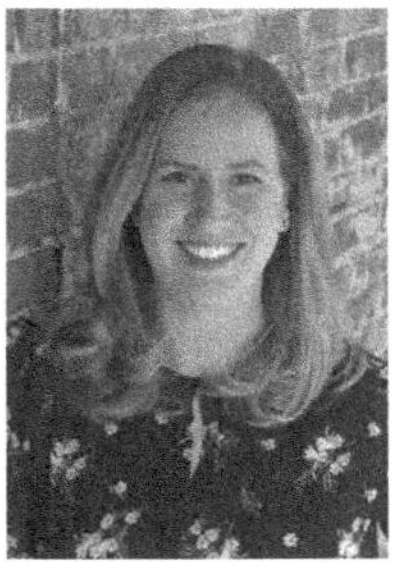

Caitlin DeWilde DVM
The Social DVM, St. Louis, MO, United States

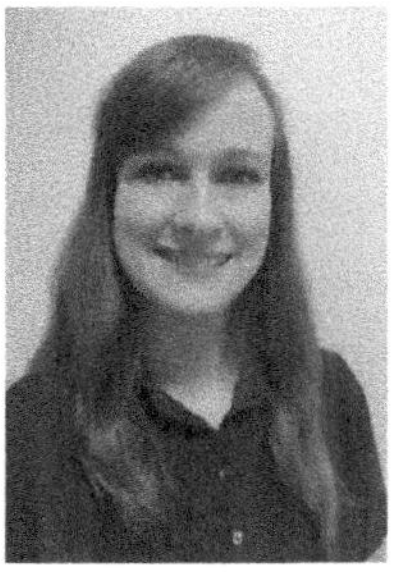

Wrenn Calcutt DVM
North Canton, OH, USA

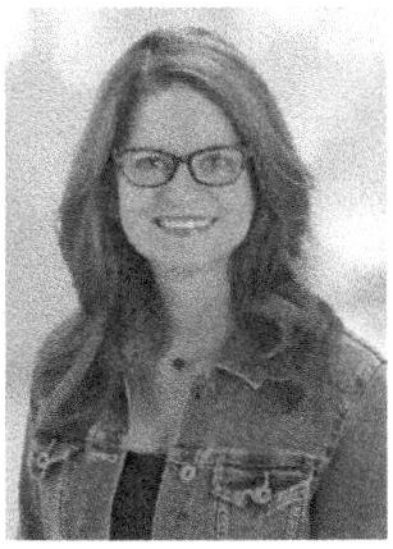

Amanda L. Donnelly DVM, MBA
ALD Veterinary Consulting, LLC, Rockledge, FL, USA

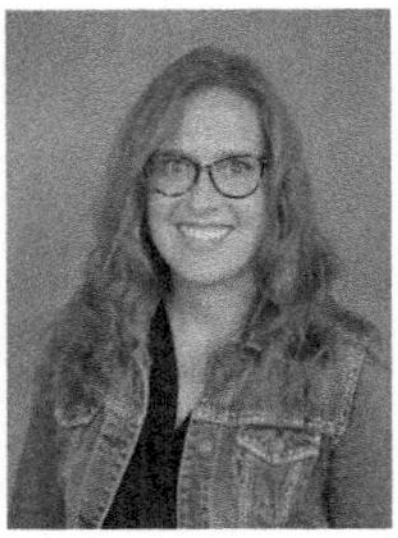

Lauren Forsythe PharmD, MBA, DICVP
University of Findlay, Findlay, OH, USA
and Foresight Pharma Solutions, LLC,
Findlay, OH, USA

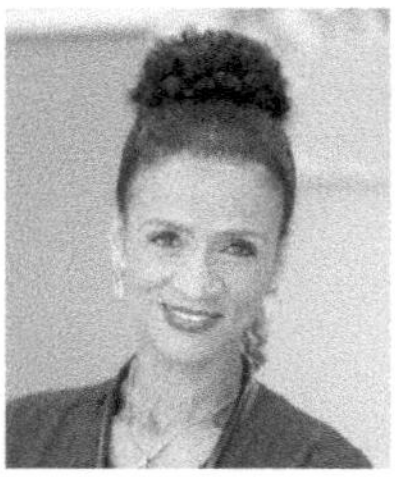

Pam Hale DVM, MBA, JM
VetLeader Coaching/Consulting Chief Medical
Officer, Marietta, GA, USA

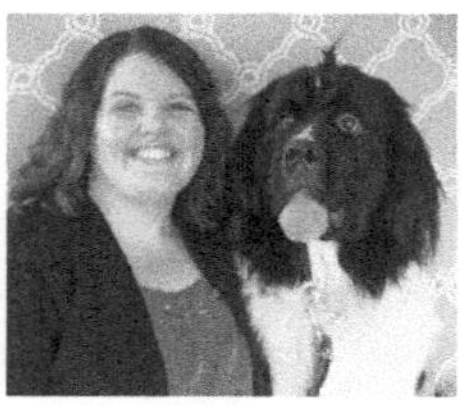

Lindsey Hedges-Gieseking DVM
Mission Pet Health, Homewood,
AL, USA

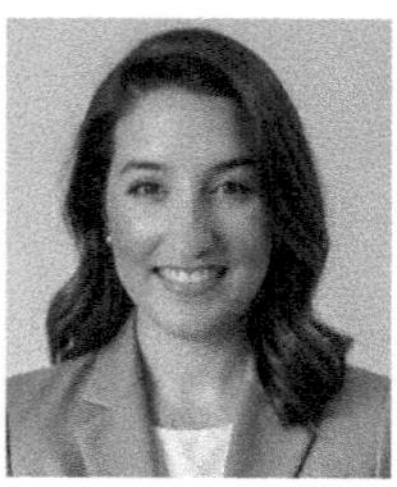

Mariel Hendricks MVEd, RVTg, FVTE
MentorVet, Lexington, KY, USA

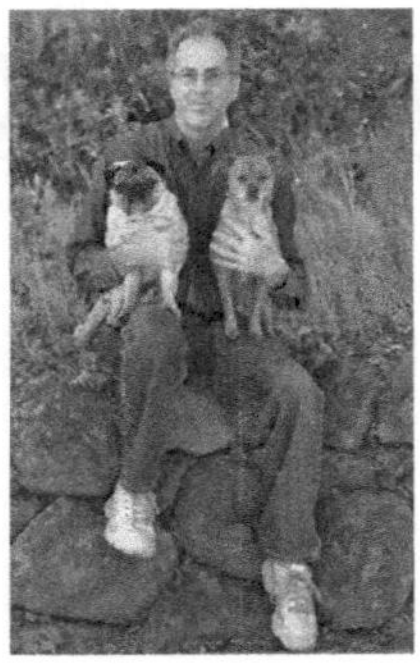

Barry Kipperman DVM, DACVIM, MSc,
DACAW
UC Davis, Davis, CA, USA and University of
Missouri, Columbia, MO, USA

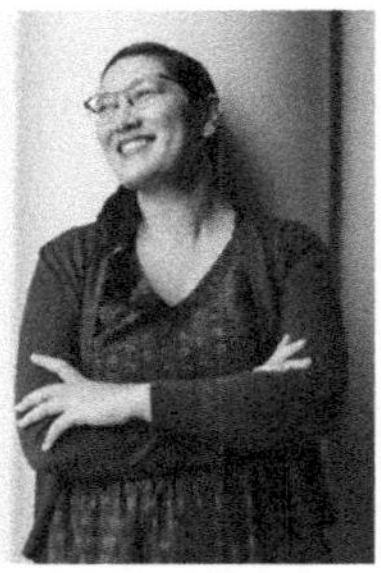

Erika Lin-Hendel VMD, PhD
Empathy at Large, LLC, San Jose, CA, USA

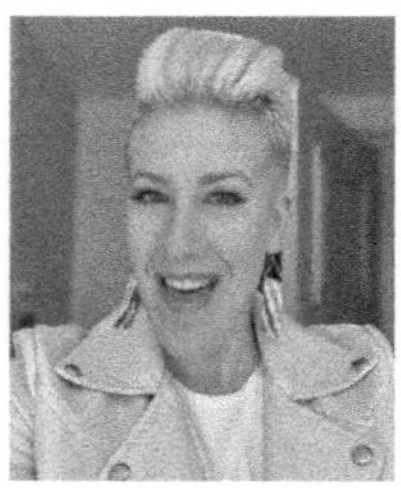

Alyssa C. Mages BS, CVT, FVTE
Empowering Veterinary Teams, Burlington,
NJ, USA; MentorVet, Lexington, KY, USA;
and Project Sticker Chicago, IL, USA

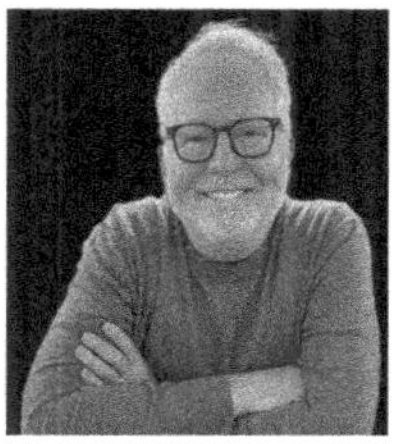

Gary Marshall DVM
Feline Practitioner, Mentor, Educator
Beaux Arts Village, WA, USA

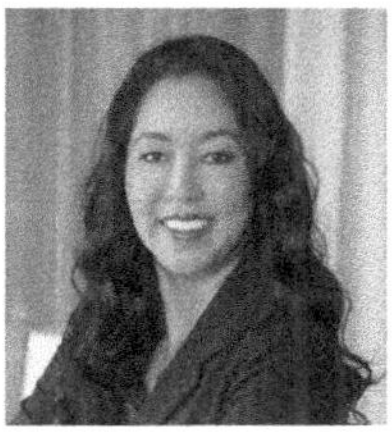

Jill Muraoka DVM
Islander Veterinary Business Consultants, LLC, Ventura, CA, USA

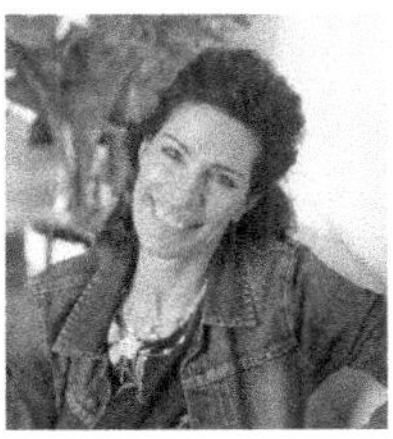

Sonja A. Olson DVM
Heartstorming Wellness, LLC, Vancouver, WA, USA

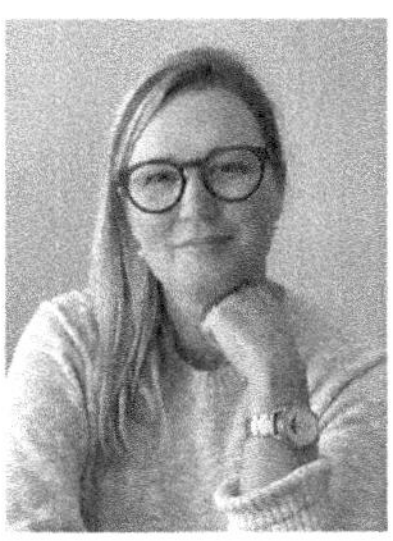

Jessica Petty EdD
Senior Director Pet Preventive Care Marketing (Boehringer Ingelheim), Nashville, TN, USA

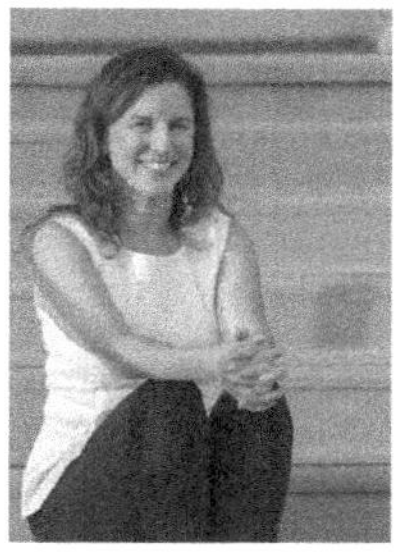

Dani Rabwin DVM
Ready, Vet, Go
Benicia, CA, USA

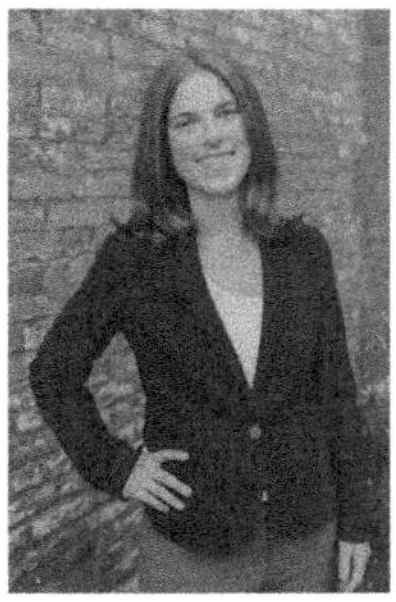

Addie Reinhard DVM, MS
MentorVet, Lexington, KY, USA

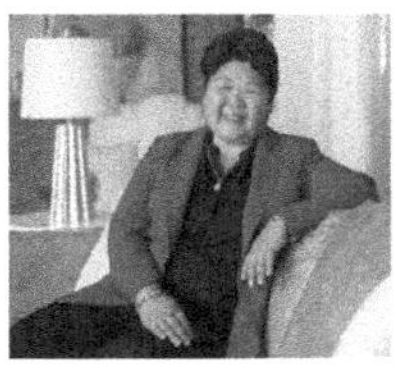

Janis Shinkawa DVM, CPA
Islander Veterinary Business Consultants, LLC, Ventura, CA, USA

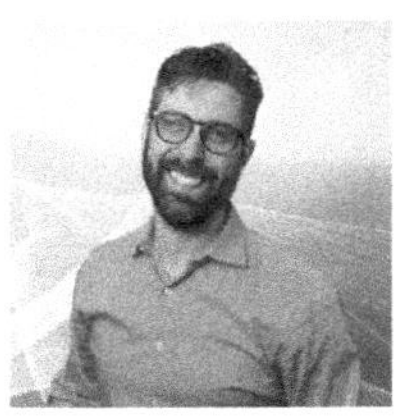

Ron Sosa CVPM, CCFP, PgD-CLD
Uncharted Veterinary Conference, Greenville, SC, USA; Syn-APT Leadership & Coaching
Fort Mill, SC, USA

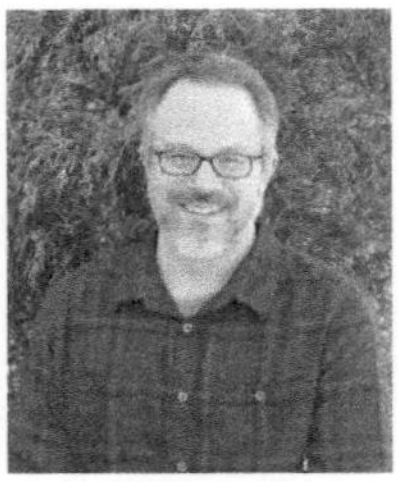

Daniel Stillwell PhD, LMFT
MentorVet, Lexington, KY, USA

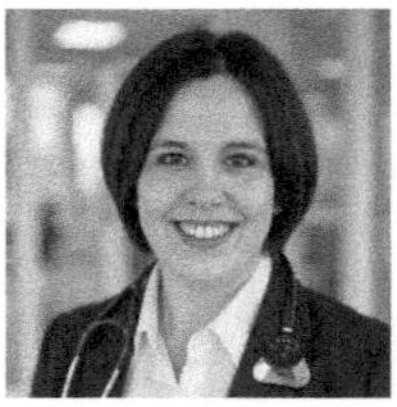

Legend A. Thurman DVM, MSL, CVBP
MRCVS
GoodVets, Chicago, IL, USA

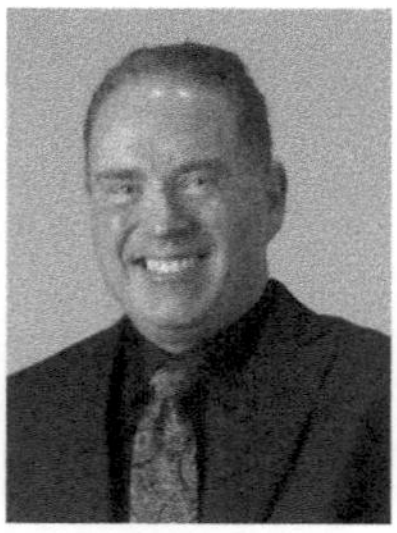

James Townend B.Admin/Econ Certified Life
Coach-Canadian Coaching Federation
Owner Operator ASD Life Coaching, Airdrie,
AB, Canada

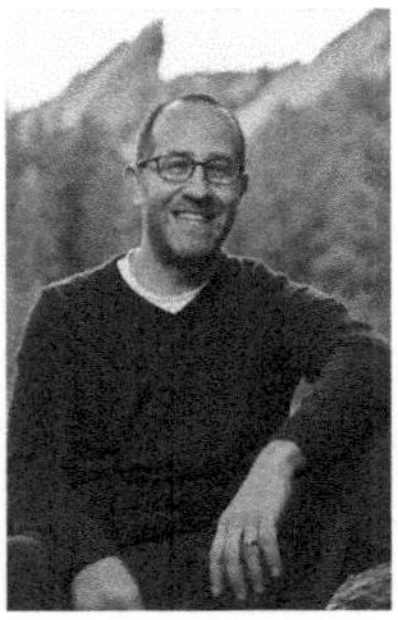

Josh Vaisman MAPPCP, CCFP
Flourish Veterinary Consulting, Boulder,
CO, USA

Foreword

Mentorship, an often-overlooked yet transformative force, quietly shapes the landscape of veterinary medicine. More often, it shows up in the in-between moments. Mentorship is a steady voice after a hard case, a debrief that turns shame into learning, a colleague who says, "I've been there. Let's figure it out together."

That is the spirit of *Mentorship in Veterinary Medicine*, edited by Dr. Dani Rabwin, a practicing veterinarian and mentorship educator whose work has helped make support for veterinary professionals more intentional and more accessible. After graduating from UC Davis School of Veterinary Medicine in 2004, Dr. Rabwin built a career in small-animal general and emergency practice, with clinical interests in abdominal ultrasound and clinical pathology/cytology. (I'm also keeping her credentials here because mentorship is strongest when it's grounded in real clinical experience.)

Dr. Rabwin's mentorship journey accelerated in 2020, when she began creating Ready, Vet, Go, a structured, cohort-style mentorship program designed to support early-career veterinarians through guided learning, community, and practical coaching. The program's philosophy is key—mentorship should be structured, consistent, and integral to team support, not left to chance or personality.

This matters because veterinary medicine is a field that is both technical and deeply human. We diagnose, treat, and manage complex chronic disease, but the most defining moments often involve people: clients making painful choices, teams navigating conflict, leaders setting priorities under constraint, and clinicians absorbing grief that can accumulate quietly over time. In both clinical and nonclinical settings, outcomes depend on trust and relationship-building.

This trust is built through psychological safety: the shared understanding that the veterinary health care team is encouraged to ask questions, admit uncertainty, report a mistake early, and name a concern without fear of humiliation. Psychological safety isn't the absence of high standards. It's what allows clinical excellence to be achieved. When a new graduate says, "I'm not sure about this ultrasound finding," the patient benefits. When a technician says, "This dosing feels off. Can we double-check?" the patient benefits. When a team member says, "I'm not okay. Can we talk?" the person, the team, and the practice benefit.

That kind of safety requires vulnerability, and vulnerability requires skill. Emotional intelligence, the ability to notice what you're feeling, regulate it, and respond with empathy and clarity, matters as much in a client's concern as it does in a post-op complication. Honesty in the mentorship process matters, too: formative feedback that is specific and kind, reflection that separates a mistake from a moral failure, and the willingness to say, "I don't know yet, but I will learn." Support is not simply reassurance. It is guidance, accountability, and follow-through, especially when the work is heavy and the stakes feel personal.

Mentorship also takes many forms, and *Mentorship in Veterinary Medicine* acknowledges that range. Sometimes mentorship is formal and includes scheduled check-ins, clear learning goals, structured case review, and coaching that complements what a practice can provide during a busy day. And sometimes mentorship is informal and includes a five-minute "how did that conversation go?" in the treatment area, a shared script before a difficult phone call, an invitation to debrief instead of an expectation to "just move on." And sometimes it is peer support: early-career veterinarians learning side-by-side, technicians mentoring technicians, associates sharing what they've learned the hard way, leaders creating space for hard truths rather than performative confidence.

Mentorship is distinct from supervision. Supervision asks, "Can you do this task safely today?" while mentorship adds, "Who are you becoming as you learn to do it and how can we help you grow?" The "we" matters. Sustainable mentorship doesn't rely on one heroic mentor, it is woven into a practice's norms. Mentorship includes how questions are welcomed, how mistakes are handled, how wins are recognized, and how people are supported from uncertainty into competence over time.

If you are mentoring someone now, thank you. You are not just shaping a skill set, you are nurturing the future of veterinary medicine. You are shaping confidence, clinical judgment, and belonging. And if you are seeking mentorship, this book is a reminder that you deserve it—not as a luxury, but as a cornerstone of excellent veterinary medicine and to help you thrive in the world's greatest profession.

Christina V. Tran, DVM
Executive Associate Dean & Clinical Professor
Roseman University of Health Sciences
College of Veterinary Medicine (proposed)

Preface

For over two decades in practice, I have watched early-career veterinarians enter the profession full of hope, skill, and compassion, only to leave their first practice or the profession entirely, far too soon. Again and again, I've heard the same story: "I didn't get the mentorship I was promised." Those words have shaped the direction of my own work and inspired this book.

As a clinician, mentor, and founder of a mentorship program and community for early-career veterinarians, I've seen what happens when mentorship is done well and when it isn't. Effective mentorship has the power to change not only an individual's experience but also the health and sustainability of our entire profession. Yet mentorship remains inconsistently defined, inconsistently delivered, and too often dependent on luck rather than design.

This book was born from the belief that we can, and must, do better. It brings together voices from across veterinary medicine and beyond to explore what modern mentorship looks like when it is intentional, inclusive, and grounded in evidence. Together, these chapters bridge the gap between theory and practice, offering mentors the tools to build programs and relationships that truly support early-career veterinarians.

The work of mentorship is never finished—it evolves alongside our profession. My hope is that this book not only informs but also sparks ongoing conversation and innovation as we continue learning together.

It has been a joy and a privilege to collaborate with so many leaders in this space. The contributors to this book have been generous with their time, patient through the process, and deeply committed to helping others grow. I am profoundly grateful for their insight and humbled by how much I have learned from each of them.

And now, as I tell my mentees: go out and have fun—you've got this!

Dani Rabwin, DVM
Editor

Acknowledgments

This book exists because of the generosity, curiosity, and commitment of many people who believe deeply in mentorship, care deeply about the veterinary profession, and believed in me enough to help bring this work to life.

I am profoundly grateful to the chapter authors who contributed their voices, expertise, and lived experience to this book. Each chapter reflects thoughtful engagement with complex issues, and together they offer a rich and practical exploration of what modern mentorship can, and should, look like in veterinary medicine.

I also want to thank the colleagues who participated in early virtual mastermind conversations in 2024, which helped shape this project in its earliest stages. Those discussions—often candid, occasionally challenging, and always thoughtful—played a critical role in refining the questions this book seeks to address. Many of those contributions came from individuals who are not listed as chapter authors, but their influence is woven throughout these pages.

My thanks as well to the editorial and publishing team for their guidance, patience, and steady support throughout a complex, multiauthored process.

This book was very much a family effort, and I am deeply grateful for their support throughout the process. My mom, Karen, has been my greatest cheerleader throughout this process, and my dad, Paul—ever the grammar police—served as a trusted unofficial editor, keeping a careful eye on clarity, precision, and the occasional errant comma. My sister, Amy, and brother-in-law, Dave, provided much-needed comic relief during stressful moments and reminded me not to take myself too seriously. My son, Zack, brought his attention to detail—and healthy skepticism of artificial intelligence—by helping to check citations. I am also thankful to my partner, Krista, whose moral support, academic perspective, and steady encouragement sustained and encouraged me from start to finish.

Finally, I am grateful to the mentors, mentees, and community of Ready, Vet, Go, whose vulnerability, generosity, and willingness to engage in honest conversation helped shape the direction of this work and gave new meaning to my professional life beyond the clinic.

The Mentorship Gap

CHAPTER 1

INTRODUCTION

Dani Rabwin

Veterinary medicine faces significant challenges that threaten both workforce sustainability and professional well-being. Nearly half of new graduates leave their first position within two years (Gates et al., 2020), with over 70% departing their initial employer within several years of graduation (Jelinski et al., 2009). When asked why, most point to the same factor: inadequate mentorship. This pattern has persisted for over a decade, and the consequences extend far beyond individual career disappointments. The systemic breakdown in early-career support costs the profession an estimated $2 billion annually (Neill et al., 2022), while contributing to alarming rates of burnout, compassion fatigue, and mental health challenges among veterinarians.

At the heart of these challenges lies a fundamental misunderstanding of what modern veterinary mentorship needs to accomplish. This chapter will demonstrate how the gap between what practices currently offer and what early-career practitioners actually need is driving talented veterinarians from their first jobs and sometimes from the profession itself. Practices often provide either informal and inconsistent traditional approaches or overly rigid programs focused primarily on clinical checklists and productivity metrics, when new graduates need structured yet comprehensive support that addresses not only medical expertise but also professional well-being, emotional resilience, and career satisfaction. Through evidence-based research and real case studies, we'll explore how mentorship must evolve beyond the apprenticeship model to create reliable, sustainable foundations for veterinary careers.

THE MENTORSHIP GAP

In the evolving landscape of veterinary medicine, a troubling pattern has emerged. Many practices proudly advertise mentorship programs, but these often fall into two problematic extremes: either overly rigid, checklist-driven approaches that ignore individual needs or completely unstructured arrangements that provide few opportunities for meaningful guidance. As one recent graduate puts it, "They promised mentorship during the interview, but what they meant was someone to ask questions to between appointments. I needed so much more than that." This sentiment reflects a more fundamental problem: mentees frequently report not receiving the mentorship that was promised during recruitment. Each early-career veterinarian requires different types and levels of support based on their prior experiences, professional goals, and personal challenges. Some may need intensive clinical guidance, while others may seek help with client communication or work–life integration (Figure 1.1).

This disconnect stems from a fundamental misunderstanding of modern mentorship needs, often leading to frustration for both the mentor and the mentee. Practices may focus on clinical skills' checklists and technical proficiency, while new graduates consistently report needing support in areas such as client communication, work–life balance, emotional resilience, and professional identity development. Research backs these concerns: mentoring programs that include communication skills' training improve confidence and client relationships (Elce, 2021),

WHAT PRACTICES THINK MENTORSHIP IS:	WHAT NEW GRADS SAY THEY NEED:
Open Door Checklists Case Rounds	Communication Support Work-life Balance Emotional Resilience

FIGURE 1.1 The mentorship disconnect.

while structured mentorship addressing work–life balance and resilience reduces burnout (Mastenbroek et al., 2015). Yet when early-career veterinarians leave, citing a "lack of mentorship," practice owners and managers often respond with genuine bewilderment. "But we were providing mentorship!" they protest, pointing to open-door policies, case rounds, or availability for questions. Multiple surveys underscore how significant this gap is, showing that lack of mentorship is one of the most common reasons new graduates leave their first job (Jelinski et al., 2009; Gates et al., 2020). The problem lies in misaligned definitions and expectations. What owners view as adequate (being available for questions) often feels insufficient to a new graduate seeking not only clinical guidance but also emotional support, professional development, and help toward navigating practice culture and team dynamics.

THE FINANCIAL COST OF FAILED MENTORSHIP

The costs of inadequate mentorship extend far beyond financial metrics—impacting veterinarian well-being, team morale, and the sustainability of the profession itself. Yet even examining the financial implications alone reveals the scope of this challenge. A comprehensive 2022 study analyzing data from 5786 associate veterinarians found that burnout alone costs the veterinary industry between $1.57 and $2.33 billion annually when including both veterinarians and technicians, representing nearly 4% of the entire industry's value (Neill et al., 2022). The study revealed that 86.7% of US veterinarians had moderate or high burnout scores, with median replacement costs of $104,000 per veterinarian—figures that encompass recruitment, onboarding, and lost productivity during an average 40-day vacancy period. These individual costs compound across the profession, with turnover costs proving nearly twice as expensive as reduced working hours, creating substantial industry-wide losses that far exceed what practices might invest in comprehensive mentorship programs.

Even more conservative models suggest that replacing a team member can cost 50–75% of their salary, depending on their specialization (Veterinary Business Matters, 2018). The VetPartners Veterinary Team Utilization Guide further underscores how improper support and poor role utilization amplify these costs, driving inefficiency and accelerating attrition (VetPartners, 2022). Ultimately, what may begin as an attempt to save time or dollars by skimping on structured mentorship ends up costing far more when staff leave and disrupt client continuity, team morale, and practice operations.

Too often, practices try to bridge this gap with money. Sign-on bonuses, while attractive, cannot substitute for meaningful mentorship. As one practice manager observed, "We can offer all the bonuses we want, but if we're not providing the support structure these doctors need, they'll take the bonus and be gone within a year." This economic reality aligns with research showing that organizational interventions are significantly more effective than individual-level approaches for addressing burnout, underscoring why practices must invest in systematic support systems rather than expecting individual veterinarians to manage professional challenges alone (Neill et al., 2022).

MISALIGNED EXPECTATIONS IN PRACTICE

The reasons new graduates leave their first jobs often trace back to unmet expectations around mentorship. Surveys over many years reinforce this point: mentorship consistently ranks as the most valuable nonmonetary feature new graduates seek when evaluating jobs (Jelinski et al., 2009). New graduates frequently cite the lack of protected time for mentorship activities, noting that promised mentorship sessions get squeezed out by busy appointment schedules. Despite having time specifically blocked for mentorship, they find these crucial sessions are often sacrificed to accommodate "emergency" appointments or to meet daily revenue targets. As one new graduate explained, "Every time my mentor and I were supposed to meet, someone would say 'But this client really needs to be seen today,' or 'We're a little behind on our monthly goals.' Eventually, I stopped even expecting the mentorship time to happen."

This short-sighted prioritization of immediate demands over long-term development carries significant consequences. While fitting in an extra appointment might help meet that day's metrics or satisfy an anxious client, this approach gradually erodes the foundation of support new graduates need to thrive. They express frustration at missed learning opportunities—from having insufficient time to discuss challenging medical cases to losing chances to scrub in with a mentor on surgeries they need to master. Many reports limited support for both clinical and professional development, while others point to the absence of clear mentorship structure or goals. Perhaps most tellingly, there's often a stark misalignment between the mentorship promised during interviews and what's actually delivered in practice. **Practice leaders who sacrifice mentorship time to meet immediate operational goals often find themselves facing much larger operational challenges when their early-career veterinarians leave, creating a cycle of increased stress, higher costs, and greater instability for the entire practice.**

SCALE AND STRUCTURE CHALLENGES

The evolution of veterinary practice ownership presents both opportunities and challenges for mentorship. Once dominated by independent clinics, the profession has undergone rapid consolidation. Corporate groups now own roughly a quarter of general practices and three-quarters of specialty clinics, representing close to half of US veterinary care market share (AAHA, 2023). Broader analyses estimate that 25–50% of all practices are now corporately managed (American Economic Liberties Project, 2025). Larger organizations may be able to leverage their scale to develop structured mentorship programs and cross-location networks, while smaller practices remain well positioned to deliver highly personalized, relationship-driven support. Regardless of ownership model, the challenge and opportunity lie in building mentorship frameworks that combine structure with the individualized guidance new graduates' need.

However, delivering personalized mentorship at scale requires thoughtful planning and resource allocation. Organizations must balance efficiency with individualization, finding ways to maintain the personal connection that makes mentorship effective while operating within broader structured frameworks. Success depends on several key elements working in concert. Organizations need to create protected time for mentorship within busy clinical schedules and to develop flexible frameworks that can adapt to individual needs. They must build systems to connect mentees with mentors across multiple locations while supporting those mentors with proper training and resources to excel in their roles. Equally important is the implementation of systems to measure mentorship outcomes, allowing for continuous program improvement and refinement (Figure 1.2).

Both large organizations and independent practices increasingly recognize the value of supplementing their internal mentorship with structured external programs. Remote mentorship platforms provide comprehensive support that complements in-house mentoring. These programs offer structured curriculum covering both clinical and nonclinical skills while providing access to

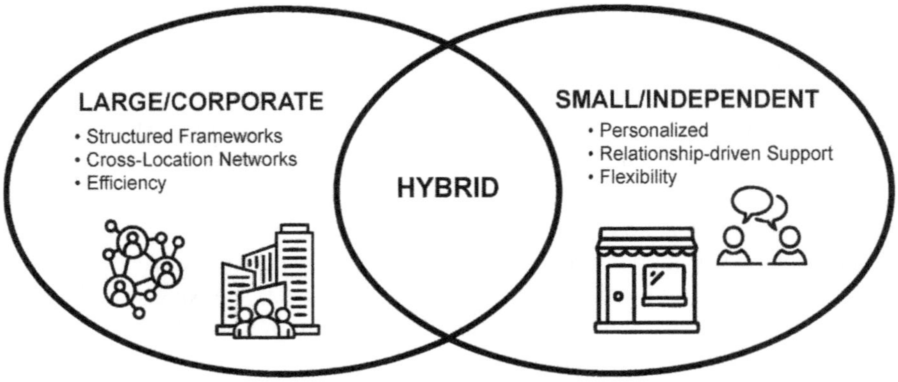

FIGURE 1.2 Balancing scale with personalization.

diverse mentorship perspectives that enrich the new graduate's development. Practice owners often appreciate that these external programs create a "safe space" where their associates can openly discuss challenges they face within the clinic. External perspectives allow new graduates to process difficult situations, develop solutions, and return to their practice with fresh insights and constructive strategies for growth. They also provide consistent support, even during practice transitions, and offer valuable objective third-party guidance that complements the day-to-day mentoring within the practice.

The key to success, regardless of practice model, lies in creating mentorship programs that combine the strengths of in-house support with intentionally designed external resources. This hybrid approach ensures new graduates receive comprehensive support while practices maintain flexibility in their mentorship delivery. When internal mentorship is enhanced by structured external programs, practices position themselves to retain talented early-career veterinarians—an investment that pays dividends well beyond the initial costs of program implementation.

A CASE STUDY: BEYOND CLINICAL SKILLS

I remember the phone call clearly. Only two years into her clinical practice, Lindsey had lost her way. She had been driven by a crystal-clear goal—to become a veterinarian. That goal had powered her through countless hours of volunteering, late nights studying, the grueling clinical year, and North American Veterinary Licensing Exam (NAVLE) preparation. But now that she had achieved it, the clarity was gone.

She struggled daily with confidence, with connecting to her clients, and found herself driven primarily by fear—fear of making mistakes, fear of failure, and fear of negative feedback from clients. Her experience wasn't unique. In fact, a 2018 well-being survey of more than 3500 US veterinarians found that two-thirds had experienced anxiety, burnout, or panic attacks within the past year, with younger veterinarians at highest risk (Volk et al., 2018). These findings echo what so many early-career practitioners describe the constant undercurrent of fear that shapes their decisions, their confidence, and, too often, their sense of whether they belong in the profession.

"It sounds like you've lost your Why," I said gently.

"I don't even know what my Why is anymore," she replied through sobs.

I offered her a challenge: "Spend some time thinking about your Why. Why did you work so hard through undergrad and vet school? What was the real point of it all? Let's talk next week and see what you've discovered."

When we spoke again, Lindsey had gained some clarity, but hadn't quite honed in on her Why. This wasn't surprising—she'd been struggling for two years. These kinds of revelations take time. After our call, I sent her a text: "Thank you so much for your openness and sharing your story and feelings. You have come so far in your professional and personal growth. You have a lot to be proud of. Our profession is lucky to have you and personally I'm grateful to know you. I'm here for you any time!"

I couldn't find Lindsey's Why for her, but I could provide the comprehensive support she needed to discover it herself. This multifaceted approach—combining emotional support, reflective dialogue, and what mentors sometimes call "cheerleading"—proves crucial for early-career veterinarians. With studies showing between 33% and 44% of new veterinarians leaving their first job within one to two years (Jelinski et al., 2009; Gates et al., 2020) and most citing lack of mentorship as a top reason for leaving, it's clear that technical guidance alone isn't enough. In one surprising survey, approximately 70% of those surveyed disagreed or strongly disagreed with the statement, "Employer is supportive and understanding when a case or procedure goes badly," and only about 26% agreed or strongly agreed with the statement, "Employer praises good work" (Jelinski et al., 2009, p. 946). In another survey, 70% of early career respondents said they would find regular sessions with a mentor to discuss things like personal well-being and professional (nonclinical) issues very or extremely helpful (Gates et al., 2020, p. 220). These findings underscore exactly what Lindsey's experience illustrates: new graduates need comprehensive mentorship that addresses their emotional and professional development alongside clinical training.

I didn't hear from Lindsey for a few weeks. Then one day, my phone lit up with a text message: "I found my Why!"

Attached was a photo of Lindsey in her surgical gown, cap, and mask. Though I could only see her eyes, I knew there was a huge smile hidden beneath that mask. In her hands, she proudly displayed the massive pyometra uterus she'd just removed—clearly infected but a testament to her success. She was ecstatic. The next photo showed her in a run with a recovering patient she had just saved.

The story came tumbling out: Lola, the patient, belonged to a sweet young man who had brought her in sick and worried. Lindsey had used her experience, training, and natural empathy to collect a detailed history, connect with the client, and make diagnostic recommendations that led to a pyometra diagnosis. When Lola's owner couldn't afford referral to an emergency clinic, it fell to Lindsey to perform a surgery she had never done before. With the guidance of another vet in the clinic, she completed her first pyometra and saved Lola's life. But she did more than that—she saved the precious relationship between a young man and his beloved dog.

"I realized my Why is to help people!" she wrote. "By helping pets, I can actually help people, and that's what I want to do."

Is a large dog pyometra surgery scary? You bet. Is it technically challenging? You know it. Was Lindsey scared? Absolutely. But the combination of finding her Why and receiving both clinical guidance and emotional support helped her overcome that fear. This transformation illustrates a crucial truth about modern veterinary mentorship: Lindsey needed both the technical mentorship to successfully perform a complex surgery she'd never done before and the comprehensive emotional support that gave her the confidence to attempt it. The intersection of clinical guidance with structured support for professional development creates resilient professionals who can overcome challenges and find lasting satisfaction in their work.

Lindsey's story exemplifies the broader crisis we've outlined. Early career veterinarians often enter practice with a wealth of clinical knowledge but struggle with confidence, purpose, and professional identity. Her journey demonstrates exactly why traditional mentorship models focused primarily on clinical and technical skills fail to address the whole veterinarian—their technical abilities, their emotional well-being, and their sense of purpose. The mentorship that helped her find her Why went far beyond teaching procedures and protocols. It provided the emotional support and reflective space that transformed challenging moments from sources of fear into opportunities for growth and discovery.

THE TRADITIONAL MODEL: STRENGTHS AND LIMITATIONS

After graduation from UC Davis School of Veterinary Medicine in 2004, followed by a rotating small animal internship at a private specialty hospital, I began my veterinary career with high hopes of honing my skills in a bustling 24-hour clinic. While I gained valuable technical expertise there, the true foundation of my career was built in the 24-hour clinic's quieter, smaller satellite practice under the guidance of Dr. Mike Buffum—"Buff."

What made Buff such an exceptional mentor was his understanding of the difference between what can be taught through books and protocols vs. what must be learned through experience and guidance. This distinction often reminds me of a recurring conversation I have with my partner, a microbiology professor. Sometimes when I ask a question or I am curious about something, she responds with, "That sounds lookupable." It's become something of a joke between us, but it highlights a crucial distinction and relates to the evolution of mentorship in veterinary medicine. Differential diagnoses, drug doses, surgical protocols, and suture patterns are "lookupable," but the art of practice—the nuanced skills that help veterinarians find meaning, joy, and sustainable fulfillment in their careers—emerges through experience, reflection, and supportive professional relationships. This distinction gets to the heart of what we mean when we talk about mentorship in veterinary medicine. It's not simply about being told what to do or having someone check your work. **Structured mentorship is about creating the conditions and relationships that allow early-career veterinarians to develop their own authentic approach to practice (Figure 1.3).**

Buff understood this instinctively. He embodied the classic mentor: an experienced practitioner who took me under his wing and shared not only his clinical knowledge but also his unique approach to patient care, client relationships, and even the business side of veterinary practice. In our semirural practice located just outside of Los Angeles, Buff taught me what he called "cowboy medicine." This wasn't a cavalier approach but a pragmatic one, grounded in delivering a complete spectrum of care to a diverse clientele—from Hollywood elites living on sprawling horse properties to everyday locals.

What made Buff's mentorship exceptional wasn't just his clinical expertise, but his understanding that becoming a veterinarian meant mastering a complex web of interpersonal skills. He had a habit—annoying at the time, but invaluable in hindsight—of pulling me out of an exam room to introduce me to his long-standing clients personally. "This is Dr. Rabwin," he'd say. "She's new, which means she knows a lot more than me, and Fluffy will be in good hands if I'm not around." With this simple introduction, he accomplished multiple goals: building client trust, boosting my confidence, and modeling humility—all while making a self-deprecating joke that put everyone at ease.

When I faced challenging situations, whether delivering bad news or admitting a mistake, Buff would role-play with me, helping me find language that felt authentic. These sessions were awkward, but practicing with him before speaking to clients made all the difference. Today, when my own mentees squirm uncomfortably during similar role-playing exercises, I'm reminded of

LOOKUPABLE	UN-LOOKUPABLE
Drug Doses Protocols Suture Patterns Statistics	Client Communication Delivering Bad News Building Trust Sustaining Joy

FIGURE 1.3 Lookupable vs. un-lookupable.

how those awkward practice sessions with Buff ultimately helped shape my own approach to difficult conversations.

Perhaps most surprisingly, Buff insisted on showing me the financial books—another task I initially resisted. Like many veterinarians, I didn't go into the profession to talk about money. I was in the business of patient care! But Buff wanted me to understand how my production as a veterinarian impacted the practice's bottom line, from the equipment we could buy to the salaries we could pay staff. This financial literacy, though uncomfortable at first, became another gift that contributed to my professional growth and well-being.

Looking back on my time with Buff, I can see both the profound strengths and inherent limitations of traditional mentorship models. The strengths were significant: the deep one-on-one relationship, the daily exposure to both clinical and nonclinical skills, and the organic way learning unfolded through real-world cases. While personal connections and comprehensive skill development remain valuable elements of effective mentorship, the limitations of this traditional model are equally important to recognize.

I was lucky—many new graduates don't have access to a mentor like Buff. The informal nature of traditional mentorship means its quality can vary dramatically depending on the individual mentor and practice setting. Many early-career veterinarians are requesting formal mentorship during their first years in practice, with recent data underscoring this. According to the American Veterinary Medical Association (AVMA), 84% of 2022 veterinary graduates indicated that the desire for mentorship influenced their job choice, ranking it above factors like location, compensation, or benefits (AVMA, 2023). Studies on the human health side demonstrate this as well, with one study finding that "Millennial and Gen Z (surgical) trainees are. . .more likely to desire clearly defined expectations with structured approaches to training" (Koti et al., 2024).

What we need today is an approach that preserves the best aspects of traditional or informal mentorship—the personal connection and the emphasis on both clinical and nonclinical skills—while adding the structure and intentionality required by modern veterinary medicine. We need purposeful mentorship that scales beyond the one-to-one relationship but maintains the depth and value of relationships like mine with Buff.

WHY TRADITIONAL MODELS FALL SHORT OF MODERN NEEDS

When I think about how veterinary mentorship has evolved, I'm reminded of a conversation with Dr. Sarah, a colleague who had just hired her first associate. "I want to do better than what was done for me," she told me. "My mentors taught me medicine, but no one taught me how to handle the emotional toll of this profession, how to set boundaries, or how to build sustainable practices. We need to do better for the next generation."

Sarah's insight cuts to the heart of the disconnect we've been examining. The traditional apprenticeship model of veterinary mentorship, while successful at passing down clinical skills, left significant gaps that have contributed to concerning patterns in our profession: alarming rates of burnout, compassion fatigue, and suicide. According to one survey, one in 11 veterinarians experienced significant psychological distress, while one in six experienced suicidal ideation (Yanke et al., 2023). The stark reality is that veterinarians are at significantly higher risk for mental health challenges compared to the general population. Studies show that veterinarians are 2.1 times more likely for men and 3.5 times more likely for women to die by suicide than the US population overall, with suicidal thoughts reported by nearly three times as many veterinarians compared to national averages (CDC/AVMA, 2015). International data echoes these findings, with UK research showing that veterinary surgeons have a suicide rate four times higher than the general population and roughly twice that of other healthcare professionals (Bartram and Baldwin, 2010). These statistics underscore the urgent need for mentorship models that address not only clinical development but also emotional well-being and professional sustainability.

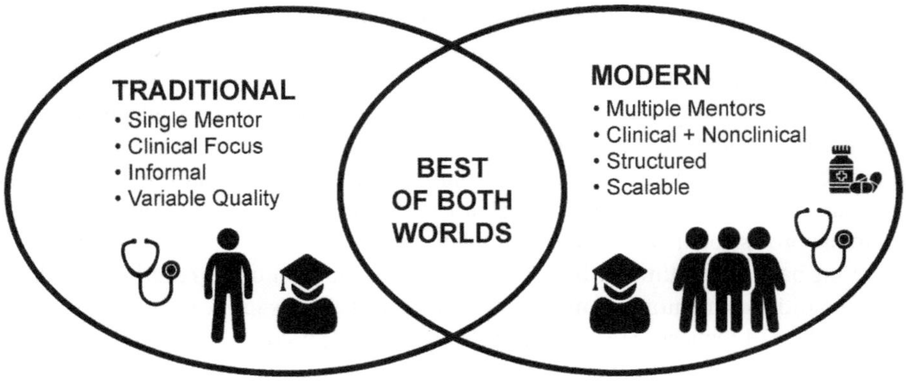

FIGURE 1.4 Traditional vs. modern mentorship.

The apprenticeship approach focused primarily on clinical skills' transmission: watching, learning, and gradually taking on more responsibility under the guidance of an experienced practitioner. This model successfully created technically competent veterinarians, but often at a cost. By emphasizing medical knowledge above all else, it left new graduates ill-equipped to respond to high emotional demands, navigate difficult client interactions, maintain work–life boundaries, or manage the business aspects of practice. Recent data suggests that 27% of veterinarians had signs of emotional exhaustion and up to 18% suffer from high to very high burnout (Yanke et al., 2023; Volk et al., 2024).

Today's new graduates are advocating for change, and this advocacy represents a positive evolution in our profession. Rather than accepting the status quo of "this is how it was done for me," they're openly discussing their needs for emotional support, work–life integration, and comprehensive professional development. According to the Merck Animal Health Veterinary Wellbeing Study IV, 17.3% of young veterinarians (≤34 years) experience serious psychological distress, compared to 11.8% for those aged 35–44, with even lower rates among older veterinarians (Volk et al., 2024). This transparency about mental health and well-being needs isn't a sign of weakness—it represents a healthier approach to professional sustainability.

Many practices have recognized these evolving needs and have attempted to modernize their support systems. However, their responses often focus primarily on clinical development—implementing structured training programs that track clinical milestones and measure financial key performance indicators (KPIs). While developing clinical competence is crucial, this narrow focus perpetuates the same gaps that have historically contributed to professional distress. As one experienced practice manager noted, "You can have an associate who performs perfect surgeries but still struggles with compassion fatigue or burns out within their first year. We need to expand our definition of what success looks like" (Figure 1.4).

THE EVOLUTION TOWARD COMPREHENSIVE MENTORSHIP

This recognition has led to an important realization: **modern veterinarians need multiple mentors and multiple forms of structured and intentional support.** This isn't a reflection of any individual mentor's inadequacy, but rather an acknowledgment of the breadth of skills required for sustainable success in today's profession. In a recent analysis of mentoring programs for medical students, Elce noted that multilevel mentoring involving both faculty and peer-peer mentoring improved personal and professional outcomes, highlighting the need for mosaic mentoring in veterinary medicine to "fulfill slightly different, although overlapping, needs of the

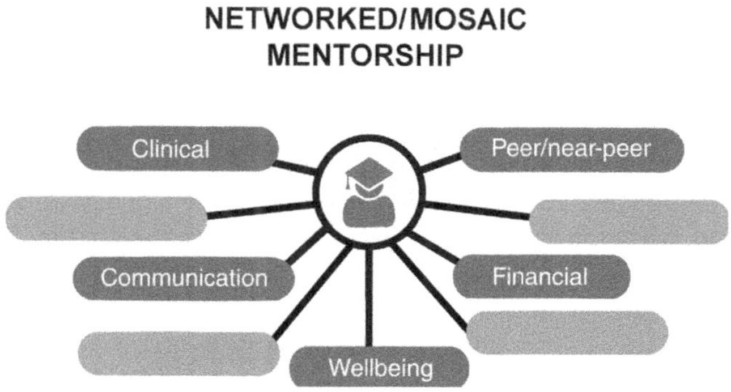

FIGURE 1.5 Mosaic mentorship.

mentee" (Elce, 2021, p. 1101). Moreover, as Freeman and colleagues demonstrated in their work developing mentee training programs, the mentee must take an active role in driving the mentoring relationship—identifying their needs, setting goals, and proactively seeking guidance (Freeman et al., 2021; Hodgson et al., 2022). Different mentors bring different strengths and perspectives, helping new graduates develop not just medical expertise but also emotional resilience, communication skills, and professional sustainability (Figure 1.5).

Combining multiple mentors with mentee-driven engagement helps practices move beyond the "see one, do one, teach one" model while retaining the valuable aspects of experiential learning. It provides a framework for addressing the full spectrum of professional development needs we've discussed—from clinical skills to emotional resilience and from client communication to work–life integration.

This approach becomes especially powerful when we consider the evolving demographics of our profession and the critical need to support an increasingly diverse veterinary workforce. As documented by Burkhard et al. (2022), in the 2019–2020 academic year, more than 75% of veterinary students were White, while less than 25% identified as part of underrepresented groups. While this represents a persistent disparity, these numbers reflect gradual progress toward increased diversity in our profession—progress that must be supported through intentional, effective mentorship approaches.

This demographic reality intersects directly with our earlier discussion about moving beyond the limitations of traditional apprenticeship models. Just as we recognized that the sink-or-swim approach to clinical training was inadequate for developing complete professionals, we must acknowledge that informal or unstructured mentorship models may unintentionally perpetuate barriers for underrepresented students. Research has shown that students from underrepresented backgrounds often benefit from structured mentorship programs that provide consistent access to mentors, clear developmental pathways, and intentional support (National Academies of Sciences, Engineering, and Medicine, 2019, p. 69).

Given current demographics, many mentees will work with mentors who don't share their background or lived experiences. This reality doesn't diminish the potential for meaningful mentorship—rather, it heightens the importance of intentionality in these relationships. The evolution we've traced from dyadic to more complex mentoring structures becomes particularly relevant here. Network mentorship and group mentorship models can help create multiple points of connection and support, ensuring that mentees have access to diverse perspectives and experiences even if their primary mentor doesn't share their background.

The mentorship models we've discussed—ranging from traditional, apprenticeship-style approaches to more structured and intentional programs—each offer distinct advantages for supporting diversity in our profession. **Informal mentorship can provide natural opportunities for connection, but structured approaches are often necessary to ensure that mentees from all backgrounds consistently receive the guidance and opportunities they need.** Peer and near-peer mentorship can add important layers of relatability and support, while experienced mentors can help open professional doors. When combined thoughtfully, these approaches create multiple points of connection and a more inclusive mentorship environment, particularly in settings where organic relationships may not naturally develop across differences.

Importantly, successful mentorship across differences requires more than just good intentions or general mentorship skills. Mentors need to combine structured approaches with cultural awareness and a genuine commitment to understanding their mentees' unique perspectives and challenges. This might mean being more explicit about expectations, more intentional about creating safe spaces for difficult conversations, and more proactive about connecting mentees with additional resources and support networks. We will discuss all of these topics in more detail throughout the book.

As the field evolves, we must remember that some things remain "unlookupable"—they must be learned through experience, guided by mentors who understand that veterinary medicine is as much an art as it is a science. The challenge lies in creating mentorship programs that can deliver these crucial experiences consistently and effectively to a new generation of veterinarians. The solution lies not in larger sign-on bonuses or more rigid protocols, but in creating flexible, comprehensive mentorship programs that address both the clinical and nonclinical aspects of veterinary medicine.

CONCLUSION

The chapters that follow will explore each element of effective mentorship in greater detail. We'll examine specific strategies for implementing structured mentorship programs and building mentorship frameworks that work at any scale. We'll dive deep into the art of supporting emotional well-being alongside clinical development, exploring how mentors can help new graduates build resilience, navigate difficult cases and ethical dilemmas, and develop the communication skills essential for veterinary practice. We'll investigate how to build trust and rapport in mentor–mentee relationships, provide effective feedback that fosters growth, and evaluate mentorship programs to ensure they're meeting their goals. Through case studies, research insights, and practical frameworks, we'll provide concrete tools for both mentors and mentees to create meaningful, sustainable relationships that evolve over time and strengthen our entire profession. By reimagining mentorship for modern veterinary medicine, we can build a future where early-career veterinarians receive the comprehensive support they need to develop into confident, resilient professionals who find sustainable satisfaction in their careers.

BIBLIOGRAPHY

AAHA (2023). Corporate consolidation and the rise of private equity. *Trends Magazine*. American Animal Hospital Association. https://www.aaha.org/trends-magazine/publications/corporate-consolidation-and-the-rise-of-private-equity/.

American Economic Liberties Project (2025). The Save Our Pets Act: stopping the corporate takeover of veterinary practices. https://www.economicliberties.us/our-work/the-save-our-pets-act-stopping-the-corporate-takeover-of-veterinary-practices.

AVMA (2023). Chart of the month: new veterinarians prioritize mentorship. https://www.avma.org/news/chart-month-new-veterinarians-prioritize-mentorship.

Bartram, D.J. and Baldwin, D.S. (2010). Veterinary surgeons and suicide: a structured review of possible influences on increased risk. *Veterinary Record* 166 (13): 388–397.

Burkhard, M.J., Dawkins, S., Knoblaugh, S.E. et al. (2022). Supporting diversity, equity, inclusion, and belonging to strengthen and position the veterinary profession for service, sustainability, excellence, and impact. *Journal of the American Veterinary Medical Association* 260 (11): 1283–1290.

Centers for Disease Control and Prevention (CDC) and American Veterinary Medical Association (AVMA) (2015). Study: 1 in 6 veterinarians have considered suicide. *JAVMA News* (1 April).

Elce, Y. (2021). The mentor-mentee relationship, addressing challenges in veterinary medicine together. *Veterinary Clinics of North America: Small Animal Practice* 51 (6): 1099–1109.

Freeman, D., Hodgson, K., and Darling, M. (2021). Mentoring new veterinary graduates for transition to practice and lifelong learning. *Journal of Veterinary Medical Education* e20210036. https://doi.org/10.3138/jvme-2021-0036.

Gates, M.C., McLachlan, I., Butler, S., and Weston, J.F. (2020). Experiences of recent veterinary graduates in their first employment position and their preferences for new graduate support programmes. *New Zealand Veterinary Journal* 68 (4): 214–224.

Hodgson, K., Freeman, D., and Darling, M. (2022). Developing mentee skills: a curriculum guide. *Journal of Veterinary Medical Education* 49 (4): 575–583.

Jelinski, M.D., Campbell, J.R., MacGregor, M.W., and Watts, J.M. (2009). Factors associated with veterinarians' career path choices in the early postgraduate period. *The Canadian Veterinary Journal* 50 (9): 943–948.

Koti, S., Xie, J., Chopra, M., and Patel, V. (2024). Surgical mentorship for next generation is changing. *ACS Bulletin* 109 (8): September.

Mastenbroek, N.J., van Beukelen, P., Demerouti, E. et al. (2015). Effects of a 1 year development programme for recently graduated veterinary professionals on personal and job resources: a combined quantitative and qualitative approach. *BMC Veterinary Research* 11: 311.

National Academies of Sciences, Engineering, and Medicine (2019). *The Science of Effective Mentorship in STEMM*. Washington, DC: The National Academies Press.

Neill, C.L., Hansen, C.R., and Salois, M. (2022). The economic cost of burnout in veterinary medicine. *Frontiers in Veterinary Science* 9: 814104.

Veterinary Business Matters (2018). The high cost of employee turnover in a veterinary clinic. Veterinary Business Matters Blog (19 July). https://veterinarybusinessmatters.com/2018/07/19/the-high-cost-of-employee-turnover-veterinary-clinic/.

VetPartners. (2022). Veterinary Team Utilization Guide. https://www.vetpartners.org/resources/veterinary-team-utilization-guide/.

Volk, J.O., Schimmack, U., Strand, E.B. et al. (2018). Executive summary of the Merck animal health veterinary wellbeing study. *Journal of the American Veterinary Medical Association* 252 (10): 1231–1238.

Volk, J.O., Schimmack, U., Strand, E.B. et al. (2024). Merck animal health veterinary wellbeing study IV. *Journal of the American Veterinary Medical Association* 262 (1): 35–47.

Yanke, A.B., Weigand, K.A., and Hofmeister, E.H. (2023). Addressing the needs and challenges of mentorship in veterinary medicine. *New Directions for Teaching and Learning* 2023: 83–93.

CHAPTER 2 Foundations

INTRODUCTION

Dani Rabwin

A practical question that every mentor faces is how do we build meaningful mentorship relationships that actually work? Too often, mentorship in veterinary medicine happens by accident—informal, inconsistent, and leaving both mentors and mentees frustrated when expectations don't align. The gap between good intentions and effective mentorship can be the difference between a thriving new graduate and one who leaves your practice or the profession entirely.

I've brought together two exceptional practitioners who understand mentorship from both sides of the equation and can guide us beyond the theoretical into actionable frameworks for your mentoring relationships. Kate Boatright, VMD, brings over 13 years of clinical experience and deep expertise in mentorship program development. She is the author of the *Veterinary Mentorship Manual* and has been actively mentoring for over eight years while speaking nationally on mentorship topics. Her systematic approach to mentorship structure provides the foundation this chapter builds upon.

Legend Thurman, DVM, an international bestselling author and policy advocate, offers a unique perspective on professional development, bringing extensive training in burnout prevention and well-being education alongside her clinical practice. Her focus on mentee skill development ensures that we're not just creating dependent relationships but also empowering new and early career veterinarians to become confident, self-directed learners.

This chapter moves beyond the hit-or-miss mentorship contributing to our profession's challenges by providing concrete guidance on identifying compatible mentor–mentee pairs, establishing clear expectations, and creating structured frameworks that protect both parties while fostering growth. You'll discover the characteristics that make both mentors and mentees successful, learn strategies for helping your mentees find additional mentorship beyond your practice, and understand how to create mentorship agreements that set everyone up for success.

This chapter is filled with valuable information you can share with your mentees, including strategies to help them take an active role in their own growth. Whether you're supporting a mentee informally or guiding them through a structured program, this information can be a conversation starter, a resource to pass along, or a framework for mutual reflection. This chapter examines mentoring relationships and skills from a broad perspective that can be applied both in the clinic and outside of it. Appendix A (Structuring Effective In-Clinic Mentorship Programs) provides expanded information on the development of in-clinic mentoring programs.

Perhaps, most importantly, this chapter will help you understand what your mentees need to develop beyond clinical skills—from communication and resilience to professional identity formation. While the chapter includes guidance your mentees can use directly, your role as mentor is to recognize these developmental needs and create space for them to flourish.

THE MENTOR–MENTEE RELATIONSHIP

Kate Boatright

The most rewarding and successful mentoring relationships are formed between individuals who invest time, energy, and effort into the relationship. Before starting a mentoring relationship, mentors and mentees should understand the characteristics that support success as well as the responsibilities they have to their counterpart and themselves.

The most important characteristics for mentor and mentee success have nothing to do with clinical techniques or experience and instead focus on interpersonal and communication skills. Table 2.1 outlines the essential skills and characteristics seen in mentors and mentees. Many of these skills and characteristics are important for both roles, which is beneficial for those who may find themselves being mentored and providing mentorship simultaneously.

Effective mentoring relationships require engagement from both mentor and mentee. The specific responsibilities of each individual will vary depending on the goals of the relationship and whether the mentorship is happening in the workplace or outside of it (see Table 2.2 for example roles and responsibilities). Responsibilities and expectations should be discussed at the beginning of the mentorship. In a formal relationship, these are included in the mentoring agreement, which will be discussed in more detail later in this chapter.

Table 2.1 Essential Skills and Characteristics of Mentors and Mentees

Mentors	Mentees	Both mentors and mentees
• Patient • Have available time • Well-developed leadership skills • Passionate • Interested in providing mentorship	• Desire to learn • Have a growth mindset • Humble • Adaptable/flexible • Engaged • Curious	• Approachable • High emotional intelligence • Problem-solving • Empathy • Active and reflective listening • Clear communication skills • Conflict resolution skills • Comfortable delivering feedback • Open to receiving feedback

Table 2.2 Roles and Responsibilities of Mentors and Mentees

Mentors	Mentees
• Provide support and guidance • Provide timely and specific feedback • Be open to mentee feedback and suggestions • Support confidence building • Model healthy boundaries and other personal wellness skills • Demonstrate communication, leadership, and other essential nonclinical skills • Help to identify resources for continued growth	• Engage in self-directed learning • Ask for help when needed • Be open to feedback and suggestions • Request feedback regularly • Provide feedback to mentor and make respectful suggestions for change • Share knowledge with your team • Practice self-care and be aware of mental health challenges • Develop interpersonal skills, such as communication and conflict resolution • Ask for the resources needed

HOW TO FIND A MENTOR BEYOND THE CLINIC

Often a mentor is assigned to the mentee in an in-clinic or formalized mentoring program. But in most other mentoring relationships, the mentee identifies a need for support, seeks out a prospective mentor, and initiates the relationship. Mentees should know what kind of mentorship theyww want and need, where to look for a mentor who can meet their needs, and how to make a strong and respectful request for mentorship (Boatright, 2024).

EVALUATE THE NEED FOR MENTORSHIP

Before seeking out a mentor, spend time in self-reflection to determine your current needs (Reinhard et al., 2023). Consider the following questions:

- What goals are you working toward, and how will a mentor help you reach them? These can be personal or professional goals.
- Consider current strengths and opportunities for improvement. Is there a specific skill or knowledge area you need support in developing?
- How much time do you have available to engage with a mentor?
- What level of responsibility are you willing to take in making the mentoring relationship successful?

The answers to these questions can help determine the type of mentoring relationship you are looking for and what type of person might be a good fit for a mentor.

EXPLORE MENTORING RELATIONSHIPS

Mentorship can happen in many different environments and be structured in numerous ways. These models vary in their level of structure, number of mentors and mentees, and location of mentoring. Identifying the best type of mentorship will vary depending on your goals. Table 2.3 summarizes the common types of mentoring relationships.

Understanding the many forms of mentorship can help to determine which model(s) can meet your needs. Mentorship models are not exclusive. In fact, many mentoring models can be complementary to each other. **Instead of thinking of mentorship as a set menu where you must choose a single model, consider it as a buffet, where you can choose multiple models simultaneously.** This is also known as mosaic mentorship (Elce, 2021).

Mentors and mentees should find a mentoring model that meets their individual needs, skills, and availability. Here are examples of how the different types of mentoring models have worked in my own career:

- As a veterinary student, I relied on support from my pre-veterinary mentors through informal, distance mentoring. The first call I made after failing my first anatomy practical was to a mentor who provided a listening ear and support.
- As a new graduate veterinarian and again when I started emergency work a few years out of school, I was lucky to have traditional, in-clinic, formalized mentorship relationships to support my clinical and professional development.
- When I no longer had a formal mentee in the clinic, I joined a virtual mentoring program so that I could continue to provide mentorship in a formalized, distance mentorship setting. This allowed me to continue to develop my skills as a mentor and enjoy the rewards active mentorship can provide.

SEARCH FOR A MENTOR

Mentors can be found in many places throughout an individual's career. Some relationships will develop spontaneously with a professor, clinician, or colleague in school, the workplace, or a professional organization. Formalized mentorship programs may be available to match you with

Table 2.3 Types of Mentoring Relationships

Variable	Types of mentoring relationships	
Level of structure	**Formal** • Has a defined structure and involves the development of clear goals, expectations, responsibilities, and regular meetings. • Often governed by a written agreement.	**Informal** • Usually develops spontaneously between colleagues. • Meetings occur on an as-needed basis. • More flexibility in the structure, but drawback is this can make finding time to meet more difficult.
Who is the mentor?	**Traditional** • This is the typical mentoring relationship where a more experienced individual serves in the mentor role while the less experienced individual serves in the mentee role.	**Reverse** • The typical mentor–mentee roles are flipped. • The less-experienced individual takes on the mentor role and can support the development of new skills and knowledge for the more experienced individual.
Number of mentors	**One** • Mentoring happens between a single mentor and a single mentee.	**Multiple or team** • More than one mentor supports a single mentee. • Each mentor provides support in different areas of personal and professional development for the mentee. • Multiple mentoring is generally less coordinated than team mentoring, where mentors collaborate.
Number of mentees	**One** • Mentoring happens between a single mentor and a single mentee.	**Group** • Multiple mentees are supported by a single mentor. • Mentees may benefit from peer support from their cohorts in addition to the support of the mentor.
Where mentorship happens	**Local/in-person** • Mentor and mentee are in the same physical location. This may be the same workplace or city.	**Distance/virtual** • Mentor and mentee are in different locations, separated by some degree of distance. • Mentor meetings and interactions happen online or by phone. • This type of mentorship widens the availability of mentors, especially in niche areas that may not be available locally.

Mentorship can take place in many forms and environments. This table summarizes the characteristics of different types of mentoring relationships. *Source:* Data from Elce (2021), Reinhard et al. (2023).

available mentors. Other relationships will take more time and work to develop but can be just as valuable.

When looking for a mentor, cast a wide net. First, determine the goal(s) of the mentorship and the type of person who can best provide support (i.e., a specialist in a field of interest, an experienced clinician to provide general support, or an industry professional who can help develop nonclinical skills). Remember that a mentor does not need to have the same professional title as you. Credentialed technicians, veterinary assistants, client service representatives, practice managers, and professionals outside of the clinic can all provide mentorship to veterinarians, and vice versa.

Mentors can be found in many places, including:

- **Veterinary schools**—Connect with faculty, alumni, and peers through events, clubs, or national organizations like Student American Veterinary Medical Association (SAVMA) and Veterinary Business Management Association (VBMA).
- **Your workplace**—Even if assigned a mentor, other veterinarians and team members can offer valuable support.
- **Local practices**—Especially useful for students exploring externships or job opportunities.
- **Professional organizations**—Many veterinary associations and specialty colleges offer mentorship programs or searchable directories.
- **Conferences**—Network with speakers, attend mentoring events, and spend time in the exhibit hall.
- **Social media**—Some veterinarians are active online and open to mentoring or answering questions.
- **Mentorship programs**—National groups like Pawsibilities VetMed, MentorVet, and Ready, Vet, Go connect mentees with trained mentors.
- **Your existing network**—Don't overlook classmates, colleagues, or friends who may be able to connect you with a mentor in your area of interest.

REQUEST MENTORSHIP

After identifying a possible mentor, create a plan to approach them and ask about their interest in establishing a mentoring relationship. Before reaching out, do some background research to ensure this person will be a good fit for your individual goals. This can also help make the mentoring request more personal, which can highlight the level of interest you have in this individual as a mentor.

An initial request for mentoring should include (see Box 2.1 for example):

- A brief introduction to who you are (i.e., name, location, current role)
- Your areas of interest/goals

BOX 2.1 SAMPLE MENTORING REQUEST

Hello Dr. Mentor,

My name is Future Mentee, and I am a small animal veterinarian in western Pennsylvania. I graduated from the University of Pennsylvania this year and am interested in learning more about exotic animal medicine. Your clinic is highly recommended by many of the veterinarians in my area. I saw on your website you offer training and support to local veterinarians who are interested in learning more about exotic animals.

I was wondering if you currently have the time and availability to take on a new mentee. If so, I would be happy to discuss more about what I'm looking for in mentorship by email, phone, or set up a virtual meeting.

Sincerely,
Future Mentee

- How you found them and why you think they might be a good a mentor
- Inquiry about interest in mentorship
- Offer to meet or provide more information about your needs

The initial request should be on the shorter side, but you should be prepared to answer questions about the type of mentoring relationship you are looking for, your ideal length, and how frequently you are hoping to meet. This information can be included in a follow-up email, phone call, or virtual meeting if your possible mentor states they are open to discussing mentorship further. Providing these types of details helps a prospective mentor to determine if they have the interest, availability, and necessary skills to support you. Maintain a level of flexibility in your ideas around what a mentoring relationship might look like so that you and your mentor can find a relationship that is mutually beneficial.

Do not take it personally if the person you approach says no. There are many reasons a possible mentor may decline your request, including available time, comfort with teaching, past mentoring experiences, and personal commitments. Consider asking if they know of a colleague who may be a good fit for a mentorship and would be willing to make an introduction.

CONSIDERATIONS FOR IN-CLINIC MENTORS

Identifying a mentor is a critical first step for in-clinic mentoring programs. **Clinics should not begin to promote mentorship before ensuring there is an available and interested veterinarian to serve in the role.** It is also critical that clinic management be willing to provide support for both mentor and mentee. For more information on the specifics of developing an in-clinic mentorship program, see Appendix A.

While there is not a set amount of clinical experience a veterinarian needs before taking on the role of primary mentor, this individual should be confident in their own clinical abilities, be efficient with their normal clinical duties, and have strong communication skills.

The responsibilities of a mentor in a formalized clinical mentorship program include:

- Provide guidance in clinical cases (medicine and surgery)
- Set schedule for mentorship and ensure meeting times are protected
- Communicate with team on plans around appointment and surgery scheduling
- Collect feedback from team members and clients on the mentee's performance
- Provide regular, timely, and specific feedback on mentee performance
- Evaluate mentee's skills and help with making action plans and goal setting
- Support confidence building
- Model healthy boundaries and other personal wellness skills
- Demonstrate communication, leadership, and other essential nonclinical skills
- Advocate for the mentee's needs with clinic management

COMPENSATION FOR MENTORS

Mentoring requires time and energy from both mentor and mentee. While many individuals mentor because they find great joy and fulfillment in supporting their less-experienced colleagues, it is not unreasonable to consider compensation for the mentor, especially in a formalized in-clinic mentorship program.

Several models have been described for monetary compensation of mentors, including (VetPartners, 2025):

- Mentoring stipends, which are a set amount provided to the mentor. This may be given as a lump sum or divided and paid over the course of the mentorship.
- Bonus structures, which provide financial rewards when mentees reach particular milestones in the mentoring program (i.e., developing particular skills, seeing a certain number of patients, or hitting a revenue goal).
- Production structure, where the mentor is paid a small percentage of the mentee's production for the clinic.
- Additional incentives, which could include a bonus received for mentee retention.

An additional consideration is that a mentor veterinarian may need to have their normal clinical duties reduced to allow time for mentoring. This may be especially important in the early stage of the mentorship period, when the mentee is likely to need the most support. This could include reduced hours in appointments and procedures to decrease the overall caseload. Alternatively, consider limiting double bookings or adding an occasional block of catch-up time during the normal appointment schedule to account for time spent mentoring during the day. Additionally, if the mentor has additional duties in the clinic, such as team training or social media management, consider delegating these duties to another team member.

Compensation should take into consideration the time and energy invested as a mentor as well as the potential for reduced income. This is particularly relevant to veterinarians paid on a production model.

ALIGNING EXPECTATIONS

Strong mentoring relationships are built on shared expectations. Before formally beginning the relationship, mentors and mentees should meet to clarify key aspects of the relationship, including:

- **Set clear goals:** Discuss what each person hopes to achieve through the mentoring relationship. These goals can include personal and professional development as well as goals that benefit your clinic or workplace.
  - Example 1: The mentee wants to improve surgical efficiency so they can perform more surgeries each shift.
  - Example 2: The mentor wants to improve how they communicate constructive criticism in a compassionate way.
  - Example 3: The mentor and mentee set a revenue goal for surgical cases in the next quarter.
- **Explore values:** Share personal and professional values to better understand each other's approach to mentorship, teaching style, and priorities.
- **Agree on a shared definition of mentorship:** Clarify what mentorship means to each of you and what a successful relationship will look like. This is essential to achieve a successful relationship.

These details can be included in the mentoring agreement, which will be discussed in more detail later in the final section of this chapter.

MENTEE SKILLS

Legend A. Thurman

Effective mentees actively engage in the mentoring relationship and regular self-reflection. Mentees who take initiative—setting clear goals, asking for feedback, and seeking new challenges—maximize the benefits of mentoring relationships (Rose et al., 2020). Veterinary students and early-career professionals in particular benefit from mentorship when navigating clinical decision-making, developing communication skills, and identifying career trajectories in an evolving field.

MENTEE SKILL DEVELOPMENT LIFECYCLE

Mentees typically progress through a lifecycle of development that includes four stages (Levinson, 1978). Throughout this cycle, mentors play an integral role in supporting mentee development (see Figure 2.1).

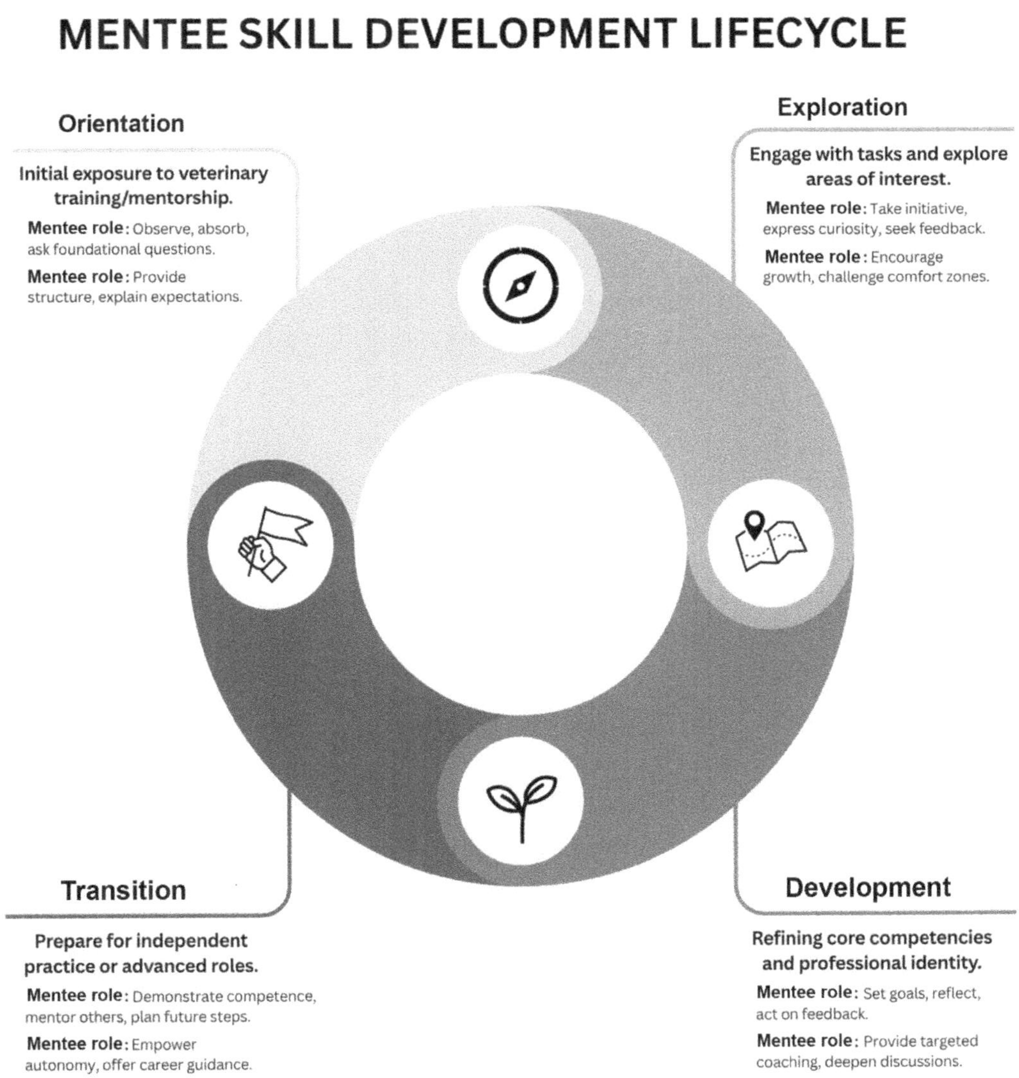

FIGURE 2.1 Mentee skill development lifecycle. This diagram illustrates the cyclical progression of veterinary mentees through four key phases of development with mentor and mentee roles highlighted for each phase. *Source:* Courtesy of Kate Boatright (2025).

STAGE ONE: INITIAL PHASE (ORIENTATION)

This is a period of observation, learning, and goal setting with the mentor. Mentees should familiarize themselves with their roles and expectations. During this stage, mentees often exhibit a high level of enthusiasm but may also encounter imposter syndrome or feelings of uncertainty.

MENTOR TIP

Help the mentee manage imposter syndrome by normalizing early-career uncertainty. Share personal stories from your own early career and collaborate with your mentee to set short-term, achievable goals.

STAGE TWO: DEVELOPMENT PHASE

Feedback is critical during this period of skill refinement. Mentees should actively seek feedback from mentors and peers to refine their skills. Mentees should begin to step out of their comfort zones and take on more challenging cases or roles during this time.

MENTOR TIP

Provide timely, specific feedback and encourage reflection. Create opportunities for mentees to stretch their abilities (i.e., leading case discussions or client communication) while ensuring psychological safety. Celebrate growth.

STAGE THREE: EXPLORATION PHASE

By this stage, mentees are more confident in their clinical and professional responsibilities. They can handle complex cases independently and may begin to mentor less-experienced peers. While formal mentor meetings may lessen in frequency, mentees should still engage with mentors to support ongoing personal and professional growth.

MENTOR TIP

Shift into a coaching role by offering strategic career guidance and opportunities for leadership development. Encourage your mentee to engage in mentoring others, which reinforces their own skills while contributing to the learning culture.

STAGE FOUR: TRANSITION PHASE

As mentees transition into independent roles or seek new career opportunities, they should reflect on their journey and set new professional goals. At this point, the mentorship relationship often evolves into a professional network where mentees continue to consult with mentors on a less formal, as needed basis.

MENTOR TIP

Support your mentee's long-term career planning by facilitating introductions within your network and discussing professional identity evolution. Affirm their readiness for independence and invite them to stay in touch as a trusted colleague and peer.

DEVELOPING CORE COMPETENCIES THROUGHOUT THE MENTORSHIP JOURNEY

As mentees progress through these developmental stages, they rely on foundational skills that support growth at every phase. The following core competencies—communication, growth mindset, well-being, conflict resolution, and feedback receptiveness—are interconnected tools that mentees should continuously develop and refine throughout their careers.

SKILL SET 1: COMMUNICATION SKILLS

Becoming a confident veterinarian and gaining client trust is not about how much information you know. Instead, it is about how you present that information to clients and colleagues. Veterinary professionals operate in high-stakes environments that demand clarity, empathy, and professionalism in communication. Both verbal and nonverbal communication influence interactions with clients, team members, and colleagues.

Mentees should continue developing core communication skills learned during their veterinary training. Table 2.4 provides examples of each of the following critical communication skills:

1. Verbal Communication and Audience Awareness
   Project professionalism through appropriate tone and vocabulary when speaking. The terminology used should be adjusted for the audience. When speaking to colleagues, assume a certain level of knowledge and provide evidence-based data, detailed diagnoses, and treatment options.

   When speaking to clients, use simple language, analogies, and visuals to explain the case. Always prioritize their understanding and emotional needs. For instance, the term *radiograph* is appropriate when speaking to a colleague but not to a client, where *x-ray* is more likely to be understood.

2. Listening Techniques
   Active listening—marked by presence, open posture, and minimal interruptions—facilitates trust and enhances understanding. It ensures that the speaker feels they are being heard.
   Reflective listening helps mentees develop diagnostic reasoning by accurately interpreting complex narratives from clients and ensuring appropriate understanding (Bachmann et al., 2020). It ensures that the listener understands information as the speaker intended.

3. Nonverbal Communication
   Subtle nonverbal cues influence how messages are perceived. Inconsistent body language or inappropriate facial expressions can undermine even well-articulated verbal communication (Archer and Miller, 2011). When speaking, develop awareness of facial expressions, posture, and voice modulation, especially in emotionally charged discussions. When listening, remain aware of the client's nonverbal cues. This can provide important information about a client's comprehension and comfort with the topics being discussed.

Table 2.4 Communication Skill Development Examples

Skill area	Learning objective	Example mentee behavior	Example mentor support
Verbal communication	Use professional language and tone appropriate for the audience	Explains discharge instructions clearly to a client using laymen terminology	Provides opportunities to rehearse client communication in rounds
Active listening	Demonstrate listening and comprehension	Minimizes interruptions and paraphrases client concerns in own words	Directly observes client communication and conveys observed behaviors
Reflective listening	Ensure appropriate understanding of what the client shared	Asks client if the information paraphrased is correct	Directly observes client communication and conveys observed behaviors
Body language	Use appropriate posture and eye contact	Maintains open stance in consultation	Videotapes client interactions to review with the mentee
Use of open-ended questions	Formulate questions that invite the client to share information beyond a yes or no answer	Utilize open-ended questions in history-taking to gain insight into client's concerns	Practices altering closed-ended questions into open-ended questions during rounds
Written medical records	Document accurately and concisely	Submits SOAP note with objective terminology	Randomly audits medical records for appropriate terminology and efficiency
Written client communication	Explains concepts clearly and at an accessible reading level	Sends email to client with answer to a follow-up question	Audits mentee's written communications and discharge instructions

4. Asking Insightful Questions and Seeking Clarification
   Asking thoughtful, open-ended questions demonstrates curiosity and encourages deeper learning. Mentees should not fear seeking clarification—from clients or colleagues—as this reflects an eagerness to understand.

5. Written Communication
   Clear, concise, and objective writing in emails, SOAP (Subjective, Objective, Assessment, Plan) notes, and discharge instructions ensures continuity of care and legal compliance. Written communication to clients should be at a reading level that is accessible to the average client and avoids jargon and overuse of medical terminology. Mentees should seek feedback on written communication early in their training to prevent ingraining poor habits.

MENTOR TIP

Support the development of crucial communication skills by demonstrating them in your own communication and providing opportunities for the mentee to utilize them in low-stakes environments, such as mock communication exercises, team meetings, and rounds. *See chapter 9 for more on mentoring communication skills.*

AVOIDING COMMON COMMUNICATION MISTAKES

Most client complaints result from a lack of communication or miscommunication (Russell et al., 2022). Mentees should remain aware of the common communication mistakes outlined in Table 2.5 and utilize their mentor's experience and guidance to recognize and avoid them.

SKILL SET 2: CULTIVATE A GROWTH MINDSET

A growth mindset positively correlates with performance and well-being in veterinary trainees. How an individual responds to challenges reflects their mindset. Those with a fixed mindset may view mistakes as failures, while those with a growth mindset use these moments as opportunities for development.

Table 2.5 Common Communication Mistakes in Clinical Practice

Mistake	Description	Example	How the mentor can help
Failing to listen	Focusing on your response instead of the client's concerns can make them feel unheard, leading to frustration or distrust.	A client explains their pet's lethargy, but the mentee interrupts with treatment options before fully understanding the timeline or concerns.	Model and role-play active listening techniques. Debrief with the mentee after appointments. Evaluate listening cues used or missed.
Overloading information	Use of medical terms or providing excessive detail can confuse or overwhelm clients, damaging rapport and understanding.	The mentee explains a diagnosis using complex terms without checking for client comprehension.	Encourage mentees to practice using analogies and plain language. Review client education handouts together and codevelop simple scripts.
Not setting realistic expectations	Overpromising or failing to explain uncertainties can cause dissatisfaction when outcomes differ from what was communicated.	The mentee assures a client that their pet will recover fully without discussing possible complications.	Share past experiences where honest communication built trust. Coach mentee on how to balance empathy with medical realism.
Ignoring nonverbal cues	Missing body language, tone, or facial expressions can result in overlooking client confusion or distress.	A client crosses their arms and avoids eye contact, but the mentee continues the conversation without checking in.	Watch client interactions together (when appropriate) or discuss observations. Teach mentees to check in based on what they notice nonverbally.
Avoiding difficult conversations	Skipping or rushing hard topics like euthanasia or finances can leave clients feeling unprepared and unsupported.	The mentee avoids discussing poor prognosis until the client presses for answers.	Provide structured communication tools (e.g., SPIKES). Role-play tough conversations and offer reassurance after emotionally charged cases.
Not providing adequate follow-up	Lack of follow-up can lead to confusion or noncompliance.	A client leaves without knowing when to return or what signs to monitor, resulting in delayed treatment.	Encourage mentees to always end visits with a summary and clear plan. Cocreate follow-up protocols or checklists as training tools.

Mentees should be encouraged to embrace a growth mindset as they navigate their professional journey (Dweck, 2006). Reframe failure as an opportunity for growth and experimentation. By providing consistent encouragement, constructive feedback, and opportunities for mentees to tackle new challenges, mentors help shift the focus from perfection to progress, reinforcing that growth is a continuous, supported process within the veterinary profession.

Embrace Challenges as Learning Opportunities

Facing challenges is inevitable in the unpredictable world of veterinary medicine. Mentees should cultivate a sense of curiosity and embrace learning opportunities, whether those are clinical skills, communication strategies, or innovative approaches to medical care. This approach broadens clinical expertise and enhances confidence and resilience. Embracing new cases, technologies, and procedures with an open mind is crucial. Mentees should reflect on experiences, seek mentorship during difficult cases, and take calculated risks to broaden their clinical exposure.

Take Control of Your Learning

Self-directed learning is essential for professional growth. This style of learning places the responsibility of learning in the mentee's hands, which increases engagement, motivation, and information retention (Freeman et al., 2022). Through this process, mentees identify their needs, set goals, and engage in learning activities that support skill development. This style of learning applies to all types of skill development—from learning to effectively manage a medical case to improving communication.

Mentors can support self-directed learning by adapting their approach to each mentee's needs. When I worked with one of my mentees on a case, I found that breaking the task into smaller steps made them feel more confident as they could slowly analyze the problem in a manner that was most efficient and supportive for their individual learning needs.

Engage in Reflection

Structured self-reflection enhances learning and can be accomplished through journaling or debriefing with a mentor. Mentees can learn from each case and interaction with clients and colleagues to enhance clinical judgment, emotional resilience, and other skills. This practice allows mentees to understand their strengths, identify areas for improvement, and make meaningful progress toward personal and professional goals.

MENTOR TIP

Foster a growth mindset in your mentee by modeling resilience, normalizing setbacks, and celebrating effort as much as the outcome. Share your own learning curves and demonstrate adaptive problem-solving. Empower your mentee to take risks, engage in self-directed learning, and reflect openly.

SKILL SET 3: PRIORITIZE WELL-BEING

Veterinary professionals face high levels of stress, which can lead to burnout and compassion fatigue. Early career veterinarians are at higher risk of reduced well-being and serious psychological distress than their experienced colleagues (Reinhard, 2023). Mentees must develop tools and strategies to maintain well-being and preserve career longevity and mental health.

These tools may include:

- Set boundaries between time in the clinic and home life.
- Develop healthy stress management tools, such as journaling, participating in debriefs with the mentor, and mindfulness.
- Maintain physical health through sleep, exercise, and nutrition.
- Maintain spiritual health by engaging in practices that support individual beliefs. This may include meditation, other grounding practices, or participating in organized religion.
- Engage in interests outside of veterinary medicine to foster identity diversification and enhance emotional resilience.
- Recognize signs of compassion fatigue and secondary trauma, including irritability, depersonalization, and sleep disturbances.
- Develop a support network of peers, colleagues, mentors, and mental health professionals.
- Develop resilience, which is the ability to recover from setbacks and continue moving forward in the face of challenges.

MENTOR TIP

Be aware of signs of burnout, compassion fatigue, and serious psychological distress as well as available resources for mental health support through your employer or profession at large. To support well-being, model healthy habits and invite mentees to engage in open discussion about their stressors and well-being. *For an in-depth discussion on how mentors can support their mentee's well-being and resilience, see chapter 10.*

SKILL SET 4: COPING WITH CHALLENGING CASES

Mentees will be challenged by managing difficult cases and emotionally charged client interactions. Critical skills for these situations include empathy, ethical decision-making, clear communication, and emotional resilience. In the moment, sensitivity, critical thinking, and the ability to maintain professionalism—particularly when emotions run high—are vital.

Emotional regulation is a key skill for managing these difficult cases. Clients may become emotionally distressed by the potential loss of a pet, financial strain, or disagreements about treatment options. In such situations, acknowledging the client's emotional state, validating their feelings, and offering support while guiding them toward appropriate medical decisions is essential.

For example, in cases where euthanasia is being considered, approach the client with care and respect. Frame the discussion around the pet's quality of life and the ethical implications, ensuring the client feels supported in making an informed decision. This may include discussing options for palliative care or making a referral to a specialist for a second opinion. Be aware of the cultural and personal beliefs of the client, as these can significantly influence their decisions.

MENTOR TIP

Provide coaching on how to navigate ethically complex or emotionally fraught cases. Encourage open discussion without fear of judgment when your mentee faces a challenging case. This creates a psychologically safe space where the mentees can articulate their concerns, explore options, and receive constructive feedback on possible courses of action. By walking through real-world dilemmas together, mentors can also share their own past experiences and decision-making processes, offering valuable insight into how they have navigated similar conflicts in practice.

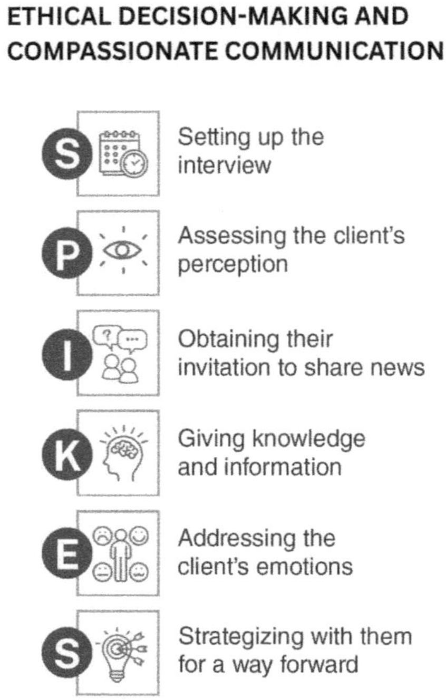

FIGURE 2.2 The SPIKES protocol. This figure presents the SPIKES framework, a structured approach used to guide veterinary professionals through delivering difficult news while upholding ethical standards and emotional sensitivity. This tool is especially valuable in mentoring settings focused on building communication competence in ethically charged clinical situations. *Source:* Courtesy of Kate Boatright (2025).

Compassionate Communication

When delivering difficult news, consider using "Breaking Bad News" communication techniques, such as the SPIKES model: Setting up the interview, assessing the client's Perception, obtaining their Invitation to share news, giving Knowledge and Information, addressing the client's Emotions, and Strategizing with them for a way forward. These techniques can ensure that the client is well-informed, supported, and engaged in the decision-making process.

Additionally, mentees should always follow-up with clients after challenging interactions to check on their emotional well-being, clarify any further questions, and reinforce that they are available for support. This approach not only strengthens the relationship with the client but also fosters a culture of empathy and trust within the veterinary practice. This can sometimes feel intimidating or overwhelming, especially after a negative client interaction (Figure 2.2).

MENTOR TIP

Help mentees prepare for difficult client communication by role-playing the conversation, discussing key client communication points, reviewing communication strategies like the SPIKES model, and helping mentees anticipate and manage client reactions.

Coping with Failure

Some cases will feel like a failure in the moment, even if no mistake was made. This perceived failure may include a misdiagnosis, surgical complication, adverse outcome following treatment, or emotional client interaction. Facing failure is an inevitable part of professional growth and learning (Mitchener and Ogilvie, 2002). Developing emotional regulation strategies, such as mindfulness, reflection, or peer support, helps mentees cope with these difficult moments. These techniques help maintain professional composure and prevent the emotional toll from affecting long-term career satisfaction.

MENTOR TIP

After a distressing case, check in with your mentee. Create time to debrief, provide emotional support, affirm their efforts, and identify strengths and opportunities for improvement. This support can reduce feelings of isolation, build resilience, and reinforce that navigating difficult ethical and emotional terrain is a shared and learnable part of the profession. *Chapter 11 explores ethical dilemmas and navigating mistakes in more detail.*

SKILL SET 5: CONFLICT RESOLUTION

Conflict is inevitable. How it is managed impacts professional growth and relationships with colleagues, team members, and clients. Mentees should learn strategies to recognize and manage conflict as it arises.

Recognizing Potential for Conflict

Disagreements between mentees and mentors may occur as mentees grow more confident in their skills and seek more autonomy. These conflicts may arise due to differences in clinical approaches, teaching styles, or expectations and can be influenced by generational differences, personality, and communication styles. Mentees must approach these conflicts in a manner that maintains mutual respect by engaging in open communication and expressing concerns calmly and professionally.

Disagreements with colleagues can arise over clinical decisions, workflows, or team dynamics. Conflict in these scenarios can be particularly challenging due to the wide variety of professional backgrounds, experiences, and perspectives between individuals.

Navigating Conflict in the Workplace

Regardless of who the conflict is with, similar strategies can be utilized:

- Use "I" statements when expressing feelings and perspectives to avoid sounding accusatory or defensive. For example, instead of saying "You always interrupt me when I'm explaining my thoughts," say "I feel that I don't always get to complete my thoughts during our discussions. I would appreciate the opportunity to explain my thought process."
- Remain open to receiving feedback and seek to understand the other individual's perspective, even when it might differ from your own. Focus on fostering a collaborative atmosphere by actively listening to others' points of view.
- Work to find common ground that can serve as a starting place to create a solution. Express genuine curiosity with questions like "Can you explain why you feel that way?" or "What led you to that conclusion?"
- Maintain a solution-focused approach to disagreements with "constructive feedback." Instead of simply pointing out a problem, propose a potential solution. This method encourages dialogue rather than confrontation. For instance, when discussing differing clinical approaches, a mentee could say, "I see the benefit of your approach, but I'm concerned about X. Would you consider trying Y to see if it might address the issue more effectively?"

- When tensions arise, use self-regulation techniques to manage your emotions. This can help to de-escalate the conflict in the moment. These strategies include deep breathing, pausing before responding, or taking a brief break from the discussion
- Remain aware of nonverbal cues—both your own and those of the other person(s) involved in the conflict. Nonverbal cues like crossed arms or an impatient tone can inadvertently escalate a disagreement. Aim for open, non-defensive body language and a calm, measured tone.
- Remember that not all conflicts can or should be resolved immediately. Sometimes, it's best to step back, reflect, and allow time for emotions to settle before revisiting the issue.

MENTOR TIP

Help your mentee create a plan for managing conflicts with clients and colleagues. This should include de-escalation followed by a plan for conflict resolution. For more information about conflict resolution, see Chapter 9, Communication Skills.

SKILL SET 6: REMAIN OPEN TO FEEDBACK

Feedback is essential to professional growth, though it can be difficult to receive. Developing a feedback mindset, which views constructive criticism as a tool for improvement rather than a personal judgment, significantly improves learning outcomes (Blanchard and Johnson, 1982; Williams and Morey, 2021).

Mentees should remain open and curious when receiving feedback, ask clarifying questions, and reflect before reacting. Staying receptive involves managing emotional responses and focusing on actionable insights. Rather than avoiding criticism, mentees should actively seek it out by asking open-ended questions, engaging informal feedback opportunities, and demonstrating a commitment to implementing what they learn by creating an action plan.

Cultural norms and personal identities can influence how feedback is received. For example, a mentee from a collectivist background may avoid open disagreement, while a neurodiverse mentee may prefer written over verbal feedback. Mentees can advocate for themselves by sharing personal preferences for how feedback is received with their mentor.

MENTOR TIP

Feedback should be provided regularly and include specific examples of both successes and opportunities for improvement. Be aware and respectful of personal preferences shared by the mentee in how feedback is delivered. *Learn more about feedback in Chapter 12.*

Responding to Feedback: Creating Goals and an Action Plan

Mentees should use feedback to establish goals and document action steps for improvement. Many goal-setting frameworks exist, and individuals should identify the best strategy for themselves. One common strategy is SMART goals, which are explored in Figure 2.3. Regardless of the strategy used for goal setting, each goal should be aligned with both personal and professional development objectives (SMART Goals: How to Write SMART Goals, n.d.).

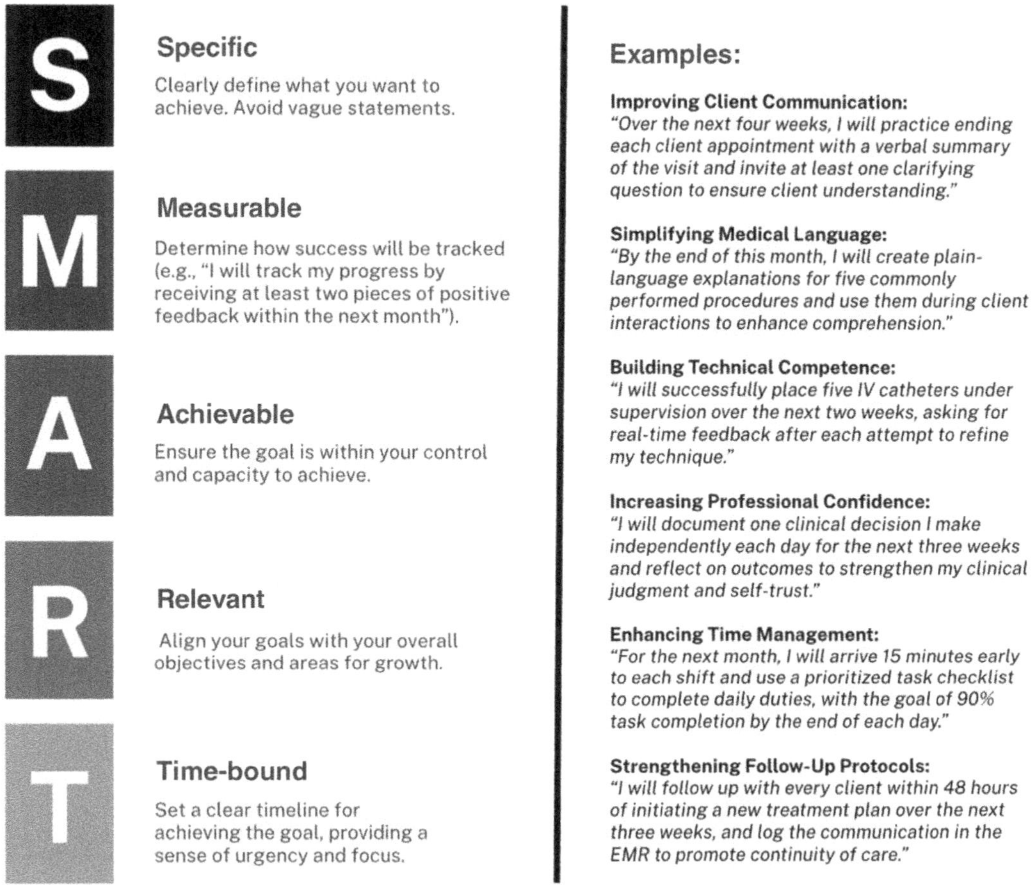

FIGURE 2.3 SMART goals. This figure outlines the SMART goal-setting framework. Examples provided focus on common clinical and professional growth opportunities. *Source:* Courtesy of Kate Boatright (2025).

An action plan is the "how to" for achieving goals. It breaks down each goal into concrete steps that are more manageable to accomplish. Tracking progress through the action plan helps show the progress you've made. To create an action plan, follow these steps:

1. Break down each goal into small, manageable tasks.
2. Assign deadlines to each task to create accountability.
3. Reassess your progress regularly to determine if adjustments are necessary.
4. Seek support if you find yourself struggling to meet any of your goals.

MENTOR TIP

Work with your mentee to establish an action plan based on the feedback you provide. Encourage mentees to set goals and then develop a list of tasks that are needed to reach the desired goal.

Mentees who intentionally develop professional skills will navigate veterinary training with greater confidence and professionalism. Structured mentorship, combined with self-awareness and reflection, enables veterinary professionals to flourish in both clinical and nonclinical domains. This section only brushes the surface of the key skills mentees should develop to engage successfully in the mentoring relationship. Each of these skills is explored in more detail later in this book from the mentor's perspective.

While developing these core competencies is essential, translating them into practice requires structure—a clear framework that guides how mentor and mentee will work together toward shared goals.

BUILDING A MENTORSHIP FRAMEWORK AND PLAN

Kate Boatright

Mentors and mentees should work together to define the mentorship's structure and primary objective(s). This information is used to create a mentorship agreement and plan that will establish boundaries and accountability for both mentor and mentee.

ESTABLISHING THE PURPOSE OF THE MENTORSHIP

Earlier in this chapter, we discussed the importance of goal setting to guide mentee learning. These learning goals are often subsets of the overall purpose of the mentorship, also known as the mentorship's objective. While not a requirement, these objectives often have benefit to the mentee, mentor, and clinic.

Example objectives include:

- Support mentee's transition into the clinic and professional development in the first year after veterinary school so the clinic can retain a new associate veterinarian.
- Guide mentee in expanding a particular skill set to expand the clinic's current service offerings.
- Provide guidance and support the mentee's development to obtain an advanced certification.

Goals can be set by either party to work toward the overall objective. Mentees and mentors may work toward several goals during the mentorship. For instance, an in-clinic mentoring relationship has the overall objective of supporting the mentee's transition into the clinic. The mentee's goals might include improving efficiency in appointments, learning new surgical procedures, and enhancing client communication skills. The mentor's goals could include providing more effective feedback or communicating expectations more clearly.

CREATING A MENTORING AGREEMENT AND PLAN

A mentoring agreement summarizes the planned structure of the mentoring relationship and serves as an accountability tool. Some clinics will have a template agreement that can be customized as needed. However, **it is important that both mentor and mentee have input on the contents of the final agreement.** Additionally, for in-clinic mentoring programs, clinic management plays a role in the success of the mentorship and should be included in the agreement. A sample agreement is included at the end of this chapter.

The mentoring agreement should define:

- Who the mentor and mentee are
- The start and end date for the relationship
- The objective of the relationship
- Roles and responsibilities of the mentor, mentee, and clinic leadership (if applicable)
- Minimum frequency of mentoring meetings
- An outline of how often formal feedback will be delivered and by who (the mentor only or the mentor and clinic management)

- What resources will be provided to the mentor and mentee
- When and how the relationship can be terminated

A mentoring plan is a companion to the agreement that more clearly defines the "how" of the mentorship. When creating a mentoring plan, consider the following questions:

- How often will the mentor and mentee meet? (Remember, the agreement defined the *minimum* frequency of meetings. In the early stages, it is often helpful to meet more frequently.)
    - How long will each meeting be scheduled?
    - When and where will these meetings be held?
    - What is expected of mentor and mentee for meeting preparation?
- How often will feedback be given? This should apply to both the progress of the mentee and allow time for the mentee to give feedback to the mentor.
- What are the initial goals for the mentee and mentor?
    - How often will progress toward these goals be evaluated?
- What resources do the mentor and mentee need to accomplish their goals?
- How often will the mentoring plan and agreement be reviewed?

The mentorship plan is meant to be more flexible than the mentoring agreement as it will develop and evolve over time. Creating two separating documents is ideal so that the plan can be easily revised without altering the more formalized agreement. Table 2.6 summarizes key differences between these documents. Specific considerations for in-clinic mentorship will be discussed in more detail later throughout this book.

Table 2.6 Comparison of Mentoring Agreement and Plan Documents

	Mentoring agreement	Mentoring plan
Purpose	Defines structure, responsibilities, and objectives.	Outlines how mentorship will be carried out day-to-day.
Formality	Formal, especially in structured mentoring programs.	Semiformal to informal.
Content	Roles, responsibilities, minimum frequency of meetings, feedback expectations, duration, and confidentiality.	Meeting logistics, preparation expectations, short-term goals, and resource needs.
Flexibility	Low. Changes require formal review.	High. Easily adjusted as the relationship evolves.
Review frequency	Quarterly or at major checkpoints.	Monthly or as needed.
Who is involved	Mentor, mentee, and clinic management (if applicable).	Mentor and mentee.
Typical format	Written document; may be included in the employment contract; to avoid needing multiple contract revisions (which can be expensive and time-consuming), consider including a mentorship clause in the contract and maintaining the agreement as a separate document.	Shared document or notes that are easily edited by both parties.
Legal review	Necessary if part of a contract; recommended for in-clinic mentoring programs.	Not needed.

REVIEWING THE AGREEMENT AND PLAN

Both the agreement and plan should be reviewed periodically to ensure that expectations are being met. The frequency of review will vary depending on the length of the mentorship.

Consider the following questions when reviewing these documents:

- Are the responsibilities outlined in the agreement being fulfilled? If not, what is missing, and what needs to change?
- Are any of the responsibilities no longer relevant to the mentorship?
- Are the meeting frequency and frequency of feedback still appropriate?
- Have all promised resources been delivered? If any are missing, what is the timeline to receive them?
- Are any additional mentoring resources needed?
- Should the relationship continue as is or are adjustments needed to the agreement/plan?

ESTABLISHING SAFETY AND CONFIDENTIALITY

Mentoring requires trust between mentor and mentee. Committing to confidentiality, nondiscrimination, and non-harassment provides a foundation for this trust. The American Animal Hospital Association (AAHA) Mentoring Toolkit includes a Safe Mentoring Pledge, which addresses these concerns (see Figure 2.4), and can be included in a mentoring agreement.

Safe Mentoring Relationship Pledge

(to be completed by mentor and mentee)

AAHA

I, ______________________________, agree to invest my time in the mentoring relationship with ______________________________ in the role of mentor/mentee. I understand that mentoring requires a safe space and agree to provide this to the best of my abilities. This includes a commitment to create an environment free of discrimination and harassment on all bases, including--but not limited to–race, ethnicity/cultural background, sexual orientation, gender identity, disability, neurodiversity, religion, citizenship/immigration status, and socioeconomic status.

Additionally, I acknowledge that information discussed between mentor and mentee is confidential and will not be disclosed to outside individuals, including employers, family members, and other professionals without the permission of my mentor/mentee. The only exception to this would be in the case of a medical or mental health emergency or a public safety risk. Mentors must disclose if they are mandatory reporters.

Mentor Signature ______________________________ Date ____________

Mentee Signature ______________________________ Date ____________

FIGURE 2.4 The Safe Mentoring Relationship Pledge, AAHA Mentoring Toolkit, American Animal Hospital Association (2024). *Source:* https://www.aaha.org/resources/2023-aaha-mentoring-guidelines/mentoring-toolkit//with permission of American Animal Hospital Association (AAHA).

UNDERSTANDING INDIVIDUAL PREFERENCES

Mentors and mentees should establish individual preferences early in the relationship to improve communication and enhance learning. Discussions should include preferred learning styles, communication modalities, and boundaries around availability.

LEARNING STYLES

Understanding how an individual learns best can help improve the mentor's ability to provide instruction. Having a preferred learning style does not mean this is the only way an individual can learn or provide instruction (Horii, 2007), but knowing preferences can help tailor how information is presented. Several learning styles are described in the literature (Horii, 2007; Storm, 2023) and summarized in Table 2.7.

In many cases, these learning styles can be combined to strengthen the way the material is presented. For example:

- Training videos support both visual and auditory learners.
- Rounds discussions can support many types of learners depending on whether the topic is discussed as a group (i.e. social learning), taught by asking a series of questions and having the mentee work through a thought process (i.e. logical learning) or giving a short presentation to the mentee (i.e. verbal).
- Preparing template discharge instructions promotes both solo and read/write learning styles.

Table 2.7 Understanding Adult Learning Styles

Learning style	How they learn best	How mentors can use this style
Visual	See the material (i.e. charts, diagrams, images)	Provide a video of a new procedure for mentee to review or perform the procedure with the mentee watching.
		Provide flowchart of clinical decision-making for a specific disease.
Auditory	Hear or listen to the material	Share a continuing education lecture recording or podcast on a specific disease process.
		Give short lectures during rounds/mentor meetings.
Read/Write	Through the written word	Provide an article or textbook.
		Encourage mentee to write template discharge instructions for specific diseases.
Kinesthetic	Physically performing a task	Mentee scrubs in to learn a procedure.
Logical or Analytical	Think through problems, answer questions, and look for patterns	Practice pattern recognition (i.e. signalment and history; pathognomonic laboratory changes).
		Ask a series of questions to guide the mentee through the thought process around a case.
Social	In a group or with a partner	Discuss topics during team meetings.
		Encourage peer mentoring relationships.
Solo	On own without interactions with other people	Encourage mentee to engage in self-directed learning.

COMMUNICATION PREFERENCES

With the growing number of communication modalities available, mentors and mentees should share personal preferences:

- Are in person or virtual meetings preferred for local relationships?
- Do you prefer phone calls, emails, or text messages for communicating between mentoring meetings or when not working in the same clinic?
- How quickly is a response expected with each communication modality?

SETTING BOUNDARIES

A final expectation that should be set in the relationship is around availability. While some mentors are happy to be available at all times and encourage their mentees to call, email, or text at any time—even if they aren't working in the clinic together—other mentors want clear boundaries between their work and personal life and prefer to set limitations around their availability. Both of these individuals can be exceptional mentors, as long as the mentee has appropriate expectations of their mentor's availability.

Mentors who don't want to be available at all times but don't articulate these boundaries can find themselves feeling resentful if the mentee contacts them while they are away from the office. This can result in reluctance to engage with the mentee and could be interpreted by the mentee as a disinterest in mentorship.

Setting boundaries around availability is also important for the mentee. Just as mentors should not be expected to be constantly available, the same is true for mentees. Encouraging mentees to set boundaries between work and personal life is an important way to support well-being.

For all mentoring relationships, mentors and mentees should spend time discussing:

- When the mentor or mentee is available for questions
- What timeline the person asking a question can expect for answers to questions that are sent asynchronously (i.e. text or email)
- How often the mentor and mentee are available for meetings

For in-clinic mentoring relationships, these additional considerations should be discussed:

- Is the mentor comfortable being contacted outside of the clinic?
- Are there certain times the mentor will not be available to field case questions?
- What resources does the mentee have for support if the mentor is not available (i.e. textbooks, online forums, other doctors)?

CONTINUAL EVOLUTION

Preferences and boundaries may change as the relationship develops and mentees become more confident in their own skills. Revisit discussions around preferred communication, availability, and boundaries at least quarterly to ensure that both mentor and mentee are satisfied. However, if something isn't working in the relationship, it should be discussed as soon as possible. Mentors and mentees should always feel comfortable requesting a discussion around any of these topics.

CONCLUSION

The mentor–mentee relationship is built on intention, structure, and mutual commitment. This chapter has outlined the essential components that transform informal guidance into purposeful professional development: identifying engaged partners who bring complementary skills and shared values, cultivating core competencies that support growth at every career stage, and establishing clear frameworks that guide the relationship toward meaningful outcomes.

Successful mentorship requires more than good intentions. It demands that mentees actively develop communication skills, embrace challenges with a growth mindset, prioritize their well-being, and remain open to feedback. It requires that mentors provide structured support, model professional behaviors, and create safe spaces for learning and reflection. When these elements work together—engaged participants, intentional skill development, and thoughtful structure—mentorship becomes a powerful catalyst for professional growth, clinical confidence, and career satisfaction. The relationships formed through this process shape not only individual careers but also the culture of veterinary medicine itself.

Mentoring Agreement Template

This agreement is established between ______________, the mentor, and ______________, the mentee.

Mentoring Timeline and Goals

The mentorship will begin on __________________ and last for _____ months.

The primary objective of this relationship is

____

____.

Mentorship Structure

Mentoring meetings will be scheduled at least ______ per week/month/quarter during the duration of this relationship.

Formal reviews will be provided by clinic management at the end of the first month and quarterly thereafter. The mentor will provide regular feedback during mentoring meetings.

Roles and Responsibilities

The mentor agrees to:

The mentee agrees to:

Clinic leadership agrees to support the mentoring relationship by:

Termination

This mentoring agreement will automatically terminate at the end of the agreed-upon timeline unless both mentor and mentee agree to extend it.

The mentoring relationship may be terminated earlier if. . .

BIBLIOGRAPHY

American Animal Hospital Association (AAHA) (2024). AAHA mentoring toolkit. https://www.aaha.org/resources/2023-aaha-mentoring-guidelines/mentoring-toolkit/.

American Veterinary Medical Association (AVMA) (2023). Wellbeing and burnout prevention resources. https://www.avma.org.

Archer, J. and Miller, N. (2011). Communication skills for veterinary professionals. *Vet Times* 41 (6): 14–16.

Bachmann, C., Roschlaub, S., Harendza, S., and Keim, C. (2020). Teaching communication skills: best practices in medical and veterinary education. *Journal of Veterinary Medical Education* 47 (4): 456–465.

Blanchard, K. and Johnson, S. (1982). *The One-Minute Manager*. New York: William Morrow.

Boatright, K. (2024). 5 steps for finding a mentor. *AAHA NEWStat*. https://www.aaha.org/newstat/publications/5-steps-for-finding-a-mentor/ (accessed 11 May 2025).

Dweck, C.S. (2006). *Mindset: The New Psychology of Success*. New York: Random House.

Elce, Y. (2021). The mentor-mentee relationship, addressing challenges in veterinary medicine together. *The Veterinary Clinics of North America. Small Animal Practice* 51: 1099–1109. https://doi.org/10.1016/j.cvsm.2021.04.023.

Freeman, D., Hodgson, K., and Darling, M. (2022). Mentoring new veterinary graduates for transition to practice and lifelong learning. *Journal of Veterinary Medical Education* 49 (4): 409–413. https://doi.org/10.3138/jvme-2021-0036.

Horii, C.V. (2007). Teaching insights from adult learning theory. *Journal of Veterinary Medical Education* 34: 369–376. https://doi.org/10.3138/jvme.34.4.369.

Levinson, D.J. (1978). *The Seasons of a Man's Life*. New York: Random House.

Mindset Works (n.d.). Growth mindset infographic. https://www.mindsetworks.com.

Mitchener, K.L. and Ogilvie, G.K. (2002). Understanding compassion fatigue: keys for working with the veterinary healthcare team. *Journal of the American Animal Hospital Association* 38 (4): 307–310.

Reinhard, A.R. (2023). Early career veterinary wellbeing and solutions to help young veterinarians thrive. *Advances in Small Animal Care* 4: 113–122. https://doi.org/10.1016/j.yasa.2023.05.005.

Reinhard, A., Bourquin, B., Bruno, N. et al. (2023). *2023 AAHA Mentoring Guidelines*. AAHA https://www.aaha.org/resources/2023-aaha-mentoring-guidelines/.

Rose, R., Pinchbeck, G., and Williams, N. (2020). Veterinary student perceptions of mentoring: a survey-based study in UK universities. *Veterinary Record* 186 (2): e16.

Russell, E., Mossop, L., Forbes, E., and Oxtoby, C. (2022). Uncovering the 'messy details' of veterinary communication: an analysis of communication problems in cases of alleged professional negligence. *The Veterinary Record* 190 (3): e1068. https://doi.org/10.1002/vetr.1068.

SMART Goals: How to Write SMART Goals (n.d.). MindTools. https://www.mindtools.com.

Storm, A. (2023). The 7 main types of learning styles (and how to teach to them). *Thinkific*. https://www.thinkific.com/blog/learning-styles/ (accessed 6 October 2025).

The Ohio State University College of Veterinary Medicine (n.d.). Client communication diagram. https://vet.osu.edu.

VetPartners (2025). Compensation for veterinary mentors [WWW Document]. Team Util. Guide. https://utilization-guide.vetpartners.org/guide/5-11 (accessed 12 May 2025).

Williams, S. and Morey, R. (2021). Effective communication in veterinary practice: how feedback improves patient care. *Veterinary Leadership Review* 9 (1): 4–12.

The New Graduate Mindset CHAPTER 3

INTRODUCTION

Dani Rabwin

One of the greatest challenges in veterinary mentorship is understanding what it feels like to stand where our mentees stand—at the very beginning of their careers, balancing excitement with self-doubt. The fears, impostor syndrome, and psychological hurdles that plague early-career veterinarians aren't character flaws to overcome—they're predictable responses to the enormous transition from student to practitioner that require intentional mentorship strategies. I wanted this chapter to capture that perspective while also showing mentors how to respond in ways that truly make a difference.

To bring these perspectives to life, I turned to Lindsey Hedges, DVM, and Wrenn Calcutt, DVM. Lindsey, now the Senior Director of Medical Learning at Mission Pet Health, has walked the path from new graduate to practice owner and has built mentorship programs that support veterinarians at scale. She opens and closes this chapter with the seasoned perspective of a mentor who believes that great mentorship is the foundation of career satisfaction. In the middle, Wrenn provides a candid look from the mentee's side—sharing what it really feels like to transition from veterinary school into practice, from improvising CIDR (Controlled Internal Drug Release) applicators to managing her first solo equine euthanasia. I wanted her voice placed here intentionally, so readers could step directly into the shoes of a new graduate before returning to Lindsey's broader guidance.

Together, they illuminate both the fears that keep many new graduates awake at night—"What if I miss something and hurt a patient?" "What if my team regrets hiring me?"—and the remarkable strengths new graduates bring to practice. You'll learn how to help your mentees distinguish between helpful preparatory anxiety and destructive impostor syndrome, how to leverage the power of supportive relationships in building confidence, and how to create environments where curiosity and vulnerability are safe. Perhaps most importantly, this chapter will remind you that new graduates don't only need your guidance—they also bring fresh energy and perspective that can reinvigorate entire teams when their contributions are welcomed and valued.

COMMON FEARS AND EXPECTATIONS

Lindsey Hedges-Gieseking

WHAT IF?

What if my clients hate me? What if I have no idea what I'm doing? What if I passed NAVLE (North American Veterinary Licensing Exam) from lucky guesses? What if my treatment doesn't work? What if these diagnostics don't give me an answer? What if my team thinks I'm incompetent? What if I miss something and hurt a patient? What if I don't know what to do in an emergency? What if my patients are better off with a more experienced doctor? What if I'm not cut out to be a veterinarian?

Here's a secret: **common fears are common**. Unfortunately, most of us don't talk about our fears enough to figure out how common they really are.

What if it's ok to admit we don't have experience or wisdom? What if it's essential to seek feedback from people around us? What if the courage to speak up about our fears is the key to developing clinical confidence?

HELLO IMPOSTOR: MY OLD FRIEND

Doubting our qualifications is a normal part of learning. When we start a new role or do something we've never done before, it's natural for our brains to question whether we have the skills and the tools to get the job done. Gaining experience is hard, so imagining "What If" helps us to think through all the possibilities on the road ahead and what we might do if something goes wrong. It prepares us with strength and courage for the bumpy road ahead.

Our inner critic is not our enemy; it is our pessimistic friend. Impostor syndrome, on the other hand, is when that friendship turns toxic. Impostor syndrome occurs when we get stuck in the idea that we *can't* answer "What if" or that we will *never* build the skills to be successful, even if we've been successful in other circumstances before (Kogan, 2020). Instead of seeing these thoughts as helpful in preparing us for the challenge ahead, we accept these thoughts as true and try to avoid letting others discover our shortcomings. Instead of building courage and strength to face our challenges, impostor syndrome stops us from even trying.

The underlying driver for impostor syndrome is the belief that other people are confident and "in the know" and we are incompetent and "in the dark." When we summon the courage to be curious instead of judgmental about these impostor thoughts, we soon learn that confidence comes not from knowing all the answers, but from being comfortable in the unknown (Wilson, 2024). Most of us are in the dark, figuring out veterinary medicine (and life) one "What if" at a time.

Impostor thought	Judgmental reaction	Explore the logic	Get curious
What if I miss something and hurt a patient?	I should only see "easy" cases to avoid mistakes.	Confidence and mastery do not come from "easy" cases. To learn, we must stretch.	Have the other veterinarians I work with missed something before? What happened? What did they learn?
What if I can't stop the bleeding during a large dog spay?	If I can't handle a surgical emergency, I shouldn't do the surgery.	The entire team is needed during an emergency. Even experienced surgeons ask for help.	Has this happened to my mentor? What did they do? How often do surgical complications happen? What is our protocol in case of an emergency? How can we practice protocols as a team?

What if my team regrets hiring me?	I am so slow, and I ask too many questions. I am a burden to the other doctors and staff.	Asking questions is essential to development and shows engagement.	Is the tension I feel within the team real? What else is happening that might be causing stress? Who will give me honest feedback? How do I feel when helping a staff member or student extern learn something new?
What if all my classmates are doing foreign body surgeries and I'm still nervous about vaccines?	I'm so far behind, there's no way I'll ever catch up. I am not getting the experience to gain confidence as a veterinarian.	What is shown on social media is not the full story. Clinical development is a personalized path influenced by many variables.	What excites me about foreign body surgeries? What did my classmate do to get that surgical experience? What resources could help me learn? How have I improved since last month?

The first step in managing your fears is to develop self-awareness to know that impostor thoughts are our well-intentioned friends that can turn toxic if they overstay their welcome. The next step is to build a trusted group of mentors to give feedback, help set realistic expectations, and cheerlead when we are challenged (Carreras, 2022). **Overcoming fears is easier when we have someone by our side giving us encouragement when we need it the most.**

TOGETHER IS BETTER

When you are facing a challenge, just having a supportive friend in your corner makes the challenge seem less daunting. In a study by Schnall et al. (2008), participants rated a hill as less steep when accompanied by a close friend compared to participants who were alone. Previous studies had proven that physiological factors like age, physical fitness, and fatigue influenced the perception of hill slant. Controlling for these factors, Schnall et al. proved that even *imagining* an encounter with someone of "great personal importance, who made them feel good and who would provide help in a difficult situation," made the hill appear less steep. The quality of the relationship was a significant finding in the study—the more positive you felt about the individual you imagined, the less steep the challenge ahead.

As mentees, our mindset about our mentors is just as important, if not more so, than the physical presence of our mentor by our side. We must trust their feedback and reassurance and let the thought of them help carry us through hard times. This is a critical cognitive step in combating fear and self-criticism—we must be open about the thoughts we are up against and arm ourselves with encouragement from our support system.

One of the reasons we get stuck in impostor syndrome is the belief that other people sugarcoat reality or that they would feel differently if they knew the "real you." The conundrum here is that the thoughts we have about ourselves are not "real"; we have the power to change our reality by changing our mindset.

When you change the way you look at things,
the things you look at change.

— Dr. Wayne Dyer

A core belief in impostor syndrome is that other people are more qualified than we are and that we are inadequately prepared for the task at hand. Logically, if other people are qualified and knowledgeable, we *should* believe them when they give us reassurance or positive feedback. Yet, we don't. And worse, when we withhold our thoughts and beliefs, we let our fear grow unchecked. We may believe that challenging their positive feedback may be seen as ungrateful, that asking for details is disrespectful, or that accepting praise without a side order of criticism will make us less driven to improve. None of these assumptions are true—fear is best conquered through self-awareness, courage, and mentorship.

Impostor thought: *"What if my team regrets hiring me?"*

Mentee: "I feel the tension within the team. What has everyone on edge? Am I doing anything that is making that worse?"

Mentor: "No, you are doing great. Performance reviews are this week, and our practice manager has a history of being harsh. She's well intentioned as she wants people to be aware so they can improve. . . but everyone feels dread before and defeated after."

Impostor Syndrome: *"There's something they're still not telling me... are people being punished because they take so much time to help me? I bet this is all my fault."*

Result: Withdraw from the team to "spare them" from having to help.

Get Curious: *"What can I do to help morale? I learn so much from the team and I appreciate the effort they put into helping me grow."*

Result: Build trust with the team and discover they love helping people learn.

Changing our mindset is challenging; it requires persistence and practice. While the mentee is ultimately responsible for making that change, mentor support is critical to success (Yanke, 2023). As mentors, it is discouraging to see your mentee stuck in fear, unwilling to accept the praise that affirms their success. However, mentors can also improve their likelihood of success with persistence and practice.

MENTOR TIPS: DELIVERING POSITIVE FEEDBACK TO COMBAT COMMON FEARS

1. **Be Specific**

   Find a feedback model that reminds you to provide specific details when giving positive feedback. Situation–Behavior–Impact is one such model that can be easy to remember and apply. For more options, read more about feedback in Chapter 12.

   Set the stage: "*Last week you mentioned that client communication with derm cases has been a struggle. I made sure to keep an eye out for new derm cases on your schedule this week so I could listen in. Is now a good time for feedback?*"

Category	Feedback	Description
Situation	*"Mrs. Smith came in with Koko yesterday; she's been a chronic atopy patient that we've all seen for flare ups through the years."*	Be specific about the facts: time, people, context, and circumstances. Be sure to remove emotions or subjective interpretations from your description.
Behavior	*"You spent the time to review the file beforehand and checked your knowledge of her history with both your assistant and Mrs. Smith. You asked Mrs. Smith's opinion on what she thought worked best in the past and what didn't work. You then set expectations for reducing flare up intensity and frequency and emphasized management vs. cure."*	Describe observable behavior while avoiding assumptions or interpretations of intent. This will take practice—it is natural to judge or create a story.
Impact	*"Mrs. Smith made a point to seek me out afterward and tell me how much she 'loves our new doctor.' She said she felt that you truly wanted to help her get a plan in place for long-term management and not just treating today's flare up. You are doing a great job—these cases are hard and can be frustrating for all of us. Your focus on improving client communication and involving your assistant more is working. I would bring my own atopy dog to you."*	Explain your thoughts and feelings. If you have received feedback from others about the experience, describe that impact and keep it factual. Resist the urge to embellish the story or read deeper into the feedback of others.

2. Acknowledge the Impostor Thoughts

Ask questions that help your mentee examine their imposter thoughts or fears. These questions may be hard to answer—if your mentee needs time to think about it, let them know when and where you will pick the conversation back up to dive deeper.

"When I say you are doing a great job, you often dismiss it as luck or redirect the praise to someone else. What do you think is behind that?"

"What evidence do you need to feel successful as a doctor?"

"What scares you about this case? What would help you feel less anxious?"

If you are suspicious that fear or imposter thoughts are holding your mentee back and they are not yet comfortable with voicing them, share a story about your own experience with your inner critic.

"As a new grad, I would lie awake at night and worry that I wasn't good enough, that I didn't know enough to help my patients. Turns out, brains lie to us sometimes when we are learning and growing. You get stronger with every case you see; not at knowing all the answers, but at figuring out all the things you don't know."

3. Allow Time for Reflection and Self-assessment

Emphasize progress over time. Evaluation of one point in time without comparing to past events can reinforce "All-or-Nothing" thinking. A common thinking error, the All-or-Nothing approach, leads mentees to believe that they are either right or wrong as an absolute. Comparing progress over time shifts the focus to the process itself, helping mentees form their own realistic expectations for success.

"How do you feel that spay went compared to your last one?"

"How are you managing your time differently this week than last week?"

4. **Set Realistic Expectations**
   What would you expect in this situation from a veterinarian who is three months into practice? How is that different from someone who has been out 1 year? 2 years? 10 years? Ask your mentee what they think they should be able to do. Is there a gap between your expectations and theirs?

5. **Dig Deeper**
   Sometimes, despite all our best efforts, mentees may continue to resist feedback. Encourage your mentee to dig deeper with a counselor, therapist, or coach outside of the clinic. Behavioral Therapy and Counseling can be life-changing, and sometimes encouragement from a mentor may be the boost a mentee needs to seek additional help.

   "The pressures that are put on us can be overwhelming, and sometimes it can feel like we're being crushed from all sides. It doesn't have to be that way, though. There are tools and skills that can help train our brains to relieve some of the pressure. Have you ever considered working with a counselor or therapist?"

Editor's Note: *Dr. Hedges highlights the fears, self-doubt, and impostor thoughts that often accompany the first steps into practice and how mentor support can make those challenges more manageable. To see how these themes unfold in real life, Dr. Wrenn Calcutt offers the perspective of a new graduate navigating the early transition from academia to clinical work. Her stories illustrate how textbook knowledge must quickly adapt to unpredictable situations and how mentorship provides both reassurance and practical strategies when "the rules" no longer apply.*

BRIDGING THE GAP BETWEEN ACADEMIA AND PRACTICE

Wrenn Calcutt

"Well, I don't think I learned what to do about this in vet school."
This was a phrase often sprinkled in my thoughts as a new graduate veterinarian. After spending eight years pursuing education and training as a doctor, we hope to be prepared for every medical case. But, inevitably, situations that do not fit the textbook arise, many of them not even medical in nature.

PROBLEM-SOLVING: I DON'T HAVE THE RIGHT TOOLS...OR DO I?

Shortly after taking responsibility for stocking and operating out of my own ambulatory vet truck, I went to an appointment for a goat client involved in breeding goats for 4H shows. The goal was to begin an estrus synchronization protocol so that the does would all come into heat in a particular date range. A crucial step of this synchronization protocol involved placing a CIDR—an intravaginal device that releases progesterone. On this particular day, I arrived at the client's farm and realized I did not have the CIDR applicator with me. I considered the impact of this mistake on my reputation, the reputation of my boss's business, and on the client's business. The textbooks never said what to do with a CIDR when you don't have the applicator. So, I had to get creative and use the foundational knowledge I had to move forward into an actionable solution.

SOLUTION: IMPROVISING WITH AVAILABLE TOOLS

Understanding the mechanics of a CIDR applicator, I fashioned an alternative using:

- A syringe casing with the ends filed off
- White tape to smooth rough edges
- A plastic balling gun (pill plunger)

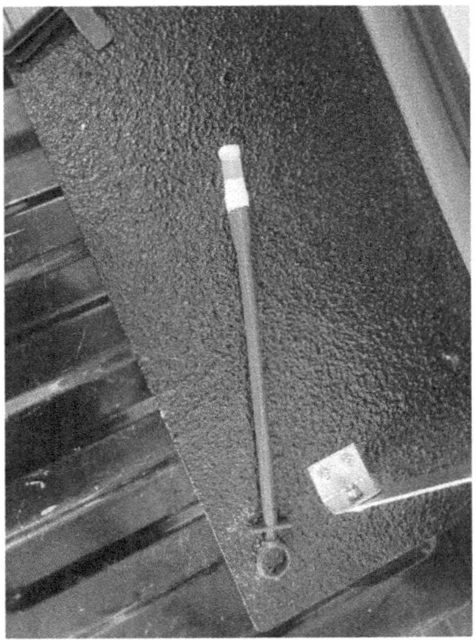

Source: Courtesy of Dr. Wrenn Calcutt.

After testing my makeshift applicator, I successfully implanted the CIDRs. My client was satisfied, and I felt a deep sense of accomplishment. It was the first of many situations I would be faced with where school knowledge was insufficient, and the ability to take what knowledge I did have and turn it into action would carry me to success. Mentors provide an example of overcoming insufficient knowledge or inadequate equipment. Their confidence and experience are the building blocks for resilience in the face of multiple challenges.

Studies support that new graduate veterinarians are experiencing the most severe levels of exhaustion and career burnout when compared with their older and presumably more experienced colleagues (Zakharenkov, 2021). Access to mentorship early in the veterinary career is a crucial part of bridging the gap between the vast information obtained in veterinary school and the challenges of real-world practice.

THE CHALLENGE OF TRANSITIONING FROM STUDENT TO PRACTITIONER

The move from vet school to practice is exciting, but it requires a shift in mindset. Instead of structured lectures and guided labs, new graduates face unpredictable cases and real-time decision-making. The daily routine will change from the past years of attending long hours of lectures and laboratories, being fully guided by instructors, to taking the lead of a team enduring long hours of active physical and mental work. I went through this transition in 2021, becoming a farm animal practitioner at a previously solo doctor practice. I then expanded the scope of my practice in 2023 by joining a 5-doctor fully mixed animal clinic. Both of these situations brought their own challenges, and the mentorship I received helped me develop resiliency and a dedication to lifelong learning. By sharing what I learned during my early career development, I want to continue creating vitalized careers for new veterinarians for many years to come.

Key Differences Between Vet School and Practice.

Vet school	Real-world practice
Structured curriculum with set objectives	Unpredictable case presentations
Exams provide clear right/wrong answers	Clinical decisions require adaptability
Perfectionism can be an asset	Perfectionism can cause self-doubt
Learning is mostly theoretical	Learning is hands-on and immediate
Guidance from experienced specialists	Leadership of an animal care team in managing cases

Source: Courtesy of Dr. Wrenn Calcutt

As the chart highlights, the transition from vet school to clinical practice isn't just a step forward—it's a shift in expectations, roles, and the nature of learning itself. This shift can be overwhelming for new graduates. A tendency toward perfectionism will magnify feelings of doubt, imposter syndrome, and exhaustion.

HOW MENTORS CAN HELP NEW GRADUATES ADAPT

CLINICAL KNOWLEDGE

Develop a Structured Schedule

Use practice management software to allow mentees to view their schedules in advance. This helps them prepare for appointments, such as:

- **Puppy wellness visits:** Reviewing vaccine schedules and common ailments.
- **Sick cases (e.g., goat with weakness, anorexia, and head pressing):** Developing differentials and considering immediate vs. send-out diagnostics. At first, scheduling extra time for these cases will allow the new graduate to consult their learning resources and build confidence in their decision-making.

For early-career veterinarians, the motivation to learn and be prepared—so essential during veterinary school—remains a powerful asset in navigating full days of wellness and sick appointments.

Implement Standard Operating Procedures (SOPs)

Having SOPs for common cases—like **otitis externa**—can guide decision-making. For example:

Otitis Externa SOP

Symptoms: Pruritic ears and head shaking

Diagnostics: Ear cytology and otoscopic exam

Treatment: Intra-aural medication + anti-inflammatory

By using this SOP, I overcame my tendency to focus solely on intra-aural medications, while neglecting to provide additional anti-inflammatory treatment to relieve pain and pruritus. Following a standardized approach helped me deliver more complete and consistent care to my patients while building my clinical confidence.

Common SOPs for General Practice		
Corneal ulcers	Diabetes	Diarrhea
Dystocia	Ear infections	Equine colic
Equine esophageal obstruction	Heart disease	Inappropriate urination
Internal/external parasites	Lacerations	Lameness
Obesity	Seizures	Soft tissue masses
Upper respiratory infection	Vomiting	Wellness visits

Clinical knowledge can be a daunting challenge. While new graduates hold the most current information from veterinary school, they may still lack the pattern recognition and clinical reasoning that comes with experience. Helping mentees in this area involves teaching them how to be active participants in their own learning and look at gaps in knowledge as opportunities to deepen their connection to their chosen profession.

SELF-DIRECTED LEARNING

1. What Self-Directed Learning IS:

   a. **Self-assessment and Goal-setting**: Rather than the mentor presenting a list of skills and procedures for the new graduate to accomplish, the mentee evaluates their own knowledge and skill gaps (e.g., understanding a particular disease, surgical technique, or client communication skill) and sets goals for themselves on a few particular areas they would like to improve. These goals should be SMART (Diehl and Galindo-Gonzalez, 2024):

      i. Specific—Well-defined, clear, and narrow goals make for the most effective planning.

      ii. Measurable—How will you gauge progress? How will you know when your goal is complete?

      iii. Achievable—Can the goal be done with the time and resources at hand?

      iv. Relevant—What need will achieving this goal meet? How does the goal fit into broader objectives?

v. Time-bound—Specify a deadline. Providing a sense of urgency reduces the risk of losing motivation or losing track of measuring progress. Deadlines can function as mile markers on a greater timeline.

b. Identifying and Seeking Resources: The mentor's role is to guide the selection of appropriate resources, steering mentees toward valuable materials and advising on how to evaluate sources critically:

i. Primary literature (research articles and case studies) and textbooks

ii. Clinical guidelines and best practices (SOPs and clinician's brief treatment algorithms)

iii. Online learning platforms (e.g., VetFolio, VIN, and Cornell ClinPath)

iv. In-person: The mentor themselves, other vets in the practice, and experienced technicians.

c. Application to Clinical Practice

i. The learner applies the information they have learned to real-world clinical cases—diagnosing conditions, performing surgeries, and managing client communications.

ii. The mentor plays a crucial role by generating these hands-on experiences and opportunities for the mentee to apply what they've learned.

iii. Based on the learner's needs, a mentor may be directly involved working collaboratively with the learner, participating in an observation role or even providing case discussion and feedback after an experience is fully complete.

d. Continuous Feedback and Adjustment: Reflection and Evaluation.

i. The mentee is encouraged to reflect on their experiences: What went well? What did not go well? Have they achieved their goal? If not, what needs to occur next?

ii. Remembering that goals should be measurable and time-bound, the mentor should provide their own evaluation of the mentee at a scheduled time. This is an opportunity to provide critique and encouragement and ensure the mentee is on the right track to achieving their goal by the deadline set.

2. What Self-Directed Learning Is NOT:

a. Being given all the answers:
Some people think that the role of a mentor in veterinary medicine is to provide all the answers to clinical questions. However, an effective mentor helps the mentee develop problem-solving skills, critical thinking, and independence. Mentorship in self-directed learning (SDL) should empower the mentee to think through challenges and <u>learn how to seek out answers,</u> rather than simply providing them.

b. Mentees learning on their own:
"Being thrown to the wolves," "Sink or Swim"—these are phrases that haunt the nightmares of all veterinary mentees. Effective learning involves collaboration with peers, seeking guidance from experts or using resources like online communities and mentors. It's about being resourceful and using <u>available support</u> when needed.

c. A free-for-all with no structure:

Another misconception is that self-directed learning is entirely unstructured or spontaneous. While it offers more freedom to create a unique mentorship path, successful SDL still requires clear planning, setting goals, and creating systems for providing evaluation and tracking progress. Without structure, opportunities for feedback will be missed and learners will lose focus or motivation.

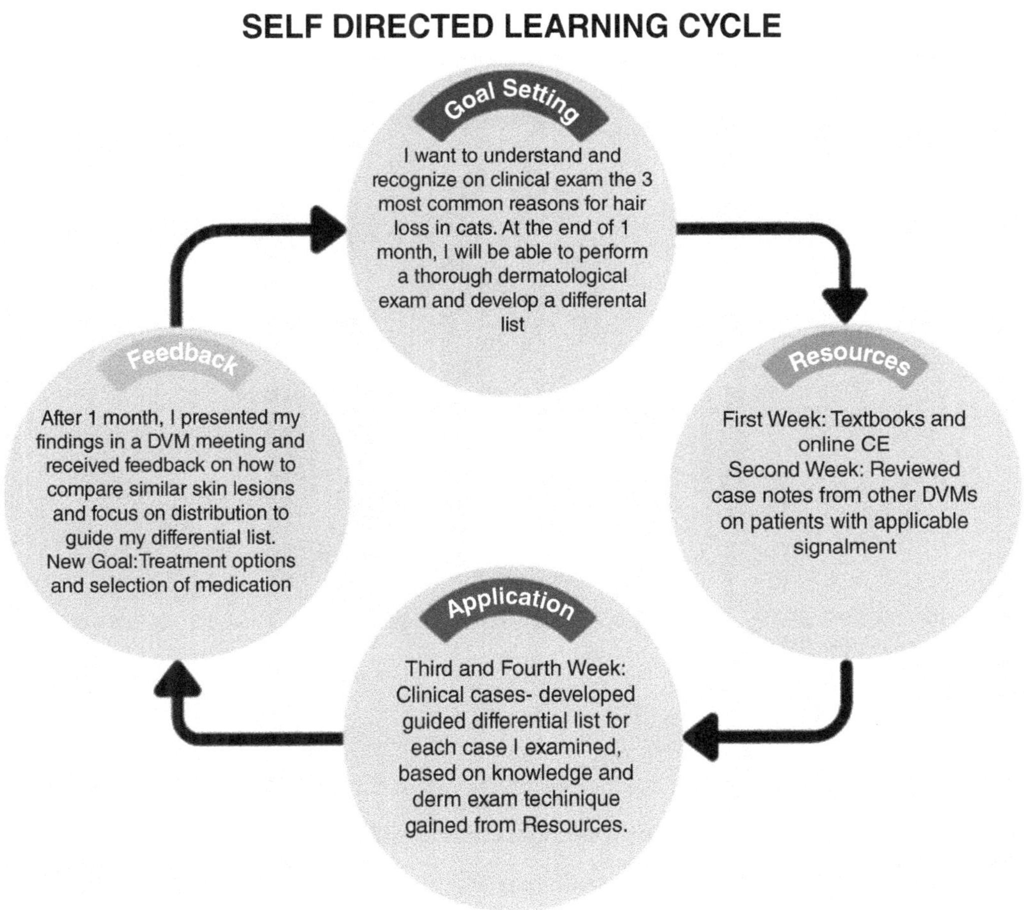

Source: Courtesy of Dr. Wrenn Calcutt (2025).

Self-directed learning requires ongoing dedication and practice, and the most fulfilling aspect was the ability to design the goals and learning process to fit my needs. This model allowed me to cover areas that caused the most stress in my daily responsibilities with a greater priority than my mentor might have given them in designing a plan independently.

NAVIGATING SOCIAL AND EMOTIONAL TRANSITIONS

Outside of clinical knowledge, new veterinarians must also navigate social and emotional changes.

1. **Building Relationships with Staff**
   - Existing staff may feel apprehensive about a new doctor's authority
   - New grads may worry about making a good impression and "fitting in" with the existing staff.

- Mentors should demonstrate how to delegate tasks to appropriate support staff. Doctors that learn how to best leverage their team are able to perform at the top of their abilities.
- Encourage new doctors to participate in clinic activities and "traditions".

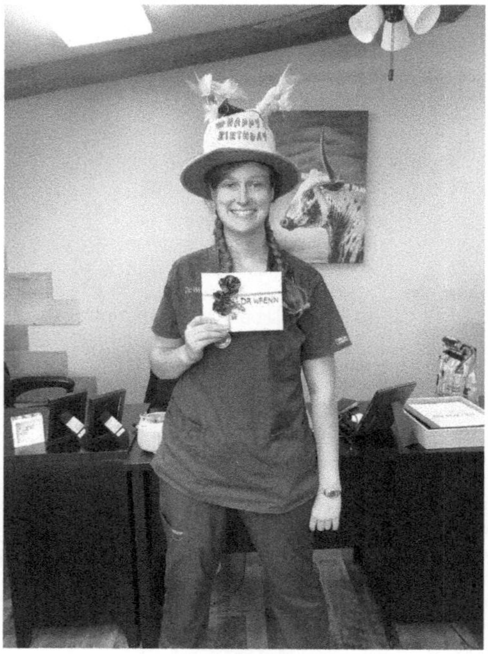

Wearing the silly hat while the entire clinic sang "Happy Birthday" made me feel included in the clinic culture.
Source: Courtesy of Dr. Wrenn Calcutt.

2. **Gaining Client Trust**

   Clients may hesitate to see a new doctor. Practices can help by:

   - Announcing the new vet in **newsletters, emails, and social media**
   - Encouraging clients to book appointments with them.
   - Having mentors publicly support the new vet (e.g., *"This is Dr. Wrenn, and I know she will provide the best care for your animals, just as I would"*).

HANDLING DIFFICULT EXPERIENCES: EUTHANASIA

One of the most challenging aspects of veterinary medicine is performing euthanasia. Euthanasia is cited as a large factor in compassion fatigue and burnout among veterinarians. A study found that 40% of veterinarians reported that their mental and physical health had been affected by euthanasia and 34% had trouble performing euthanasia because of personal distress (Dow et al., 2019). While school covers the technical aspects (drug dosages, venous access, and auscultation), real-life challenges that may not be taught include:

- **Safety concerns:** Large animals can fall unpredictably, small animals that appear heavily sedated may suddenly react and bite or scratch unexpectedly.

- **Emotional burden:** Being the final point in the human-animal bond
- **Unexpected events:** The patient doesn't become sedated from the initial protocol, the vein ruptures while trying to administer IV medication, and owners experience a rapid change in emotions.

Personal Reflection

During my first solo equine euthanasia, I felt confident that I knew how to perform the procedure and the expected series of events. But in actually focusing on obtaining and maintaining venous access and monitoring the administration rate of pentobarbital, I failed to reposition myself to a safe distance as the horse began falling, and I was battered by its head and neck as it fell. Thankfully, the blow shoved me stumbling to the side rather than a more serious outcome. When I informed my clinic mentor, we had a constructive conversation on the importance of not only being prepared with knowledge but also forming that knowledge into an action plan and following through!

MENTORSHIP MOMENT: ROLE-PLAY

Although every case, client interaction, and outcome is unique, practicing different combinations of these variables through simulated scenarios can provide a feeling of familiarity when a new doctor faces a similar scenario in the course of their daily work. The new graduate might be familiar with this style of teaching, as many veterinary schools integrate "simulated client" interactions into the curriculum as a foundation for broader professional skills. Through role-playing interactions, mentors can provide feedback not just on clinical knowledge but also on body language, phrasing, and managing appointment flow. This provides an opportunity for mentors to address specific areas of communication difficulties the doctor might be having or even just put some finishing "polish" on communication in general.

Personal Reflection

Through role-play sessions, I developed several critical phrases that strengthened my communication and diminished my worries about not knowing what to say or do in sensitive situations:

- When starting an appointment with a client who is uneasy about seeing "the new doctor": "Hello Mrs. Jones! My name is Dr. Wrenn, and I am the **newest member of the vet team** here. I have looked through Spot's history so that I can be familiar with his particular medical needs. Tell me more about your concerns with him today. . .."
- When ending an appointment: "**Thank you so much for bringing Fluffy in today**. I am happy to be a part of their care." This phrase has allowed me to end the majority of my appointments on a positive note by bringing the focus back to the patient. **For clients that are afraid of being judged for the condition their animal is in or what treatment they can afford, it has been meaningful for me to thank them for the very brave act of bringing the animal in for care.**
- When delivering news that a diagnostic we hoped would give a definitive diagnosis has unclear results: "Regarding Bella's Lyme testing today—her test has come up negative. I know we were looking forward to a solid answer to the cause of her symptoms today, **but by having ruled out Lyme disease, we can focus our next steps** on the other potential illnesses we have discussed."

- When a client has financial constraints: "Taking the cost of today's visit into consideration, would you share with me an amount that you are able to use for Skittles' care today? I ask because this will **help me focus your resources** into the very best care we can provide for Skittles."
- When performing euthanasia: "I'm very sorry for your loss. I can tell that you love Patches very much. Do you have a favorite memory of Patches?" I try to circle back to this when ending the euthanasia appointment "Please take time to remember the good things with Patches, like the first time he learned to play fetch, and **let those memories comfort you in the coming days**."

  It took multiple practice sessions to find the phrasing that worked best for me, and as I have practiced, these phrases now come to me naturally.

  Social and emotional challenges are part of the veterinary experience because they are part of the universal human experience. Taking time to reflect on the emotions that are intertwined with our daily work strengthens the bond between a mentor and mentee.

Do the best you can until you know better. Then when you know better, do better. —Maya Angelou

This wisdom captures the essence of effective mentorship—a journey of mutual growth where both experienced veterinarians and new graduates commit to continuous improvement and adaptation. Advances in medical research and treatment options are continually changing the landscape of veterinary medicine, and your particular style of mentorship can change too.

Consider these actionable strategies to develop and refine your approach to mentoring new veterinarians:

- Think back to when you were a new doctor: What were some of your biggest challenges? How were you supported during this time? Or, if you felt you weren't supported, what characteristics would you have wanted in a mentor?
- Use a structured mentorship model with regularly scheduled intervals for constructive feedback and reflection to maximize your efficiency. A schedule allows for the mentor's time to be protected from being overwhelmed and also makes the mentee feel valued with time that is dedicated solely to their development.
- What core values or "culture" do you desire for your clinic? How are these values encouraged among support staff, doctors, and clientele? What role do you expect the new doctor to play in upholding or expanding these values?

  Transitioning from veterinary school to real-world practice presents new graduates with both exciting opportunities and significant challenges. A holistic approach to mentorship in all facets of "real-world practice" will empower new graduates to bridge the gap between their foundational knowledge and the daily challenges of veterinary practice.

Editor's Note: *Dr. Calcutt's experiences underscore just how steep the learning curve can feel when moving from school into practice—and how creativity, resilience, and mentor support are essential to finding solutions in the moment. Building on this lived experience, Dr. Lindsey Hedges turns our focus to the unique strengths that new graduates bring with them: curiosity, adaptability, and the awe of doing something for the first time. By recognizing and leveraging these qualities, mentors can create environments where new graduates not only survive but also thrive the transition.*

LEVERAGING THE STRENGTHS OF NEW GRADUATES

Lindsey Hedges-Gieseking

It's your first day in practice. You have endured four years of veterinary school, preparing for this moment—the honor to be called "Doctor." Your heart is full of excitement, your gut is full of nervous energy, and your brain is full of somewhat unorganized facts that are primed and ready for practical application.

Experienced veterinarians: When was the last time you were filled with awe? When were you last excited (or nervous) for a "first?" First spay, first gastropexy , first diabetic, first lanced abscess? Awe and wonder are contagious. For some, that contagion never goes away and everyday in practice is like that first day. For most, routine sets in with experience, and we swap out awe for autopilot.

Bringing a new graduate into your practice is one of the best ways to reconnect the entire team to the wonder of veterinary medicine and to appreciate the awesome small moments each day, even in the routine cases. However, as mentors, we must guard against slipping back into the routine and becoming annoyed with questions or irritated at having to slow down the normal process. As we prepare our teams to support new graduates, we must be vocal about the opportunity we have ahead of us—we are building the foundation of someone's career, and we will learn as much as we teach, if we stay open to the process (Boatright, 2022).

START IN THE INTERVIEW

Many new graduates interview a practice based on the hospital's strengths—what value does the *hospital* bring to the new graduate's early career development? What experience can this mentee gain in their first year in practice? It's assumed that because new graduates lack experience, they have yet to develop their own strengths. They may have an inkling of what they like and dislike, but it's assumed that it's up to the mentor to help the mentee build and hone their skills from a relatively blank slate.

If we were interviewing an experienced veterinarian, **curiosity, open-mindedness, willingness, and adaptability to change** would be strengths that separate a "great" candidate from a "good" candidate. We don't stop to consider the fact that nearly every new graduate has all these characteristics and more. The "blank slate" is a strength in and of itself—if we frame it as such for our mentees and our teams.

Here are a few interview questions to help you and your future mentee recognize the strengths they will bring to the team:

- Tell me about a case you've had in clinics that you couldn't wait to learn more about. What sparked your interest, and how did you research the topic?
- What do you love about veterinary medicine?
- Have you encountered any situations in clinics or externships where the doctor took an approach that was different than what you expected or were taught? What did you learn in that situation?
- What does mentorship mean to you? If you made a medical error, how would you want your mentor to respond?
- Our days can sometimes be unpredictable; how do you manage unexpected changes in your schedule? What if a CSR puts a same day work-in on your schedule that you feel is highly complicated or advanced?

SET THE STAGE WITH YOUR TEAM

It's critical to emphasize the strengths and opportunities on the path ahead for the entire team from the moment we celebrate hiring a new grad.

> *Dr. New Grad is joining our team in June! When they interviewed, they were so impressed how everyone involved them, asking questions and explaining procedures even in the middle of a busy day. They especially liked that the CSRs and assistants were just as involved as the doctors and technicians in their interview. At this month's staff meeting, we will talk about planning for Dr. New Grad's arrival and I would love to hear everyone's thoughts on how to get them started on the right foot.*

Generating team excitement results in a positive feedback loop between the team and the new grad. Ground the positivity in reality—there will be hard times, there is so much to learn, mistakes will happen, and growing isn't easy. However, there is always someone on the team who can relate, and it is a privilege to be able to help a new team member through their learning journey. **New graduates rejuvenate team culture and strengthen the sense of purpose within the team, even before their first day in the hospital.**

One way to help the team prepare is to create "Introduction Cards" during a staff meeting. Encourage your team to share what they write with each other. The bonding and team building opportunity that is created with this activity can strengthen culture and unite the hospital within the common purpose of mentorship. During the new grad's first week, have the team introduce themselves and give their introduction cards to the new doctor. The new grad's excitement at learning about their new team will reinforce the collective strengths of the team. Mentors can also refer to those cards and redirect their mentee's questions to team members to build trust, encourage collaboration, and role model delegation.

Intro cards can be as simple as 3×5 index cards where each team member writes:

- Name and role
- Month/year they started at the hospital
- Years they've been in veterinary medicine
- Favorite thing to teach
- A procedure they want to see or something they want to learn
- What they are "known for"
- One silly, embarrassing, or memorable thing they learned in their first year in veterinary medicine

Here's an example:

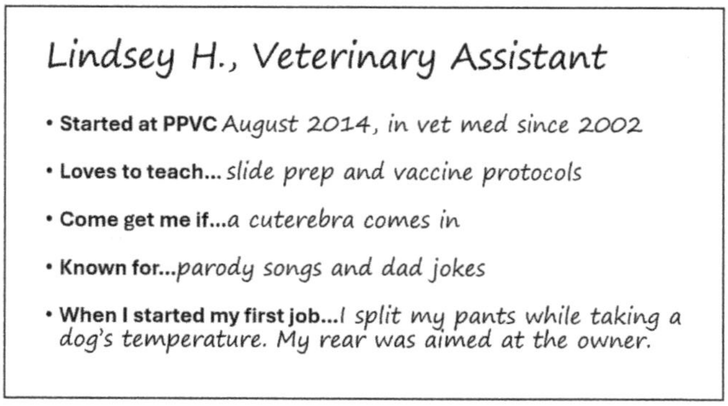

MUTUAL MENTORSHIP

New graduates approach every situation with a fresh perspective. From day-to-day operations to new diagnostics and therapeutics, everything is new, so anything is possible. Mutual mentorship recognizes that while mentors offer wisdom, context, and leadership development skills they have just as much to learn from their mentees about new approaches, medical advancements, and technology (Stanford, n.d.). New graduates may be open to sharing these ideas from day one, or they may store them up for a few weeks/months before all their feedback comes tumbling out at once.

Sometimes our knee jerk response can be to outline all the ways our mentee's suggestions won't work, using our good intentions to help ground them in reality and adapt to our hospital's standards. This can break trust and lead to fewer ideas shared in the future. On the other side of the spectrum, sometimes we give new graduates free reign to experiment with change, which can disrupt the balance within the team and lead to tension or change fatigue. Mutual mentorship requires balanced, open discussion, where both sides can explore the inherent risks and benefits of new ideas and ultimately choose a path that allows for learning and growth (Walti, 2025).

Here are a few tips for balancing mutual mentorship effectively:

1. **Define the Problem.** Mentees may offer a solution before fully considering the problem because they are excited about the positive impact the change will have. Spend some time walking backward from the solution to get to the heart of the problem. "Five Why's" is a great tool to try when defining the problem.

   Example: *We should purchase a video otoscope.*

   Why? *When we used a video otoscope in school, it allowed us to fully visualize the tympanic membrane and flush out debris. We used it on every case with otitis.*

   Why? *The cases that were sent to the teaching hospital were the worst of the worst. The dermatologist said they were the last attempt at treatment before surgical referral for a TECA-BO (Total Ear Canal Ablation and Bulla Osteotomy).*

   Why? *A lot of times owners had been using common ear medications for years, causing resistant infections and sometimes not treating the underlying cause of the allergies.*

   Why? *Some dogs had otitis media or otitis interna, or there was a wax plug or foreign material blocking topical medication from reaching full efficacy. The video otoscope helped us in those cases. Others had food allergy, and they hadn't had a long enough food trial or did not use a fully hydrolyzed food.*

   Why? *Allergy cases are hard; client education, treatment compliance, and scheduling follow-up are a lot to juggle.*

   Now define the problem: *Allergy cases are complex and managing chronic recurrent otitis can be frustrating for everyone involved.*

2. **Make an impact list.** Who does this problem impact? Have you asked them for their input on the problem and what they might do to fix it *before* choosing your first step?

   Managing chronic recurrent otitis impacts the doctors, assistants, technicians, CSRs, and, importantly, our patients and clients.

   After asking the team what they do with chronic ear infections, we find out that one of the doctors has developed an ear-cleaning handout that helps clients understand the importance of ear flush. One of the assistants loves teaching clients how to clean ears and uses a medication syringe when showing them how to pull up ear meds and make sure they get enough medication in the canal.

3. **Start Small.** If your new graduate has a big idea, ask them what their first step might be and start there. What is a 10% solution to the problem they see?

   After talking with the team, we decided to start using the ear flush handout with all otitis cases. We also ask the assistant who loves ear cleaning to demonstrate her client education approach during the next staff meeting so that everyone can learn from her. During the same staff meeting, the practice manager shares the number of patients we have seen in the last three months with "otitis externa" in their problem list and how many of them had a two week recheck recommendation when medications were dispensed.

4. **Build Momentum.** Celebrate the small wins. Track changes that happen from the initial experiment. Once the people impacted by the problem are aware of the issue, have your mentee build momentum toward their original solution.

   At the next staff meeting, the team celebrates that the total number of recheck appointments for patients with otitis has doubled since last month. Of those patients seen for recheck appointments, 30% had persistent infections.

   After the meeting, you and your mentee ask the practice manager to explain how equipment is purchased and what due diligence is needed to justify the return on investment. Your PM is supportive and asks that your mentee reaches out to your local dermatologist for recommendations on video otoscope brands and implementation recommendations for general practice before the meeting.

CONCLUSION

Adding a new graduate veterinarian to your team infuses awe and wonder into your hospital. Their curiosity, willingness, and open-mindedness can reinvigorate the team and reconnect everyone to the remarkable moments in veterinary medicine. Yet this transition also brings predictable hurdles: impostor syndrome, self-doubt, and the challenge of translating textbook knowledge into real-world problem-solving under pressure.

Effective mentorship embraces both realities. It means helping mentees distinguish helpful preparatory anxiety from destructive self-criticism, providing structured learning opportunities through SOPs and self-directed goals, and creating safe spaces where questions strengthen rather than diminish credibility (Evidence-Based Mentoring, 2025). Set the stage early with team involvement, thoughtful onboarding, and ample opportunities for mutual mentorship. With a renewed sense of purpose, your entire team will learn as much as they teach, building a foundation of mentorship throughout the practice.

BIBLIOGRAPHY

Boatright, K. (2022). Mentoring and coaching new veterinary graduates. *Today's Veterinary Practice* (14 July). https://todaysveterinarypractice.com/personal-professional-development/mentoring-and-coaching-new-veterinary-graduates/ (accessed 8 April 2025).

Carreras, S. (2022). Imposter syndrome in veterinary medicine. *MentorVet* (28 November). https://www.mentorvet.net/articles/imposter-syndrome-in-veterinary-medicine (accessed 8 April 2025).

Diehl, D.C. and Galindo-Gonzalez, S. (2024). *SMART Objectives*. Ask IFAS – Powered by EDIS https://edis.ifas.ufl.edu/publication/FY1327 (accessed 30 March 2025).

Dow, M., Chur-Hansen, A., Hamood, W., and Edwards, S. (2019). Impact of dealing with bereaved clients on the psychological wellbeing of veterinarians'. *Australian Veterinary Journal* 97: 382–389. https://doi.org/10.1111/avj.12842.

Evidence-Based Mentoring (2025). Mentoring as mutual growth: new study highlights benefits for adult mentors. *Evidence-Based Mentoring*, 26 June https://www.evidencebasedmentoring.org/ (accessed 8 April 2025).

Kogan, L.R., Schoenfeld-Tacher, R., Hellyer, P. et al. (2020). Veterinarians and impostor syndrome: an exploratory study. *Veterinary Record* 187 (7): 271. https://doi.org/10.1136/vr.105914.

Schnall, S., Harber, K.D., Stefanucci, J.K., and Proffitt, D.R. (2008). Social support and the perception of geographical slant. *Journal of Experimental Social Psychology* 44 (5): 1246–1255. https://doi.org/10.1016/j.jesp.2008.04.011.

Stanford VMware Women's Leadership Innovation Lab (n.d.). Mentoring: creating mutually empowering relationships. *Voice & Influence* https://womensleadership.stanford.edu/resources/voice-influence/mentoring-creating-mutually-empowering-relationships (accessed 8 April 2025).

Walti, J.P. (2025). *A Definitive Guide to Implementing Reciprocal Mentoring for Mutual Growth. PushFar* https://www.pushfar.com/article/a-definitive-guide-to-implementing-reciprocal-mentoring-for-mutual-growth/ (accessed 8 April 2025).

Wilson, G., Nuttall, T., and Shaw, D.J. (2024). Imposter syndrome in veterinary education? How knowledge and confidence affect treatment of canine atopic dermatitis. *Journal of Veterinary Medical Education* https://doi.org/10.3138/jvme-2023-0167 53 (1): 75–84.

Wong, B.M. and Headrick, L.A. (2021). Application of continuous quality improvement to medical education. *Medical Education* 55 (1): 72–81. https://doi.org/10.1111/medu.14351.

Yanke, A.B., Weigand, K.A., and Hofmeister, E.H. (2023). Addressing the needs and challenges of mentorship in veterinary medicine. *New Directions for Teaching and Learning* 2023: 83–93. https://doi.org/10.1002/tl.20571.

Zakharenkov, I. (2021). *Younger Vet Professionals Are More Vulnerable to Burnout. Veterinary Integration Solutions* https://vetintegrations.com/insights/veterinary-burnoutage/ (accessed 4 February 2025).

CHAPTER 4

Human-Centered Mentorship

INTRODUCTION

Dani Rabwin

Mentorship in veterinary medicine is often framed around performance: clinical competence, productivity, efficiency, and professional advancement. While these elements matter, they represent only a narrow slice of what mentorship actually requires in practice. Veterinary medicine is a relational profession, grounded in emotional labor, ethical complexity, and sustained human connection—between colleagues, clients, and communities, as well as between mentors and mentees. As a result, mentorship cannot be reduced to skill transfer or evaluation alone. It must account for the human beings involved.

This chapter explores mentorship beyond performance metrics, focusing instead on relationship, shared power, difference, and responsibility. Drawing from lived experience, advocacy, leadership, and cross-disciplinary perspectives, the authors examine how mentorship shapes belonging, confidence, identity, and long-term sustainability in the profession. When mentorship prioritizes assimilation over authenticity, it often reproduces existing norms and inequities. When it centers humanity, it creates conditions for trust, growth, and resilience—for individuals and for the systems they inhabit.

Erika Lin-Hendel, VMD, PhD, brings a foundation rooted in student advocacy, suicide prevention, and global One Health work. Their perspective reflects years of engagement with veterinary learners and early-career professionals navigating systems that have not always been designed with their safety or well-being in mind. Ron Sosa, CVPM, CCFP, PgD-CLD, contributes a leadership lens shaped by decades in veterinary management and his work in neuroinclusive leadership, burnout prevention, and human-centered organizational design. Together, they ground the chapter in principles of ethical, relational, and inclusive mentorship.

The chapter then turns to two personal narratives that bring these concepts into sharper focus. Gary Marshall, DVM, an experienced feline practitioner and former Vice President of the American Veterinary Medical Association (2024–2026) explores generational differences in mentorship and how shifting values, expectations, and stressors shape mentor–mentee relationships across career stages. James Townend, a financial and life coach with extensive experience supporting professionals navigating communication, collaboration, and burnout, offers an external but deeply relevant perspective on neurodiversity and mentorship.

Taken together, these voices invite readers to reflect not only on how mentorship is delivered but also on who it serves—and how mentorship can move the profession toward greater connection, equity, and sustainability.

BEYOND PERFORMANCE: THE HUMAN WORK OF VETERINARY MENTORSHIP

Erika Lin-Hendel and Ron Sosa

Mentorship in veterinary medicine is often framed as a structured process of skill acquisition, professional development, and performance evaluation, with institutions or authority figures positioned as the primary drivers of growth. Yet veterinary practice is inherently relational and emotionally complex, shaped by interactions between people, animals, environments, and systems across diverse contexts. Mentorship, as a result, extends beyond technical competence into the realm of human connection, culture, and power. Rooted in long-standing traditions of knowledge transmission and professional lineage (Irby et al., 2020), mentorship shapes not only how veterinarians learn but also how they are perceived, supported, and afforded opportunity. These dynamics make mentorship a deeply personal and culturally mediated experience—one that warrants closer examination through the lens of difference and inclusion.

We must therefore consider the ethical framework of mentorship in a holistic way that considers the human beings involved, not just the medicine. Mentorship requires attention to the whole person rather than medical competence or productivity alone. **At its best, mentorship expands capacity rather than enforcing conformity**. Yet many traditional models prioritize fitting mentees into existing systems, often rewarding assimilation over authenticity.

When mentorship is reduced to shaping someone into what already exists, we are no longer supporting growth—we are reproducing norms. But people are not products. They are complex, evolving individuals whose identities, values, and lived experiences influence how they learn, lead, and practice medicine. Effective mentorship holds space for that complexity and supports mentees in developing as professionals and as humans. When we mentor the person rather than the output, we create the conditions for meaningful growth—both for individuals and for the systems they inhabit.

Take a moment to reflect on the early influences in your professional development. Who were the people who shaped how you learned and practiced? Did their backgrounds and experiences resonate with yours, or did you have to sift through advice to find what fit? Did you feel seen in those relationships? When people reflect on mentorship and the individuals who shaped their practice, the experience is often deeply personal—and at times includes assigned mentorship relationships that had to be endured or overcome.

When we were invited to explore mentorship through a lens of diversity and difference, we reflected on how our own approaches to mentorship were shaped by the absence of resonant mentorship in our early careers. Much of our learning occurred through lived experience rather than formal mentorship. We found ourselves in a form of "patchwork quilt" or mosaic menteeship—sifting through information and examples to identify what aligned with our values and needs. These experiences shaped our commitment to inclusive, human-centered models of leadership and mentorship.

Because veterinary medicine lacks the diversity present in many other medical professions (Quicksall, 2024), differences between mentors and mentees can have an outsized impact on how mentorship is experienced. As the profession evolves, mentorship theories and practices must support the thriving of all members of the veterinary team (Quicksall, 2024). **Differences in background, identity, and lived experience are not barriers to effective mentorship; they are opportunities for innovation.** As in natural systems, diversity contributes to resilience and adaptability, and diverse teams often produce better outcomes (Quicksall, 2024).

Veterinary medicine cannot claim stewardship, advocacy, or service to communities without explicitly engaging with diversity, equity, and inclusion—examining who is included, who is excluded, and how power and access shape those outcomes. Mentorship is one of the primary mechanisms through which diversity, equity, and inclusion are either reinforced or undermined in practice. When mentorship fails to account for difference, it often reproduces existing inequities within the profession. When mentorship is intentional, inclusive, and human-centered, it becomes a powerful site for equity, belonging, and leadership development—shaping not only individual careers but also the future of veterinary medicine's service to animal, agricultural, and environmental health.

Veterinary medicine's earliest roots can be traced to the Code of Hammurabi (3000 BCE), long before the establishment of the first veterinary schools (MSU CVM, 2019). This long lineage of service to the human–animal bond is carried forward through mentorship, as mentors spark curiosity, purpose, and commitment in future professionals. We invite readers to approach mentorship with creativity and intention, considering its expansiveness across history, culture, and difference.

A CURRENT ASSESSMENT OF THE VETERINARY MENTORSHIP ECOSYSTEM

Effective mentorship in veterinary medicine requires more than clinical guidance; it demands an understanding of the educational, financial, and social contexts that shape new graduates' experiences. This section examines the current mentorship ecosystem to inform mentors seeking to support recruitment, retention, and long-term professional sustainability.

The critical importance of mentorship in veterinary medicine for recruitment, retention, and overall satisfaction is well established (Jelinski et al., 2009; Gates et al., 2021). Inadequate mentorship contributes to turnover, and the challenges of the early graduate period remain a key focus for mentorship development within the profession (Jelinski et al., 2009; Gates et al., 2021; Kastelic and Ogilvie, 2025).

As a field that places significant emphasis on medical practice and production management, veterinary medicine must not overlook a core component of ethical mentorship. In a profession already impacted by mental health challenges, it is essential to consider how individuals' lives and external experiences influence professional development (Tomasi et al., 2019; Volk et al., 2020; Hilton et al., 2023).

One of the most common differences within mentor–mentee pairings is generational. This essential transmission of knowledge is critical for the long term sustainability of any field or work place (Peet et al., 2010). Mentors should recognize clear differences in satisfaction and stressors between new graduates and established veterinarians (Volk et al., 2020), with younger graduates often more vulnerable to burnout (Reinhard, 2023). Decreased satisfaction is thought in part to relate to financial pressures associated with educational costs and higher debt-to-income ratios. Recent changes to educational loan policies will continue to affect new graduates (Bartels, 2025), and veterinarians from marginalized identities carry a higher loan burden (Marcano and Mages, 2025). These compounded financial stressors create meaningful power differentials within mentorship relationships, particularly as they relate to job security. Mentors in private practice should remember that new graduates have recently navigated the cumulative stressors of veterinary school, the NAVLE, and major personal milestones simply to enter the profession.

Most new graduates enter practice from academically based mentorship environments. Veterinary academia demonstrates high variability in the presence of trusting mentoring relationships (Yanke et al., 2023), and multiple publications document verbal abuse and discrimination within academic settings (BVA, 2019; Chung and Armitage-Chan, 2022; Summers et al., 2023; Barnes et al., 2025). Declining NAVLE scores, veterinary school accreditation concerns, and legal conflict around residency further highlight systemic challenges (Wogan, 2025, Won and Larkin, 2025). Gaps in mentorship accessibility—particularly for new graduates—have contributed to the growth of mentorship training programs and companies over the past decade. Veterinary colleges are also developing more intentional mentorship initiatives (Freeman et al., 2022), alongside internal company-based programs. Together, these developments underscore the evolving nature of mentorship in the field and the importance of mentors understanding their mentees' prior experiences and how these may shape the relationship. relationship. Additionally, reciprocal and collaborative mentorship across generational experience is being regarded as a more effective compared to traditional hierarchical models (Olufunmilola and Quinlan, 2024).

Beyond generational and career-stage differences, mentors and mentees must also consider how lived experience influences mentorship dynamics. Publications from veterinary industry leaders describe how discrimination and marginalization affect both individual professionals and the profession as a whole (Greenhill et al., 2013; Tran, 2024; Marshall, 2025). These resources should be integral to mentor and educator development. Where veterinary-specific research is limited, literature from other medical fields, community-focused research, and organizational advocacy groups offer valuable insights. Marginalized cohorts within veterinary medicine have formed affinity organizations to address gaps in belonging and representation. Supporting these organizations increases the likelihood that comprehensive mentorship will be accessible across the profession.

As one of the least diverse medical fields (Martínez, 2024; Quicksall, 2024), veterinary medicine cannot ignore the impact of discrimination in the workplace (Tan and Fogelberg, 2024). This is particularly critical during periods when sociopolitical conditions disproportionately affect specific cohorts within the profession. Educational, research, and regulatory systems are navigating shifting legislative and policy landscapes, alongside changes in healthcare access, with disproportionate effects on those earlier in their education and careers.

Veterinary medicine also exemplifies global interconnectedness and adaptability—from food production and safety to zoonotic disease, global trade, and One Health. This perspective highlights the field's resilience and creativity. Within veterinary medicine, mentors can harness these strengths to support relationships and communities that enable teams to succeed both personally and professionally amid ongoing challenges.

THE IMPACT OF VISIBLE AND INVISIBLE DIFFERENCES ON MENTORSHIP

Mentorship that fails to consider power dynamics, intersectionality, and cultural differences will often fall short of empowering both individuals within the relationship. Because mentors typically hold greater decision-making authority and career stability, mentees are more likely to experience harm or unintended consequences related to health, finances, and career trajectory. Ethical mentorship therefore requires awareness of this imbalance and recognition of how a mentor may unintentionally become a barrier within a person's career.

Addressing the ways discrimination—both intentional and unintentional—contributes to cycles of harm that prevent people from entering, thriving in, or remaining in the profession could fill an entire book. With that limitation in mind, mentors are encouraged to engage with existing resources that support colleagues from marginalized backgrounds and promote cultural humility (Yeager and Bauer-Wu, 2013; AAHA, 2023; Tran, 2024; Marshall, 2025).

Mentorship often begins with good intentions: guidance, support, and a desire to help someone grow. Intention alone, however, does not mitigate impact. Without thoughtful awareness, even well-meaning mentorship can cause harm.

That harm rarely begins with overt exclusion. More often, it is subtle—embedded in unspoken expectations that success looks, sounds, dresses, and works a particular way. When mentors, even unconsciously, shape mentees into the dominant culture of the profession, they communicate that difference must be edited out to belong.

This dynamic is especially damaging for mentees with invisible or marginalized identities. Mentorship can shift from relationship to performance. The pressure to conform is rarely named and is often framed as "professionalism," "fit," or "readiness." These coded terms are rooted in legacies of exclusion and sameness, rewarding masking, code-switching, assimilation, and burnout while gatekeeping access to growth and leadership (Quicksall, 2024).

It is time to shift our collective understanding of mentorship. **A mentor is not a gatekeeper; they are a steward.**

Gatekeeping mentorship measures success by how closely a mentee conforms to the system. Stewardship-based mentorship measures success by how well the system adapts to meet the evolving needs of its people. A gatekeeper asks, "Are you ready for this world?" A steward asks, "What kind of world are you building, and how can I walk alongside you?".

This shift is structural. Stewardship acknowledges the existence of power in mentorship relationships and uses it intentionally to open doors without requiring mentees to diminish themselves. It prioritizes mentoring *with*, rather than *over*, and places the human before the outcome.

When mentorship is approached through stewardship, inclusivity becomes intentional rather than aspirational. Roles and expectations are clarified, pathways for repair are cocreated, and mentees are invited to bring their full selves into the relationship. Mentorship becomes a relationship rather than a one-way transmission of wisdom.

The question we must continue to ask is this: **Is our mentorship making room or making people disappear?**

HOW CAN HARM SHOWS UP IN MENTORSHIP?

- Unexamined power dynamics undermine communication.
- Masking, code-switching, and emotional bypassing lead to burnout.
- Microaggressions and overt racism are bullying.
- Saviorism and supremacy operate as gatekeeping.
- Unchecked bias often escalates into prejudice.
- Favoritism erodes trust and engagement.

The Wheel of Power and Privilege (Figure 4.1) illustrates how visible and invisible identities shape access to power and opportunity in ways that are often unspoken but influential within mentorship relationships.

Ethical mentorship, oriented toward the success and flourishing of the next generation, requires mutual care for individual well-being and the broader veterinary community. Mentors and mentees alike hold opportunities for advocacy within workplaces and institutional structures. Through this shared responsibility, environments can be cultivated that support professional growth, sustain enthusiasm for veterinary medicine, and strengthen service to the human–animal bond.

The following sections offer perspectives related to particular cohorts within veterinary medicine. This list is not comprehensive, but rather a starting point for further exploration. Where possible, community spaces that foster connection, allyship, and mentorship are highlighted. Two focused perspectives from additional contributing authors address common differences encountered in veterinary medicine: generational experience and neurotype.

RACE AND ETHNICITY

Veterinary medicine is one of the least diverse professions in healthcare, making attention to race and ethnicity within mentorship critical (Quicksall, 2024; Stanton and Miller, 2025). Although data are limited, many new graduates are likely to have experienced discrimination during training, requiring postgraduate mentorship to actively rebuild trust with senior clinicians (Barnes et al., 2025).

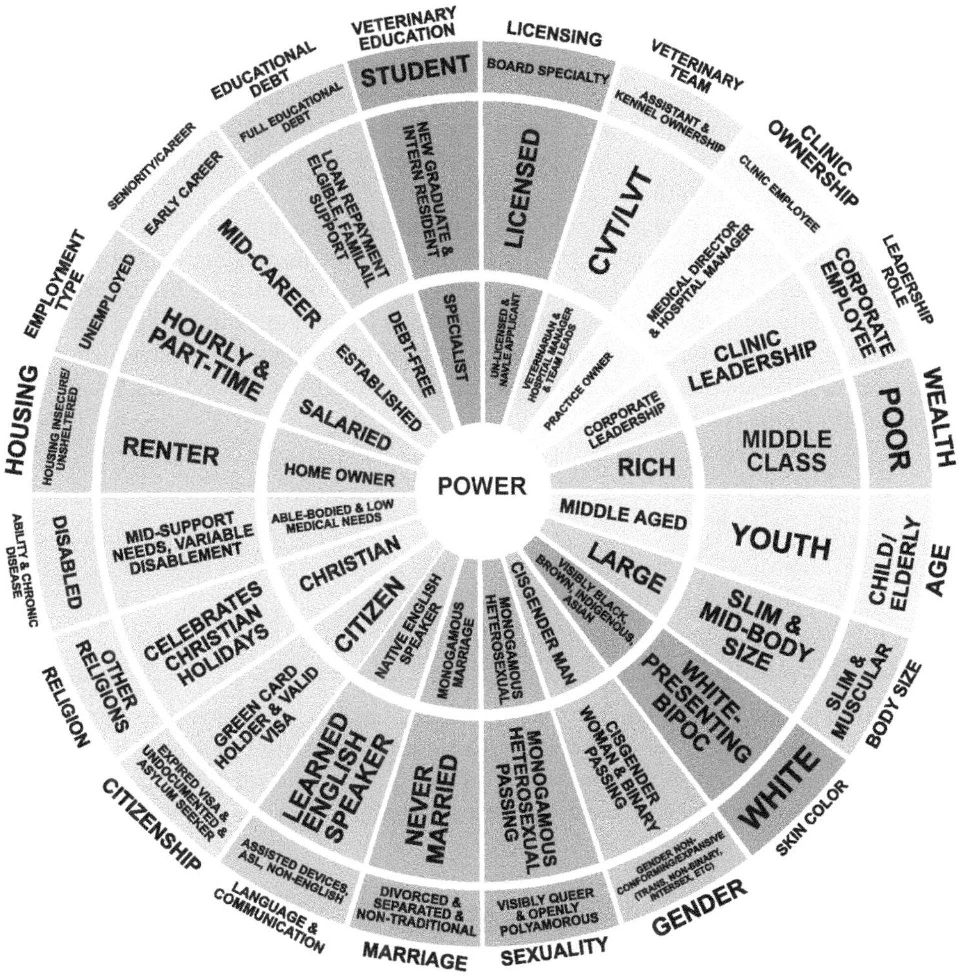

ADAPTED FROM: *Tessa Watkins, Sylvia Duckworth, Canadian Council for Reguees, and Olena Hankivsky, PhD.*

FIGURE 4.1 The wheel of power and privilege.

Issues of identity, human rights, and racial profiling materially shape the external realities that Black, Indigenous, and People of Color (BIPOC) veterinary professionals navigate. These experiences add emotional labor beyond the inherent demands of veterinary medicine and may occur both outside the hospital and within clinical environments.

Within mentorship relationships, these experiences can affect psychological safety and trust. Building rapport may require intentional space for nonmedical conversations and openness to discussing discrimination when a mentee chooses to share. Mentors should be prepared to receive feedback without defensiveness and to respond compassionately and consistently when mentees experience discrimination from clients or colleagues.

VETERINARY COMMUNITY RESOURCES

MCVMA; Pawsibilities; BlackDVM Network; NABV; AAVMP; LatinxVMA; JVMA
https://mcvma.org/wake-up-vet-med/

GENDER

Veterinary medicine is a majority-women field and is projected to become increasingly women-led (Lin-Hendel, 2025a,b). Gender dynamics therefore remains an important consideration within mentorship. Sexual harassment and abuse can occur from both clients and colleagues (Stewart, 2018; Shoichiro and Yukawa, 2022), and mentorship programs must be prepared to recognize and respond appropriately.

Ethical mentors must engage intentionally in understanding policies impacting members of our field that often vary across gender. When in positions of leadership, one can question or advocate for policies supporting access to gender-affirming and reproductive healthcare, equitable short term disability insurance, and parental leave policies. Fundamentally, now more than ever, mentors must engage intentionally in reflecting and preparing to respectfully navigate mentorship with mentees of different gender background from themselves—including trans, nonbinary, and gender-nonconforming colleagues.

VETERINARY COMMUNITY RESOURCES

WVALDI; PrideVMC Gender Identity Bill of Rights

FAMILIAL CARETAKING

Caretaking responsibilities—whether for children, aging parents, or others—are often overlooked in professional development. These responsibilities affect time, energy, and availability, and mentorship that ignores them may unintentionally penalize those who carry this load. Checking in about caretaking stressors, when a mentee chooses to share, supports engagement, and acknowledges the whole person.

SEXUAL ORIENTATION AND RELATIONAL STATUS

LGBTQ+

Mentorship that fosters belonging must be explicit rather than performative. Mentors must do more than say "you're safe here." Safety is demonstrated through consistent advocacy, respect for pronouns, and preparedness to respond to discrimination. A mentee cannot thrive in an environment where they feel compelled to hide their identity.

VETERINARY COMMUNITY RESOURCES

PrideVMC; Lab Coat No Closet

RELATIONAL STATUS

Conversations about relational status benefit from clear boundaries and consent. Respecting a mentee's comfort around personal disclosure supports trust without assuming access to private life.

RELIGION

Mentors should be prepared to recognize and support religious practices, including needs related to observance or holidays, and to respond appropriately to bias or discrimination when it occurs.

SOCIOECONOMIC STATUS

Assumptions of access to mentorship and advancement can reinforce economic inequities. Financial instability may limit participation in externships, travel, or lower-paying opportunities, particularly for students and early-career veterinarians. Mentors must remain aware of financial power differentials and avoid perpetuating toxic or unsustainable expectations.

VETERINARY COMMUNITY RESOURCES

VIN Foundation Student Debt Center; Not One More Vet, Inc. Grants

GENERATIONAL DIFFERENCES

Differences in communication styles, values, and expectations can create tension within mentorship relationships, particularly within hierarchical or corporate structures. Clear conversations about preferences, goals, feedback, and learning approaches allow these differences to become sources of reciprocal learning.

A deeper exploration of generational mentorship dynamics is provided in an upcoming section by Dr. Gary Marshall.

VETERINARY COMMUNITY RESOURCES

Pawsibilities

DISABILITY AND CHRONIC DISEASE

Disability encompasses a spectrum of visible and invisible differences that may be developmental, acquired, temporary, or variable. In professional and educational settings, disability is often framed narrowly around accommodations. We encourage mentors and mentees to engage with disability justice models that emphasize accessibility and support, recognizing that environments themselves can be disabling and that accommodations are not burdensome. Accessibility can be a design feature rather than a negotiation.

Supportive mentorship can play a critical role in helping mentees access the accommodations and resources they need. Many disabled individuals have been required to self-advocate throughout their educational, professional, and healthcare journeys, while those with newly acquired or recently diagnosed disabilities may still be learning to identify their support needs. Collaborative, proactive mentorship can reduce unnecessary barriers and isolation.

Chronic illness often involves fluctuating energy, pain, and cognitive clarity. Mentees may be managing invisible challenges while attempting to meet expectations designed without their bodies in mind. Flexible pacing, nonlinear growth, and honest check-ins are not optional accommodations—they are necessities.

VETERINARY COMMUNITY RESOURCES

Facebook group: Veterinarians with Chronic Illnesses

NEURODIVERSITY

Neurodiversity is included within the broader classification of disability and encompasses differences in neurocognitive functioning and social–behavioral processing. These differences are common within the general population and veterinary teams; for example, adult ADHD prevalence is estimated at 3.1% (Ayano et al., 2023). Conditions such as attention deficit hyperactivity disorder (ADHD), dyslexia, dyscalculia, dyspraxia, and auditory processing differences are therefore likely to be present across veterinary workplaces.

Neurodivergent differences can influence communication styles, sensory and social bandwidth, motivation, focus, engagement, and information processing during learning. Without awareness, these differences may be misinterpreted as lack of effort, disengagement, or poor fit.

Mentors can support neurodivergent mentees without requiring disclosure by adopting inclusive mentoring practices. Being specific with instructions, inviting mentees to summarize their understanding, and routinely checking in about overwhelm or overstimulation can reduce friction and support learning for all mentees (Lin-Hendel, 2025a,b). These approaches benefit mentorship broadly, while creating conditions in which neurodivergent individuals are more likely to thrive.

VETERINARY COMMUNITY RESOURCES

Facebook Groups: Veterinary Association for Neurodivergence; Squirrel! (Veterinarians with ADHD); Neurodiverse Vets Squirrel!

Visit: https://www.vetlife.org.uk/neurodiversity/

MENTAL HEALTH

Mental health conditions influence how individuals process feedback and navigate expectations. Human-centered mentorship prioritizes care rather than cure and avoids shame-based responses. Psychological safety is built through consistency, compassion, and nonpunitive responses—particularly following medical or emotional trauma.

VETERINARY COMMUNITY RESOURCES

Not One More Vet, Inc.; VIN Support Groups

NATIONALITY AND CITIZENSHIP STATUS

I am a first-generation Asian American. I was raised in and live within the immigrant community, and I have made my home in a borderland state. While driving to a shift at 6:00 a.m., I encountered traffic on the freeway due to the remnants of a spontaneous immigration checkpoint on the highway. I was breathless, taking in a line of fifteen empty cars—the remaining evidence of people taken to a series of privately owned detention facilities. Within these facilities, there are reports of denied medical care, lack of adequate food and water, and other systemic human rights violations.

On that day, I needed to be held and supported by my team to move through the acute emotional distress of what I had witnessed, while still ensuring that clients and patients received the best medical care available. I had to focus on my responsibility to practice medicine while also experiencing fear of detention, and grief for friends with detained family, and those who have died in detention. If I had been a mentee at a more

> *vulnerable stage of my career, I am not sure I would have felt safe enough to get through the day. These are the kinds of experiences a mentor needs to be prepared to support someone through. —Erika.*

Veterinary medicine is a global field that includes individuals with diverse citizenship and immigration statuses. Mentors and leaders must be prepared to support team members affected by external events related to licensing to practice (Wogan, 2024), how colleagues may be impacted by current immigration policy and enforcement, and recognize how these stressors impact wellbeing and psychological safety at work.

VETERINARY COMMUNITY RESOURCES

Foreign-Trained Veterinarians in Preparation for Licensing in North America (Facebook group)

Editor's Note: *Generational difference is one of the most common—and often least examined—sources of tension in veterinary mentorship. In the following section, Dr. Gary Marshall reflects on decades of mentoring across generations and offers a lived example of what human-centered, curiosity-driven mentorship can look like in practice.*

THE POWER OF GENERATIONAL DIVERSITY IN VETERINARY MEDICINE: A MENTOR'S PERSPECTIVE

Gary Marshall

Do you have time for coffee? This message popped up on my phone and instantly put a smile on my face. It was from Christine, a mentee who was in town on a short break from her residency training at a large midwestern veterinary school. We met more than a dozen years ago shortly after her sister started working at my feline practice as a local undergrad student hoping to get into vet school. At that time, Christine was interested in human medicine. It didn't take long for her to realize her true passion was actually vet med. Her first experience in veterinary medicine then began at my feline practice, just as her sister's had.

When Dr. Dani Rabwin asked me to contribute to this book for the Generational Differences Section the first thing I asked was "why me?" I assumed the answer would be that I'm the only practicing baby boomer she knows. But that wasn't it at all. She said she wanted people to know more about my mentoring "secret sauce"! I had no idea what she was talking about, but it motivated me to figure it out.

For over 35 years, I've had the privilege of mentoring aspiring veterinarians—pre-vet students eager to break into the field, exhausted but determined veterinary students, and early-career veterinarians finding their footing. I've seen trends come and go, technology transform the way we practice, and societal shifts change the expectations placed upon us. But one constant has remained: the richness of our profession is rooted in its people, and the true strength of veterinary medicine comes from the diversity of experiences and perspectives across generations.

Veterinary medicine, like any field, is shaped by the people who practice it. Each generation has its own challenges, strengths, and perspectives, shaped by the world they grew up in:

- **The traditionalists** (born before 1946): These veterinarians were trained in an era of paper records, handwritten SOAP notes, and limited specialization. They often emphasize self-reliance, hands-on learning, and a deep respect for experience gained over time. Many built their practices from the ground up, often working tirelessly to serve their communities.
- **Baby boomers** (born 1946–1964): Many in this generation worked their way through vet school with minimal debt and entered a profession where independent practice ownership was the primary career path. They are known for their work ethic, dedication to mentorship, and belief in personal sacrifice for professional success.
- **Generation X** (born 1965–1980): The bridge between the old and new, Gen X veterinarians embraced the introduction of digital recordkeeping, the rise of corporate practices, and increasing specialization. They value work–life balance more than their predecessors, often leading the charge for flexible work schedules and mental health awareness in the profession.
- **Millennials** (born 1981–1996): This generation entered the field with a different set of challenges—soaring student debt, corporatization, and changing client expectations. They are digital natives who prioritize mentorship, collaboration, and a sense of purpose in their careers. They have driven conversations about wellness, work—life integration, and inclusivity in veterinary medicine.
- **Generation Z** (born 1997–2012): The newest members of the profession, Gen Z veterinarians are entering with a highly developed sense of social justice, environmental consciousness, and an expectation of technological integration. They value efficiency, clear communication, and workplaces that align with their values.

When Christine showed up at my house, I brewed a pot of coffee and we each chose our favorite pastry from the assortment she had brought. Our quick "catch up" stretched to three hours. After talking through everything that had transpired for her over the four months since our last visit and updating her on my recent visits to UK veterinary schools, I asked her if she thought there was such a thing as a "secret sauce" in the relationships she has had with mentors more than twice her age. I was surprised when she answered without much hesitation, that the entire time she has known me, she always felt seen not as another millennial, or lumped in with all the others interested in vet med, or as someone's sister, but as an individual with completely unique hopes and fears and circumstances. She felt seen. She felt heard. She felt cared for.

If I had to pinpoint the most important skill I've developed over decades of mentoring, it wouldn't be my ability to give advice or teach surgical techniques. It would be the ability to listen.

True mentorship isn't about molding someone into a miniature version of yourself. It's about helping them discover their own path, their own strengths, and their own version of success. And the only way to do that is to listen—really listen.

I've mentored students who thought they wanted to be equine surgeons but discovered a passion for public health. I've worked with young veterinarians who believed they had to own a practice to be successful, only to realize they thrived in academia. I've sat with burned-out professionals who sought permission to step away from clinical work to attempt to find fulfillment in industry, research, or advocacy.

Listening means not assuming you know what's best for someone just because you've been in the field longer. It means asking questions like:

- "What excites you about this work?"
- "What challenges feel the most overwhelming right now?"
- "If you could design your perfect career, what would it look like?"
- "If you could live anywhere, what would that place look like?"
- "What does success look like to you—not to your professors, parents, or peers, but to you?"

A valid follow-up question directly after each of these should be the simple "why"?

There are challenges to mentorship relationships between individuals of different generations. These differences have also taught me some of my most valuable lessons. The most important one being that every generation brings something unique to the table, and when we listen—truly listen—to each other, we create a profession that is stronger, more innovative, and more compassionate. I believe the "secret sauce" of mentorship isn't just dispensing wisdom; it's learning what's best for each mentee—often by connecting them with others who can help shape their specific journey. And the most important ingredient to mix in to facilitate truly meaningful connections, in my opinion, is to really get to know each other.

One of the greatest misconceptions about mentorship is that it's about having all the answers. Another ingredient that I feel makes that mentorship "secret sauce" special is that effective mentorship isn't about knowing everything—it's about connecting mentees with the right people equipped to help with parts of their journey that aren't in your wheelhouse.

Over the years, I've learned that sometimes, the most valuable thing I can do for a mentee is introduce them to someone else.

- A pre-vet student unsure about their career path? I connect them with a veterinarian in an unconventional role—maybe a zoo vet, a public health official, or a pharmaceutical consultant—so they can see the breadth of opportunities available.
- A vet student struggling with imposter syndrome? I introduce them to a recent graduate who has walked the same path and come out stronger on the other side.
- A new veterinarian feeling overwhelmed? I pair them with a seasoned practitioner who understands their concerns but also knows how to help them navigate the early years without burning out.

These connections are often where the real magic happens. A single conversation with the right person can change the course of a career.

So what do we do with this information as mentors? Can understanding broad generational differences actually help us help each other?

I definitely resonate with parts of the Baby Boomer description above. And there are traits from other generations that I admire—and even wish I possessed. I suspect many of us feel the same way, regardless of when we were born.

By getting to know people from different generations, mentors and mentees can better understand how certain traits and mindsets were shaped by lived experience. When we take the time to learn how historical context influences perspective, we're more likely to judge less, respect more, and build stronger working relationships.

A profession that spans multiple generations isn't just interesting—it's essential for long-term success. Here's why generational diversity benefits veterinary medicine:

1. **Shared Wisdom and Institutional Knowledge**

   Older generations carry decades of hands-on experience. They've seen diseases that are now rare, survived economic downturns, and built lasting relationships with clients. Their mentorship helps newer veterinarians avoid mistakes and can pick them up and support them when mistakes happen (and mentors can share how they made similar mistakes). Veterinarians, who have spent decades in practice, are well suited to pass along knowledge of the profession's rich history.

   When I was a new grad, and encountered panic inducing situations, whether they involved a disgruntled client, a coding patient, or a demographic shift in the community, and I saw my mentor shift gears, not panic, and adapt to these situations seemingly effortlessly, it trained me to be that person to my mentees. "Global pandemic? Don't freak out. We can get through this!"

2. **Fresh Perspectives and Innovation**

   Younger veterinarians bring new ways of thinking. They embrace technology, challenge outdated norms, and push to establish sustainable boundaries. Their influence is what has led to telemedicine, digital medical records, and shifts in client communication strategies.

   When a Gen Z staff member is in an environment to comfortably ask their mentor: "what if. . .," wonderful things begin to happen. "What if we could automate last minute reminders to send text messages instead of having our the CSRs call everyone? Would you like me to research options?"

3. **A Stronger Professional Community**

   When generations collaborate, veterinary medicine becomes a more welcoming, inclusive profession. Older vets help younger ones navigate challenges, while younger vets help older colleagues adapt to new trends and technologies. This cross-pollination of ideas makes the profession more resilient.

   I can't emphasize this enough. This also takes the most effort I believe. Our comfort zones are bubbles of sameness. Intentionally seeking those that aren't like us (generation, gender, heritage, geography, orientation. . .) takes hard work. State veterinary medicine association boards have traditionally been homogeneous groups. In Washington State, we have been working for years to create a board that looks more like our membership, than an AARP commercial. It is working. The profession, and the people that are part of it, will be better off for it.

4. **More Comprehensive Patient Care**

   Diverse teams make better decisions. A multigenerational team in a clinic means blending time-tested diagnostic skills with modern treatment options. It means leveraging both experience and innovation to provide the best possible care.

   Baby Boomers were performing cystocentesis procedures for decades without the aid of ultrasound guidance. This terrifies many Millennials. Sharing how this can be done safely, where both parties are open to learning and safe from criticism, can add new tools to each other's toolbox.

5. **A Sense of Legacy and Purpose**

   When older veterinarians take the time to mentor, they leave a lasting impact. When younger veterinarians engage with their mentors, they help carry forward the values and knowledge that defined the profession.

   When a Gen X Medical Director truly shows interest and invests time in a younger new grad veterinarian, what that mentee experiences is more likely to be modeled and passed on to the next generation of new grads to come through that clinic.

Embracing generational differences will always make mentor–mentee pairings, veterinary hospital teams, university communities, and mentorship network cohorts stronger. The mix of experiences, new ideas, resilience, and fresh energy creates an environment where learning never stops.

The best veterinary teams, the most fulfilling careers, and the strongest mentorship relationships all have one thing in common: they are built on mutual respect and a willingness to learn from one another.

Christine and I were both a bit surprised, but not shocked, that three hours had passed by so quickly. This isn't the first time that's happened. As we got up to say our goodbyes, we simultaneously said "I needed that" to each other. I'm optimistic that our time together had a small effect to motivate and energize her to push through the final months of her residency. I know that it motivated, energized and truly nourished me to continue to carve out time for those that I've had the fortune to cross paths with on my journey through veterinary medicine. Long lasting relationships like the one between Christine and I, highlight the final component vital to the "secret sauce" of mentorship. It's best for them to simmer for a good long time. Not all mentoring relationships need to, or are able to, extend over a long period of time, but I truly feel the best ones are ongoing. My earliest mentors, twice my age, invested years, even decades, in my life. This modeling enabled me to see the value in investing in those much younger than me. I'm very confident that Christine will strive to mentor future generations herself. The profession benefits when this positive cycle continues.

As a mentor, my greatest joy isn't in seeing my mentees follow my exact path (thank goodness, because none have). It's in seeing them find their own way—sometimes with my guidance, sometimes through connections I've facilitated, and sometimes simply because I've given them the confidence to trust themselves.

Generational diversity in veterinary medicine isn't a challenge to overcome; it's an asset to embrace. If we commit to listening, learning, and encouraging each other, we can build a profession that is not only skilled and compassionate but also deeply connected across generations.

Editor's Note: *Neurodiversity reflects the reality that there is no single "normal" or ideal way for human brains to process, interpret, and respond to the world. Differences in sensory processing, communication, and social interaction are part of natural human variation. Because social behaviors—such as eye contact, facial expression, and verbal communication—are also shaped by culture and relationships, neurodiversity has meaningful implications for veterinary mentorship and workplace dynamics. In the following vignette, James Townend—an autistic coach, financial advisor, and professional mentor outside of veterinary medicine—offers perspectives that illuminate how neurodivergent experiences intersect with mentorship in our field.*

BEYOND LABELS: NEURODIVERSITY AND COLLABORATIVE MENTORSHIP

James Townend

As an autistic person, I have had to learn appropriate social mannerisms as to how to act in situations like euthanasia. Recently, a friend of mine who had to euthanize her dog was so upset she couldn't sign the papers. The veterinarian explained euthanasia was the humane thing to do, as her dog was diabetic and in liver failure. I signed the papers for my friend. I didn't cry and wasn't upset, because what the vet said made sense to me. Afterwards, as I continued to support my grieving friend, I found myself mentally spent looking for an exit.

When I talked to my therapist I asked her if I was a bad person because I didn't cry or feel anything inside. Yet when another friend told me the story of when her dog died I cried and felt knots in my stomach. I asked my therapist how that could be, how I could have different emotional reactions to similar situations. She told me I was wired differently and that I was showing cognitive empathy in the one case but my emotional connection with the other person contributed to me feeling more. She explained that as an autistic I have different emotional ranges that can vary based on context. That in the one situation I did the best I could and that I wasn't a bad person.

Before I was diagnosed, I would often "mask:" behave in a way I learned was considered the "right" (socially acceptable) thing to say even when I didn't relate to it or understand. This became feeling like I had to hide who I really was, or made me feel like a fraud. It wasn't until I heard an interview with John Schneider who has an autistic son, refer to it as a special gift. That was the first time I had heard being autistic as a special gift and I thought to myself that truer words couldn't have been said.

We are all wired differently, but at times we internalize the label or how others (even loved ones) promote what is "right and wrong" behavior, and label ourselves as wrong rather than different. Those who are on the spectrum including myself should not be afraid to be who we are. I think all special gifts should be embraced and understood.

Most of my life I went undiagnosed and this resulted in issues in all of my relationships. It led to autistic burnout, job instability and a lack of balance in my life. Misunderstandings and miscommunication frequently resulted in relationship breakdowns and stressful work scenarios, but with experience I have developed successful strategies and understanding to help navigate daily interactions.

I had a business coach for neurodiverse individuals, Martin, who helped me understand some simple communication tools that I have found to be the most effective. At our first session, Mark facilitated a discussion where we both were honest with each other about our style, what we expected from each other and to be open with each other. Something essential was that it was a partnership: it wasn't setup as one of us in charge or knowing more than the other. We approached it as a chance to learn and grow and help each other become better versions of ourselves, we didn't label ourselves as "neurotypical" and "neurodiverse" we were just Martin and James. This to me exemplifies what a mentor/mentee relationship should be about: mutual respect, trust, understanding and communication. We didn't label ourselves in our partnership, we accepted and respected each other as people. When it comes to any mentorship relationship whether it is rooted in business or a veterinary one, I think the key is to not have any preconceived ideas or assumptions about each other and enter into it as an opportunity to help yourself and help someone else grow.

MENTOR TIP

Many individuals are not diagnosed until adulthood. It is better for mentors to lead a dialogue around communication needs to understand goals, feedback and communication needs, and support. Your mentees should not have to disclose neurodiverse conditions to you.

Whether neurodiverse or neurotypical I have found that understanding your why is the most important thing, once you, yourself can understand why you are doing something the easier it is to communicate with others. Knowing the right questions to ask and how to ask them is key, neurotypicals and neurodiverse people process information differently. This is also important in building the mentor/mentee relationship as it opens an effective communication between both, creating a comfortable safe space for both to communicate will enhance the working dynamic if you both understand why the other reacts or expresses themselves in the way that they do.

When our reactions are looked at with a lens that can involve misconceptions, experiences around other's interpretation of responses led to anxiety ridden and stress around how one is "supposed" to react in this situation, which can result in distraction or emotional shutdown. As this pertains to a mentor/mentee dynamic, I would refer to this as "bedside manner."

A veterinarian on the spectrum might not show or express outward empathy and compassion in a scenario that may be perceived insensitive or clinical when interacting with a patient or colleague. Or perhaps a mentee's response may be interpreted as challenging the mentor. When mentoring an individual on the spectrum it is important to ask questions about the why or their response, to use curiosity rather than assumptions. If they are like me, and answer in a literal and logical manner explaining why being able to use a certain language to display understanding, compassion and empathy is important. Additionally, mentors may need to help mentees process how they feel about a difficult case or experience over time rather than immediately.

MENTOR TIP

If your mentee responds in a way that you disagree with, or that you have an emotional response to, pause first. Before your reaction of judging or correcting, ask at least 3 curiosity based questions. "Can you expand more on that?" "Would you feel comfortable sharing more about what you were feeling and thinking?"

Asking questions and understanding someone else's why and helping them understand their own why. It doesn't matter whether you are neurotypical or neurodiverse we all have our own unique why as to the reason we are doing something and for me I can't grow and become the best version of myself if I am not honest with myself and understand myself, just like I can't help others do the same thing if I don't understand these same things about them.

In my role as a financial advisor, I tell my clients that they didn't need to be honest with me, they needed to be honest with themselves in order for me to help them help themselves. This is true for a mentor/mentee relationship as well, if you as a mentor don't understand how your mentee processes information or what their motivation is how can you help them maximize their potential? Alternatively as a mentee how can you expect your mentor to help you if they don't understand these things about you and if you don't understand each other how can you both flourish and achieve your goals.

I believe that any successful professional partnership is based on collaboration. In my experience as an autistic professional that work relationships break down when we don't understand and communicate with each other, when we put labels on an individual, my hope is that we labels are removed when identifying each other that we don't see each other as "neurotypical" or "neurodiverse" that we see each other as people.

FOUNDATIONS OF HUMAN-CENTERED MENTORSHIP

This section introduces the foundational framework for human-centered mentorship, which serves as the through line for this chapter. The concepts explored here provide shared language for understanding the experiences discussed earlier and for applying ethical, inclusive mentorship practices throughout the sections that follow.

Human-centered mentorship is a compassion-driven model designed to support mentorship across backgrounds while offering tools to examine experiences we may have encountered, witnessed, or contributed to harm within mentor–mentee dynamics. The goals of this approach are to support prevention, repair, and restoration following negative experiences in education and work and to reduce the risk of discrimination distorting mentorship relationships.

Human-centered mentorship begins with a shift from hierarchy to humanity, from output to experience, and from compliance to consent. Rather than reinforcing rigid professional roles, this model emphasizes reciprocal relationships grounded in shared responsibility. At its core are five essential pillars of interpersonal relationships: the need to be seen, to be heard, to have lived experience validated, to be respected in one's autonomy, and to be kept from harm.

THE FIVE PILLARS OF HUMAN-CENTERED MENTORSHIP

- To be seen
- To be heard
- To be validated for lived experience
- To be respected in autonomy
- To be kept from harm

Human-centered mentorship draws from principles of universal design used in physical and workplace environments (Rose et al., 2013, Tan and Fogelberg, 2024). Applied to mentorship, these principles help anticipate diverse needs from the outset, ensuring that inclusion is built in rather than retrofitted (Quicksall, 2024). Universal mentorship principles reduce the risk of discriminatory missteps and prioritize responsiveness when harm occurs, rather than relying on retroactive or experimental approaches.

To see and hear someone is not a passive act; it is a commitment to presence. Validation requires acknowledging another person's reality, even when it differs from our own. Respecting autonomy means mentoring with, not over, others, and adopting a posture of "do no harm," particularly when offering guidance or feedback.

MENTOR TIP: CREATING CONSENT AND INVITING OPT IN

- "Are you ready to talk about this case?"
- "I'd like to give you some feedback on ___. Would now be a good time?"

This includes honoring a mentee's "no" or stated support needs without penalty. When environments feel unsafe, curiosity shrinks, participation declines, and the ability to integrate new skills is impaired (Quicksall, 2024). Safety and respect are the foundation on which professional growth stands.

Human-centered mentorship is not prescriptive; it is cocreated. Its purpose is to serve the people within the mentorship relationship in a mutually agreed-upon way. This includes collaboratively designing mentorship experiences with clear expectations, defined roles, and strategies for repair when missteps occur. Flexibility is essential, as growth is rarely linear and progress will look different for each individual.

Cultural differences and the intentional use of space must also be considered. What feels neutral to one person may feel disrespectful or dishonoring to another. Eating lunch atop a freezer used to store remains or storing personal belongings next to equipment used to clean urine and fecal material communicates disregard for cultural and professional meaning—experiences both Ron and Erika have encountered. When spaces and practices that hold meaning for others are not respected, psychological safety erodes and learning suffers (Quicksall, 2024).

Finally, mentorship must be grounded in continuity. We are not mentoring only for today, but for those who come after. Whether a mentee remains within an organization or moves beyond it, the mentor's role is to support their evolving story, not merely their current role. What we normalize today becomes what is inherited tomorrow. Human-centered mentorship creates environments that are inclusive by design rather than by exception.

SUPPORTING MENTORS ACROSS POWER AND IDENTITY DIFFERENCES

Mentoring across difference—particularly when mentors themselves hold marginalized identities—requires a level of self-awareness and intentionality that is often absent from traditional mentorship models. The assumption that mentorship is a one-way act of guidance fails to account for the emotional labor, power dynamics, and identity navigation that many mentors continuously manage. Whether mentors share marginalized identities with their mentees or are mentoring across lines of difference, **mentorship does not exist outside systems of inequity. It exists within them.**

This section is informed by work that recognizes inequity as structurally embedded rather than incidental, including Ron's forthcoming book, *Rewriting the Rules*. Through a human-centered mentorship lens, the focus here is not on assigning blame, but on understanding how mentorship can shift from burden to empowerment when care, accountability, and equity are intentionally built into the relationship.

WHEN MENTORS HOLD MARGINALIZED IDENTITIES?

For mentors who hold marginalized identities—by race, gender identity, disability, sexuality, class, or other lived experience—mentorship is rarely limited to offering professional guidance. It often becomes an act of advocacy, translation, and protection. Mentors may feel pressure to "be the example," to create pathways where none existed, or to shield mentees from harms they themselves endured. While this responsibility can be deeply meaningful, it is also exhausting.

Imposter syndrome, shaped by persistent underrepresentation, may surface as doubt about one's legitimacy as a mentor despite deep expertise and lived knowledge. Relational pacing may feel misaligned. Many marginalized mentors are hypervigilant in coded environments, reading emotional cues as a survival skill rather than a mentorship preference. Traditional mentorship frameworks often fail to account for these realities.

Overcompensation is a common adaptive response. Mentors may overextend, overdeliver, or become "the safe one" in unsafe systems. Others may withdraw emotionally to avoid reentering trauma cycles triggered by mentee experiences or institutional resistance. These responses are not personal failures—they are survival strategies within inequitable systems.

COMMON PRESSURES MARGINALIZED MENTORS CARRY

- Imposter syndrome despite expertise
- Hypervigilance in coded environments
- Overextension and emotional labor
- Emotional withdrawal as self-protection
- Pressure to represent or protect others

Supporting marginalized mentors requires rejecting linear, one-size-fits-all expectations of mentorship. Flexibility in pacing, the use of asynchronous feedback, visual tools, and alternative formats can reduce cognitive and emotional overload. Designing mentorship around capacity rather than conformity acknowledges the realities these mentors navigate daily.

Psychological safety must extend to mentors as well as mentees. Safety for mentors means they are not penalized for naming bias, advocating for structural change, or needing space. It includes recognizing and valuing what marginalized mentors often bring to mentorship relationships: emotional intelligence, pattern recognition across complex systems, the ability to hold dual realities, and the courage to speak into tension.

Environmental context also matters. Who is in the room? Who holds power? Are mentors from marginalized groups expected to represent an entire identity or honored as individuals with boundaries and agency? Human-centered mentorship plans for difference rather than demanding resilience in spite of it.

WHEN MENTORS ARE SUPPORTING MARGINALIZED MENTEES

For mentors who are not from marginalized groups but are mentoring individuals who are, the expectation is not perfection, but presence, accountability, and willingness to grow. It is easy to fall into performance allyship, where intention is centered over impact, or to become paralyzed by fear of saying the wrong thing. Avoidance, however, causes as much harm as missteps.

The first step is recognizing when mentorship occurs across a power gap. This may involve racial, cultural, linguistic, socioeconomic, neurocognitive, or gender-based differences. Subtle signals matter. Masking, code-switching, withdrawal after feedback, or hesitation to disagree are often adaptations to environments not built for the mentee—not personality traits.

Barriers arise when mentors unintentionally impose majority-norm expectations around communication style, ambition, eye contact, or "fit." Without shared context, feedback can land as judgment. Hesitation may be misread as disinterest, and quietness as disengagement, obscuring competence and insight.

Effective support requires shifting from advice-giving to cocreating clarity. Use plain, accessible language. Set expectations collaboratively. Offer context for decisions and feedback. Recognize the courage it may take for a mentee to say no, ask for help, or disagree with someone in power—and treat those moments as strength rather than insubordination. Supporting across difference is not a one-time act; it is an ongoing practice grounded in consistency and trust.

ACCOUNTABILITY WITHOUT SHAME

Accountability is not synonymous with punishment, and when it feels that way, mentorship fails. This is particularly true for mentees from marginalized backgrounds who may carry internalized shame from discrimination, microaggressions, exclusion, or the absence of representation in leadership and mentorship.

When feedback activates shame, it can trigger withdrawal, over-apologizing, or overcompensation. These responses are often invisible to the mentor and misinterpreted as defensiveness or fragility, when they are more accurately understood as trauma responses.

The mentor's emotional response matters deeply in these moments. Dismissive reactions—such as "you're too sensitive" or "we're all human here"—may seem benign but often function as emotional bypassing. This invalidates lived experience and pushes mentees further into silence, perpetuating harm rather than interrupting it.

Human-centered mentorship reframes accountability as an act of care rather than control. It emphasizes repair, context, and agency so that correction builds capacity instead of diminishing confidence.

REPAIR LANGUAGE THAT BUILDS TRUST

- "I may not have gotten that right, and I want to try again. Is that okay?"
- "Thank you for trusting me with that perspective."
- "Your experience matters, even if it's hard for me to hear."

When rupture occurs, name it. Invite reflection without shame. Offer space without withdrawing support. Accountability must be mutual, culturally aware, and adaptive. Public feedback may feel humiliating for someone from a collectivist background; abrupt conversations may trigger fight-or-flight responses for someone with a trauma history. This does not mean avoiding accountability—it means delivering it with intention.

Human-centered mentorship asks us to learn how to walk together without erasing difference. When power is acknowledged and care is practiced deliberately, mentorship becomes a space where both mentors and mentees can show up fully and thrive.

EMPOWERMENT OF THE MENTEE

This section centers the mentee and is written from a place of fierce protectiveness. It reflects Erika's more than 15 years of student advocacy within and beyond formal veterinary organizations, including work in suicide prevention and direct support of student communities during periods of crisis, both locally and globally. The vision underlying this section is a profession in which no student or early-career veterinarian feels alone and where support from the industry is not conditional, inconsistent, or withdrawn during moments of vulnerability.

Human-centered mentorship requires acknowledging that many students and new graduates enter professional spaces already carrying the impact of past harm. Empowerment, in this context, is not about teaching resilience in isolation; it is about restoring agency, confidence, and safety so that learning and growth are possible.

Most veterinary students experience mosaic mentorship during training, learning from multiple professors, clinicians, and supervisors across varied clinical environments. These settings often emphasize conformity, narrowly defined performance outcomes, and accelerated timelines. Differences in faculty-to-student ratios, access to specialists, and clinical rotations mean that graduates leave training with uneven confidence across medical domains.

Learning environments may also lack adequate accommodations or resources to support diverse learning and information-processing styles. In many cases, peer-to-peer or informal support becomes the primary source of stability. Compounding this, punitive or shame-based interactions with senior clinicians—sometimes occurring publicly—can cause lasting damage to confidence, enthusiasm, and professional identity.

Two foundational assumptions are important for mentors to hold when working with new graduates:

- Mentorship in practice will feel fundamentally different from mentorship during training.
- Some mentees may be actively recovering from toxic mentorship experiences.

PROTECTION WITHOUT NORMALIZING HARM

FOUNDATIONAL PRINCIPLE: DO NO HARM

"Do no harm" is central to medical oaths across One Health professions. It must also guide how we treat one another—especially those entering the field.

This section rejects the normalization of harm under the guise of a "tough industry." What is often framed as resilience-building is more accurately understood as intergenerational trauma perpetuated through neglect, humiliation, or abuse. Veterinary medicine is not unique in this; similar patterns exist across high-intensity, care-based professions, including human healthcare and social work.

Medical innovation and excellence do not emerge from fear-based environments. They arise from practitioners who feel safe enough to remain curious, engaged, and creative. For mentors, this level of cultural and self-reflection is essential if the profession is to continue evolving.

For mentees, it is critical to understand that abusive behavior disqualifies a mentor from being a legitimate evaluator of your worth, capability, or character. While an individual's medical expertise may hold value, discrimination, verbal domination, manipulation, or shame-based teaching reflect the mentor's limitations—not the mentee's potential.

Until these systemic failures are addressed through clearer accountability around who is entrusted to teach and lead, mentees must be empowered to extract what is useful, protect themselves from harm, and build alternative sources of safety and support.

AGENCY, SELF-ADVOCACY, AND DISCERNMENT

Empowerment includes developing the ability to recognize problematic mentorship behaviors and to understand options for response. These challenges most often arise in de facto mentorship relationships—those formed by circumstance rather than choice—such as shared workplaces or required supervisory structures.

Problematic Mentorship Behaviors

- Tone policing
- Antagonism toward questions or feedback
- Dismissiveness of concerns
- "I had it hard too—so should you" narratives
- Lack of availability or responsiveness

- Impatience or inflexibility
- Rigid right/wrong framing
- Teaching through shame or humiliation

Self-advocacy from a perceived subordinate position is inherently challenging, particularly for mentees from marginalized backgrounds. Institutional responses to discrimination may differ markedly from stated values. Mentees should be prepared for imperfect responses while recognizing that scrutiny and evaluation often flow downward, not upward.

Preparation and clarity can reduce harm. Understanding expectations, policies, and available support structures at the outset of a mentorship relationship increases agency and safety.

QUESTIONS THAT SUPPORT SELF-ADVOCACY

- How does this mentorship relationship affect my evaluation or position?
- How are concerns addressed if challenges arise?
- Is a facilitator or third party available?
- What are the expectations around constructive feedback?
- How are incidents of client discrimination handled?
- Are advocates permitted during evaluations?

MENTEE TIP

Humanizing mentors while respecting their bandwidth can support connection:

"I have a question about a case—when would be a good time to talk?"

Asking for what you need is not a failure of competence. Understanding how you best receive and integrate information—through notes, visuals, observation, repetition, or pacing—is a critical professional skill. Recovery time after emotionally charged cases may also be necessary before engaging in feedback conversations.

RESILIENCE AND ITERATION

Working under conditions of discrimination creates hostile workplaces and carries a significant personal and emotional cost. Mentor–mentee relationships should function as sources of advocacy and support, helping to mitigate external harms that do not belong in the practice of medicine.

For mentees, a foundational goal is developing resilience—defined as the ability to recover from or thrive following a negative experience (Lowe, 2025). This process is incremental and nonlinear, much like acquiring clinical skills.

Reflection can help mentees assess whether environments support or undermine learning and well-being.

REFLECTION PROMPTS FOR MENTEES

- Am I experiencing discrimination, and how is it affecting my engagement?
- Does this environment support my professional goals?
- Do I have sufficient time and space to integrate learning?
- Are sensory, physical, or health needs being met?
- Do I feel safe asking for support?
- Is my mentor willing to advocate for me?

Finally, mentorship does not need to be confined to single relationships. Expanding mentorship across multiple trusted individuals—within or beyond an organization—reduces risk and increases resilience. Organizations should consider how mentorship can be woven into daily interactions rather than limited to formal programs alone.

CONCLUSION

Mentorship in veterinary medicine does not occur in a vacuum. It is shaped by power, identity, institutional culture, and the lived experiences that both mentors and mentees bring into the relationship. Throughout this chapter, we have explored how visible and invisible differences influence mentorship dynamics, how harm can be unintentionally perpetuated through traditional models, and how a human-centered approach offers a more ethical, sustainable path forward. Human-centered mentorship asks us to move beyond technical guidance alone and toward relationships grounded in safety, consent, accountability, and respect for autonomy. It recognizes that effective mentorship is not defined by conformity or endurance, but by the conditions that allow people to learn, grow, and remain engaged in the profession.

For mentors, this requires ongoing self-reflection, humility, and a willingness to adapt—especially when mentoring across differences or navigating systems that were not designed with equity in mind. For mentees, empowerment comes from discernment, self-advocacy, and the understanding that abusive or discriminatory behavior is not a measure of their worth or potential. When mentorship is approached as a shared responsibility rather than a hierarchy, it becomes a site of repair rather than harm and of possibility rather than attrition. The future of veterinary medicine depends not only on clinical excellence but also on our collective ability to foster mentorship relationships that are humane, responsive, and worthy of the next generation entrusted to them.

BIBLIOGRAPHY

AAHA (2023). Mentorship Guidelines. https://www.aaha.org/resources/2023-aaha-mentoring-guidelines/guidelines-contributors/ (accessed 1 December 2025).

Ayano, G., Tsegay, L., Gizachew, Y. et al. (2023). Prevalence of attention deficit hyperactivity disorder in adults: umbrella review of evidence generated across the globe. *Psychiatry Research* 328: 115449.

Barnes, K.H., Johnson, S., Liu, C.-C., and Aulakh, K.S. (2025). Prevalence of mistreatment in veterinary medical education: a survey of 3rd year veterinary students at a single university. *BMC Medical Education* 25 (1): 305. https://doi.org/10.1186/s12909-024-06610-9.

Bartels, T. (2025). Changes to federal student loans come into focus. https://vinfoundation.org/changes-federal-student-loans-come-into-focus/ (accessed 19 November 2025).

BVA (2019). Report on discrimination in the veterinary profession. https://www.bva.co.uk/media/2991/bva-report-on-discrimination-in-the-veterinary-profession.pdf (accessed 19 November 2025).

Chung, G.H. and Armitage-Chan, E. (2022). Student experience and ethnic diversity: the experiences of underrepresented minority students at a veterinary university in the United Kingdom. *Journal of Veterinary Medical Education* 49: 363–371.

Freeman, D., Hodgson, K., and Darling, M. (2022). Mentoring new veterinary graduates for transition to practice and lifelong learning. *Journal of Veterinary Medical Education* 49 (4): 409–413.

Gates, M.C., McLachlan, I., Butler, S. and Weston, J.F. (2021) 'Experiences of employers, work colleagues, and mentors with new veterinary graduates and preferences towards new graduate support programmes', *New Zealand Veterinary Journal*, 69(1), 38–50. https://doi.org/10.1080/00480169.2020.1805373

Greenhill, L.M., Davis, K.C., Lowrie, P.M. and Amass, S.F. (eds) (2013) *Navigating Diversity and Inclusion in Veterinary Medicine*. West Lafayette, IN: Purdue University Press. https://doi.org/10.2307/j.ctt6wq4j2

Hilton, K.R., Burke, K.J., and Signal, T. (2023). Mental health in the veterinary profession: an individual or organisational focus? *Australian Veterinary Journal* 101 (1–2): 41–48. https://doi.org/10.1111/avj.13215.

Irby, B.J., Abdelrahman, N., Lara-Alecio, R. and Allen, T. (2020) 'Epistemological beginnings of mentoring', Irby, B.J. et al. (eds) *The Wiley International Handbook of Mentoring*. Hoboken, NJ: Wiley. https://doi.org/10.1002/9781119142973.ch2

Jelinski, M.D., Campbell, J.R., MacGregor, M.W., and Watts, J.M. (2009). Factors associated with veterinarians' career path choices in the early postgraduate period. *Canadian Veterinary Journal* 50 (9): 943–948.

Kastelic, J. and Ogilvie, T. (2025). Mentorship has never been more important in the veterinary profession. *The Canadian Veterinary Journal* 66 (4): https://www.canadianveterinarians.net/about-cvma/latest-news/mentorship-has-never-been-more-important-in-the-veterinary-profession/ (accessed 29 November 2025).

Lin-Hendel, E. (2025a). Accommodations and accessibility for autistic veterinarians. *Clinician's Brief* https://www.cliniciansbrief.com/article/veterinarian-retention-autism-accommodations (accessed 28 December 2025).

Lin-Hendel, E. (2025b). Chapter G. In: *Diversity, Equity, and Inclusion in Veterinary Medicine* (ed. K. Marshall), 67–79. Hoboken, NJ: John Wiley & Sons.

Lowe, S.R. (2025). Embracing complexity in resilience research. *Nature Mental Health* 3: 391–392.

Marcano, V.C. and Mages, A. (2025) 'The impact of socioeconomic privilege on the demographic makeup of veterinary teams', *Veterinary Ophthalmology*, 1–8. https://doi.org/10.1111/vop.70091

Marshall, K. (2025). *Diversity, Equity, and Inclusion in Veterinary Medicine*. Hoboken, NJ: John Wiley & Sons.

Martínez, M. (2024). Understanding the why: the need for diversity, equity, and inclusion in veterinary medicine. *Veterinary Clinics of North America: Small Animal Practice* 54 (5): 753–765. https://doi.org/10.1016/j.cvsm.2024.06.009.

Michigan State University, CVM (2019). Hammurabi and hippocrates: veterinary medicine BCE. https://cvm.msu.edu/vetschool-tails/hammurabi-and-hippocrates-veterinary-medicine-bce (accessed 19 July 2025).

Olufunmilola, A. and Quinlan, D.A. (2024). The lost art of intergenerational mentorship in health services research and teaching in pharmacy: the CRoME lab example. *Currents in Pharmacy Teaching and Learning* 16 (9): 102122.

Peet, M., Walsh, K., Sober, R., and Rawak, C.S. (2010). Generative knowledge interviewing: a method for knowledge transfer and talent management at the University of Michigan. *International Journal of Educational Advancement* 10: 71–85.

Quicksall, M.S. (2024). Inclusive mentorship for the next generation of veterinary professionals. *Veterinary Clinics of North America: Small Animal Practice* 54 (6): 869–880. https://doi.org/10.1016/j.cvsm.2024.07.014.

Reinhard, A.R. (2023). Early career veterinary wellbeing and solutions to help young veterinarians thrive. *Advances in Small Animal Care* 4 (1): 113–122.

Rose, D., Meyer, A., and Gordon, D. (2013). *Universal Design for Learning: Theory and Practice*. Wakefield, MA: CAST Publishing.

Shoichiro, Y. and Yukawa, M. (2022). A survey assessing the prevalence of in-hospital violence against veterinary nurses working in small animal hospitals. *Open Veterinary Journal* 12 (4): 430–433.

Stanton, M.A. and Miller, A. (2025). Addressing five explanations for the lack of racial and ethnic diversity in veterinary medicine in the United States.

Journal of Veterinary Medical Education e20240128. (Epub ahead of print).

Stewart, P (2018). #MeToo in vet med: shining a light on sexual harassment and assault. https://www.dvm360.com/view/metoo-vet-med-shining-light-sexual-harassment-and-assault (accessed 26 December 2025).

Summers, O.S., Medcalf, R., Hubbard, K.A., and McCarroll, C.S. (2023). A cross-sectional study examining perceptions of discriminatory behaviors experienced and witnessed by veterinary students undertaking clinical extra-mural studies. *Frontiers in Veterinary Science* 10.

Tan, J.-Y. and Fogelberg, K. (2024). Understanding implicit bias and its impact in veterinary medicine. *Veterinary Clinics of North America: Small Animal Practice* 54 (5): 813–824.

Tomasi, S.E., Fechter-Leggett, E.D., Edwards, N.T. et al. (2019). Suicide among veterinarians in the United States from 1979 through 2015. *Journal of the American Veterinary Medical Association* 254 (1): 104–112. https://doi.org/10.2460/javma.254.1.104.

Tran, C.V. (2024). *Diversity, Equity, and Inclusion in Veterinary Medicine, Parts I & II. Veterinary Clinics of North America: Small Animal Practice*. Elsevier.

Volk, J.O., Schimmack, U., Strand, E.B. et al. (2020). Executive summary of the Merck Animal Health Veterinarian Wellbeing Study II. *Journal of the American Veterinary Medical Association* 256 (11): 1237–1244. https://doi.org/10.2460/javma.256.11.1237.

Wogan, L. (2024). US state eases access for foreign-trained veterinarians. *Veterinary Information Network News* https://news.vin.com/default.aspx (accessed 28 December 2025).

Wogan, L. (2025). NAVLE pass rates ticked up in 2024. *Veterinary Information Network News* https://news.vin.com/default.aspx (accessed 1 December 2025).

Won, C. and Larkin, M. (2025). Proposed class action by veterinary interns brought against veterinary schools and hospitals alleging antitrust conspiracy. https://www.avma.org/news/proposed-class-action-veterinary-interns-brought-against-veterinary-schools-hospitals-alleging (accessed 2 December 2025).

Yanke, A.B., Weigand, K.A. and Hofmeister, E.H. (2023) 'Addressing the needs and challenges of mentorship in veterinary medicine', *New Directions for Teaching and Learning*, 2023, 83–93. https://doi.org/10.1002/tl.20571

Yeager, K.A. and Bauer-Wu, S. (2013) 'Cultural humility: essential foundation for clinical researchers', *Applied Nursing Research*, 26(4), 251–256. https://doi.org/10.1016/j.apnr.2013.06.008

Yukawa S, Yukawa M. A survey assessing the prevalence of in-hospital violence against veterinary nurses working in small animal hospitals. Open Vet J. 2022 Jul-Aug;12(4):430-433. doi: 10.5455/OVJ.2022.v12.i4.2. Epub 2022 Jul 8. PMID: 36118730; PMCID: PMC9473370.

Building Veterinary Leaders

CHAPTER 5

INTRODUCTION

Dani Rabwin

Mentorship is never just about teaching medicine. The most impactful mentors are those who help shape careers, not only through clinical instruction but also by modeling professionalism, offering emotional support, and creating opportunities for growth. That broader role—what happens beyond teaching—is the focus of this chapter.

The challenge is that these aspects of mentorship are often the most ambiguous. How do you balance being a role model with being authentic about your own struggles? When should you challenge a mentee vs. offer comfort? How do you open doors through your network without creating dependency? These questions matter because the answers determine whether mentorship produces confident, independent professionals and leaders or creates relationships that limit rather than liberate.

I invited Pam Hale, DVM, MBA, and Jessica Petty, EdD, to contribute because each brings a unique lens to this essential topic. Pam starts us off by exploring the day-to-day responsibilities of mentors: being role models, guiding career development, and opening doors through networks while maintaining healthy boundaries. Drawing on decades of experience as a veterinarian, practice executive, and leadership coach, she provides practical guidance for helping mentees grow into more confident and capable professionals.

Jessica then shifts our focus to the organizational level, examining how formal structures, leadership pipelines, and workplace culture shape mentorship outcomes. Her doctoral research on how organizational support impacts women leaders in the animal health industry, combined with her extensive experience in industry leadership, challenges us to consider the systemic factors that can either amplify or undermine individual mentorship efforts, particularly when it comes to equity and advancement.

Together, their insights remind us that mentorship is as much about fostering resilience, opportunity, and leadership as it is about transferring knowledge. This chapter will help you understand how to be the kind of mentor who shapes not just what mentees know, but who they become as professionals and leaders.

BEING A ROLE MODEL

Pam Hale

Veterinarians naturally become role models, often without even realizing it. Whether you are in a formal leadership position or not, your words, actions, and attitudes are being observed by new graduates, junior colleagues, and support staff. As a mentor, your role expands beyond teaching technical skills. You are also modeling how to navigate the profession with integrity, humility, and resilience.

THE POWER OF ROLE MODELING

A role model is someone whose behavior is observed and often emulated. In veterinary medicine, this includes those with formal leadership titles—medical directors, lead veterinarians, and hospital managers—but it also includes those without any official authority. A technician who mentors others with generosity, a client service team member who leads with kindness, or a veterinarian who models ethical decision-making in everyday interactions, all of these are powerful role models. This is the beauty of being a role model; anyone can be one!

As a mentor, your impact is often subtle but far-reaching. Mentees are watching how you handle difficult clients, how you talk about your team, how you recover from mistakes, and how you set boundaries. These moments can leave a lasting impression—sometimes more than any formal teaching. Being a good role model means not trying to be everything to those around you but rather being an excellent source of information and inspiration.

In my experience, I have had many people who I considered role models and held them in high esteem. There are also those I did not even realize were my role models until later in my career. The behavior that cemented someone as a role model for me has been the selfless leader who can also teach how to set boundaries for self-care. These are people who provide a listening ear yet challenge me to find solutions on my own. I have seen role models who maintain an open-door policy while not tolerating abuse of that privilege.

> **MENTOR TIP**
>
> Think about someone who shaped your own professional development. What did they model that stuck with you? Now reflect: What are you modeling today in your words, actions, and choices?

LEADING BY EXAMPLE

Mentorship is a form of leadership. Whether you hold a formal title or not, you are leading by example. Mentors who model honesty, compassion, humility, and professionalism give mentees a powerful framework for how to show up in their own careers. Some days, leadership looks like navigating a difficult case with calm. Other days, it means admitting a mistake or showing how to advocate for team well-being. These everyday choices teach mentees how to build careers rooted in both competence and character.

Effective mentors as role models demonstrate:

- **Integrity:** Speaking truthfully and following through on commitments
- **Resilience:** Bouncing back after errors or difficult days
- **Empathy:** Listening to team members and clients with compassion

- **Boundaries:** Knowing when to say no and modeling self-care
- **Humility:** Admitting mistakes and giving credit to others

I often speak on leadership and how titles initially identify someone as a leader. However, there are instances when the leader with the title is not actually the person influencing the team or achieving results. **I believe genuine leaders see their title as helpful but not defining.** Leadership requires understanding the business and what success looks like, then determining the best way to achieve those results.

As a leader, you must have a strong conviction and belief in your team. This will be required to bring a vision to fruition. A leader in veterinary medicine should encompass empathy, self-awareness, and the ability to help make decisions that move the team forward. Apply these same qualities in your role as a mentor as well.

BEING AVAILABLE—WHILE SETTING BOUNDARIES

Mentors are often busy professionals. You may be running a hospital, leading a team, or juggling multiple roles. Time with mentees may be limited, but how you handle those interactions matters more than how many you have. Your mentee will appreciate your willingness to take on this role; it is important to show that you are able and willing to participate in either a formal or informal mentorship setting. Even if you are caught off guard by being asked to be a mentor, your mentee likely sees something in you that inspires them to have the "promise of proximity" and learn from you being around the right people for the right reason (Coleman, 2019).

Set expectations for the mentorship relationship early. Will you meet regularly? Should your mentee email you between sessions or wait for scheduled times? Mentorship doesn't require constant availability—it requires intentional presence. **Being reliable, thoughtful, and respectful of your own bandwidth models healthy boundaries for your mentee.**

MENTOR TIP

Modeling time boundaries is valuable in itself. By showing that your time is structured and respected, you demonstrate professional self-care and invite your mentee to do the same.

CONSIDER THE SCENARIO

Your mentee is discouraged because a recent medical case went poorly, and they received limited feedback from their team leader. They reach out to you for guidance, but you're juggling leadership responsibilities and can't respond immediately.

If you've established clear expectations upfront, both you and your mentee know how to handle this situation:

- Your mentee understands that urgent needs may arise, but immediate responses aren't always possible
- You know to acknowledge their message quickly, even if you can't have a full conversation right away
- Your mentee doesn't interpret a delay as rejection or lack of care
- You set aside dedicated time as soon as reasonably possible

This scenario illustrates why setting boundaries and expectations early prevents misunderstandings and maintains a healthy, collaborative relationship. Both parties give each other grace while still providing meaningful support.

INSPIRING GROWTH THROUGH CONNECTION

Mentorship becomes truly transformative when it's built on mutual trust and authentic connection. While informal role models can inspire from a distance, formal mentorship allows for deeper conversations, targeted feedback, and real-time support. As a mentor, you will act as a coach, sometimes speaking in a supervisory manner to your mentees. A mentor isn't a "best friend" or fortune teller. Instead, you are a leader who will provide objective advice while helping them find their best path with their own skill set.

Be transparent about your own journey. Share what worked, what didn't, and how you learned through adversity. This helps mentees normalize challenges and builds psychological safety. **Mentors don't need to be perfect—they need to be human, honest, and invested**. There is inspiration in sharing resilience in past or present events. In fact, knowing that a mentor has struggled yet persevered is inspiring! This creates relatability with your mentee while helping them avoid placing you on a pedestal.

Establishing clear structure and expectations within the mentoring relationship amplifies these benefits. Working together allows you to identify shared values. While not strictly necessary, establishing a foundation of similar professional values and approaches to veterinary practice strengthens the relationship. It is also helpful to understand each other's ethics to ensure effective interactions. Having defined structure also allows for a specified time frame, which creates urgency for communications, updates, and check-ins. Finally, clear boundaries can be established for when interactions occur, time of day, and length of discussions.

PROVIDING EMOTIONAL AND CAREER SUPPORT

Mentorship will typically center on providing support in mentees' professional endeavors. Your conversations will tend to involve workplace challenges, providing recommendations on best paths to achieve certain goals, and expanding critical thinking while helping mentees uncover unexplored avenues. As a mentor, you should also challenge mentees to view situations through a different lens, leading to both academic and professional growth (Byars-Winston and Dahlberg, 2019).

Your support as a mentor may take many different forms. While there are times you may just need to provide a listening ear and validate an experience, there are instances where you will need to provide direction or more input. Mentees may find themselves stuck when they struggle to articulate their needs, so you will have to uncover the particular problem through active listening, probing questions and supportive exploration. This requires tremendous trust within your mentoring relationship as well as calling for you to be an intuitive mentor.

MENTOR TIP

Supporting a mentee isn't always telling them what to do. The best mentorships involve allowing mentees to forge their own pathways through problem-solving, establishing their vision, and articulating different objectives.

CHALLENGING YOUR MENTEE

While you aim not to be overbearing or overly critical as a mentor, do not shy away from challenging mentees. In fact, challenging decisions and actions should be employed on a regular basis. Use open-ended questions that require your mentee to share the situation, display their critical thinking and problem-solving skills, and determine if they are satisfied with their own process.

Of course, in most cases, there is room for you to coach your mentee, and the approach often depends on what type of coaching is needed. Here, you may share a different perspective to help mentees learn alternatives to their problem-solving process. As a mentor, it is good practice to always present different perspectives for your mentee, as it will be helpful in the moment as well as in the future. Growth happens when challenges arise. Mentees will face times in their careers that will test their resilience. As a mentor, you are tasked with preparing them for the ups and downs of a professional career, which requires difficult learning experiences.

CONSIDER THE SCENARIO

Your mentee reaches out to you to discuss what they determined to be negative interactions with their team leader. Your mentee feels that their team leader did not set aside time to work with them, coach them, or make themselves available when they needed help. During a conversation, the team leader stated, "I trust your decisions and ability to handle different situations." Your mentee expresses that they did not feel supported or heard in this conversation and still needed more input from their leader.

You allow your mentee to share their feelings from this, including feeling directionless, left to their own devices and their call for help ignored. However, as a mentor, you also suggest the team leader's perspective. As you are in a leadership role, you advise that their team leader may be overwhelmed in their role. By telling your mentee that they "trust their decisions," it should build confidence in them. Their leader does have trust in their ability to handle situations and make decisions. You can explain that your mentee can give their leader grace as their boss is trusting in their choices and critical thinking. This is a perspective that your mentee had not considered, and with this different point of view, they are able to move past their initial thoughts of the leadership lacking direction and support.

MENTOR TIP

It is not your role to agree with, soothe, coddle, or cater to mentees. By playing the devil's advocate, you will challenge ingrained patterns, ask thought-provoking questions, and inspire breakthroughs. Many lessons may not occur without these tough conversations.

GUIDING CAREER DEVELOPMENT

Beyond providing emotional support and challenging thinking, mentors play a crucial role in helping mentees navigate their professional paths. Career development conversations often emerge naturally from the trust you've built through other interactions. Below are some of the key competencies that make up strong career coaching in a mentorship context:

Essential Career Development Coaching Skills

(Adapted from Carruthers, 2023)

Foundation Skills

- **Active listening** without judgment
- **Gauge receptiveness** to feedback
- **Be introspective** in your coaching approach

Adaptive Skills

- **Share experiences** without dominating the conversation
- **Recognize and verbalize** your mentee's value
- **Show appropriate empathy** when needed

Responsive Skills

- **Discern when to provide** empathy vs. tactical input vs. affirmation
- **Adjust your approach** based on mentee's varying needs
- **Fulfill multiple roles** as situations require

Professional career development coaching requires you to master this combination of skills. The key is learning to read each situation and respond with what your mentee needs most in that moment.

Determining Career Aspirations

During this phase of mentoring, you can help mentees by uncovering their career aspirations. More likely than not, you have been sought out as a mentor due to sharing a similar field of study or profession with your mentees. Your mentee may be considering how to better learn to navigate the politics of the business world than to work with someone who has achieved leading roles and operated successfully. If a veterinarian is considering a board certification in specialty medicine, finding a mentor who has achieved that certification would be prudent for them. However, even if you are outside of a mentee's chosen profession, you are also of assistance. Remember, a mentor can be anyone who has shown success, is a role model, or has leadership experience.

This is your opportunity as a mentor to understand exactly what your mentee hopes to accomplish and tailor your guidance accordingly. Some mentees will have broad goals—they want to explore—while others will be laser-focused on a specific achievement.

CASE STUDY **SUPPORTING CAREER ADVANCEMENT**

One mentee expressed their goal of becoming a senior level director or regional medical director. Over several months, we worked together as they prepared to apply for an upcoming position in their company. Their preparation included enrolling in business certification courses, achieving success in their current role managing one veterinary hospital, and networking with colleagues to establish themselves as a "leader amongst leaders" and advocate for veterinary teams. This comprehensive professional development support proved effective—they are now under serious consideration for the new role. This example shows how mentors can help mentees create concrete action plans that align with their career aspirations.

Maintaining Professional Boundaries

Mentorship focuses on professional and career development—work duties, education, career paths, and business outcomes. As a mentor, it's important to keep conversations centered on these professional topics. While you can offer advice on work–life balance, it's best to avoid delving into personal relationships or intimate details of your mentee's private life.

Clear boundaries protect both you and your mentee. Discussing sensitive personal matters can burden you as a mentor and may have unintended consequences. If conversations start moving into inappropriate territory, redirect them back to professional topics. Such conversations can be detrimental to reputations, worsen personal relationship dilemmas, and place you as a mentor in a compromised position.

However, don't confuse workplace interpersonal issues with off-limits personal topics. Mentees often need help navigating workplace personalities, improving communication with colleagues, or interpreting interactions with supervisors. These "workplace personal" conversations are exactly what mentorship should address—they're professional challenges that happen to involve interpersonal dynamics.

GUIDANCE RATHER THAN CODEPENDENCE

Considering that a professional path may not go as planned or even happen at all, it is not your role as a mentor to be the mapmaker of another person. Mentees should come with a good understanding of what they want to be and what they want to do. Their achievements thus far can be taken into account as they discuss each step with you as their trusted mentor. The burden should not be too heavy by expecting you to have all of the answers or give a definitive outline. Each career trajectory is different.

As a mentor you may have similar experiences, provide input, contacts, and coaching; however, **the real work in mentorship is done by the mentees**. Therefore, it is critical that your guidance does not create codependence. Career progression is not always linear nor easily attained. Your role as a mentor can help mentees rebound when the best-laid plans do not materialize, are delayed, or are completely derailed.

Most career professionals have experienced roadblocks that undoubtedly will be experienced by your mentees. These roadblocks will come in the form of other people, poor preparation, lack of opportunity, or unpredictable missteps. In your mentorship, you can teach resilience as this discouragement can cause a range of emotions from annoyance to extreme emotional distress. This trait isn't to be confused with "being strong." There are times when strength isn't the answer, but a plan to get up, regroup, make new plans, and begin again is in order. Your role as a mentor will be a great asset during these obstacles.

MENTOR TIP

Resilience is a trait that all professionals will need as they learn to navigate the workplace and set goals for themselves. Do you have examples of your own efforts of overcoming disappointment, loss, and acts of sabotage? Share these examples with your mentee.

KEY TAKEAWAYS FOR MENTORS

- Challenge your mentee's thinking and be willing to play devil's advocate to teach alternative viewpoints
- Remain flexible in your coaching style and approach
- Help identify your mentee's aspirations and support their path to achieving goals
- Guide without creating codependence—let mentees do the real work
- Maintain professional boundaries while still addressing "professional personal" workplace dynamics.

FACILITATING NETWORKING AND PROFESSIONAL OPPORTUNITIES

One of the most valuable gifts a mentor can offer is access to their network and guidance on building professional relationships. Depending on your mentee's career stage, they may be inexperienced in building a network of colleagues and collaborators, as well as identifying professional opportunities. If the mentee is newly graduated, their main source of networking professionals will, in all likelihood, be other recent graduates. In mentorship, career support of mentees may take the form of helping with connections in the mentor network.

However, you should not be used only as a stepping stone or, worse, a pawn by your mentees. It takes years to build a trusted network of colleagues—professional and personal. As a mentor, it is wise to protect those connections initially to prevent misuse and overuse. When sharing your network connections, you must be able to trust that the connections will not be abused, that your mentee will not overstep you as the mentor, or, worse, reflect poorly on you in the mentor network. A collegial network is a career-long and sometimes lifelong endeavor of a trusted community. These connections should be respected by mentees. When you connect your mentee to a colleague, this should be seen as a privilege and treated with sincere gratitude. Your circle of professional contacts is sacred.

BUILDING A PROFESSIONAL NETWORK

Professional networks are built over many years. They should be valued and held closely. Thus, in sharing any contacts from your network with a mentee, you demonstrate trust in your mentee of the highest regard. Networks are built from present and past work relationships, peers, casual acquaintances, introductions, memberships in organizations, and chance meetings. Many networking opportunities are built through other networks. As a mentor, you can help your mentees build a network from sharing your own and by encouraging mentees to venture out into organizational meetings with the goal of making 2–3 networking contacts.

Key Networking Venues

- Social media platforms
- Continuing education conferences
- Professional associations and organizations
- Workplace team projects and collaborations
- Alumni functions and events

This present age with many social media outlets makes it easy to reach out to known colleagues. As a mentor, you should instruct your mentee on the best etiquette in contacting a potential contact.

Social Media Networking Best Practices

- **Be protective** of your contacts and time on social media
- **Keep posts professional**, especially on career-focused platforms
- **Avoid inflammatory comments** that may turn off potential contacts
- **Follow company social media policies**, especially during work hours
- **Use good judgment** when connecting with people through shared networks
- **Remember that complete strangers** can still expose you to unscrupulous characters

Your mentees, like most professionals, must attain continuing education to maintain licensure. These conferences can be excellent networking opportunities, as many similar professionals gather in one place for several days. Conferences offer both formal sessions and informal evening events for building connections. However, these meetings can be overwhelming! Advise your mentees to be strategic—they may not want to be seen networking with competitors if it signals they're job hunting. Remind them that sometimes it's just about gathering business cards or QR codes for future reference. They should come prepared with 2–3 planned networking goals.

Professional associations are another valuable networking avenue. As a mentor, you're likely a member of relevant organizations, making this a natural way to help your mentees get involved. Association meetings connect dedicated professionals who share similar experiences and challenges. Encourage your mentees to attend icebreakers, evening events, and breakout sessions where they'll meet empathetic colleagues willing to share their journeys. You may even attend these same meetings and facilitate introductions to key people in your network.

PROFESSIONAL DEVELOPMENT AND GROWTH

Professional development and growth are key areas where you can assist mentees in their careers. Growth can involve learning new skills, improving existing ones, or venturing into a completely new career path. Today's learning options include online courses, in-person training, formal university programs, vocational courses, and continuing education conferences.

When choosing development opportunities, discuss your mentee's goals. Are they seeking leadership skills, project management training, or specialized medical knowledge? If they're aiming for specific roles like director, regional manager, or chief of staff, choose programs with intentionality. Training programs have financial and time costs, so clarity about desired growth requires planning.

Professional development also occurs organically in the workplace—often the most valuable growth happens on the job. New mentees will have many opportunities to work in teams, establish new processes, train employees, or learn business enhancements. Encourage your mentees to embrace each opportunity, even if it seems challenging. These experiences build knowledge, stature, and leadership skills.

MENTOR TIP

Encourage mentees to seize opportunities when employers offer to pay for professional development. They should take advantage even if it doesn't seem immediately relevant to their goals. When an employer invests in an employee's growth, there's intent to prepare them for future roles. Guide mentees not to be shortsighted and turn down learning opportunities simply because they see only one path to success.

Remember that professional growth is lifelong and full of twists and turns. The mentee is responsible for their growth with your support. Your role is to guide without controlling. Help them explore short-term and long-term goals, but ditch the "5-year rule"- keep goal setting flexible with room for spontaneity and unexpected opportunities.

Be careful not to impose your ideas on a mentee. It's a delicate balance of providing guidance while allowing independent thinking. Offer ideas for growth avenues and let them choose. Listen more than you talk; be a sounding board. Stay objective with empathy, but encourage without enabling. Seek first to understand their needs, and share appropriately without forcing disclosure.

A NONLINEAR PATH

Help your mentees understand that professional development isn't a straight-line process. Many people believe that if you just work hard enough, put in time, have grit, and meet the right people, successful progression will happen automatically. This is rarely the case.

As a mentor, prepare your mentees for careers that proceed in stops and starts. The next position may be lateral or even a step back in title. Help them see these moves not as setbacks, but as steps in experience. Titles don't always define a position's authority or indicate true progression. As the quote says, "We rent titles, but own our character" (Ducket, 2023). Titles simply provide opportunities to influence an organization and advocate for clients and teams.

Support your mentees in understanding that ambition should benefit everyone around them, not just themselves. Remind them that ego can derail good decisions, so they should look at opportunities from all angles. Professional development is multifaceted, and the most successful paths often involve unexpected turns.

Mentorship extends far beyond teaching technical skills. As we've explored in this section, your role as a mentor encompasses being a role model, providing emotional and career support, and facilitating professional opportunities. Through your actions, you model integrity and resilience. Through your guidance, you help mentees navigate the many twists and turns in their professional life. Through your network—which should be held sacred—you open doors to new possibilities.

The most rewarding aspect of mentorship is watching your mentees develop confidence in decision-making and discern what their strengths are and how to use them. Your goal is not to instill any particular trait or create a copy of yourself, but to allow mentees to do the best for themselves and their work lives. When empathy and mutual grace flow as freely as dialogue, you create a relationship that benefits both parties and strengthens the entire profession.

Remember, effective mentorship is about deftly coaching your mentees through challenges while being human, honest, and invested. Your willingness to share your journey, including the struggles and setbacks, gives your mentees permission to be resilient without placing you on a pedestal. In doing so, you help shape not just individual careers, but the future of veterinary medicine.

Editor's Note: *The day-to-day work of mentorship—modeling resilience, offering honest feedback, opening doors—happens in individual relationships. Yet mentorship also exists within a larger system. Organizational culture, leadership pathways, and even unconscious bias shape the opportunities mentors and mentees can access. To explore this broader context, in the following section, Dr. Jessica Petty draws on her research and industry leadership experience to examine how organizations can better support mentorship, and how intentional structures can help build a more equitable pipeline of veterinary leaders.*

MENTORSHIP AS A LEADERSHIP PIPELINE

Jessica Petty

A crisis of leadership is a symptom of organizational failure. Building a pipeline of leaders sounds perfectly logical on paper—but, in practice, with daily demands and competing priorities, it often falls to the bottom of the list. Focus typically returns only at a critical inflection point—when employee turnover rises, morale sinks, or toxic culture takes hold—sparking a renewed search for engaged and capable leaders.

An uncomfortable truth in the medical and academic world is that strong clinical skills don't always translate into effective leadership. Balancing human needs with the practical business demands of a veterinary practice can often feel at odds. Getting tossed into the deep end is one way to learn, but it usually comes with missteps and stubbed toes (Figure 5.1).

Building a pipeline of prepared, effective leaders requires both time and investment. Mentorship has proven to serve this endeavor well, with research showing that participating in a formal mentor relationship results in a 50% higher incidence of promotion (Ibarra et al., 2010). Crucially, the key word is *formal*. When early-career professionals are left to identify a mentor on their own, the impact is diluted. Organizations that support mentees with time allowances, resources, and connection opportunities create the structure necessary for real development. Building a foundation for a robust mentorship program includes three essential ingredients: leveling the playing field for mentorship access, (re)defining what makes a leader, and actively listening to what mentees need in order to succeed—both individually and as part of the organization.

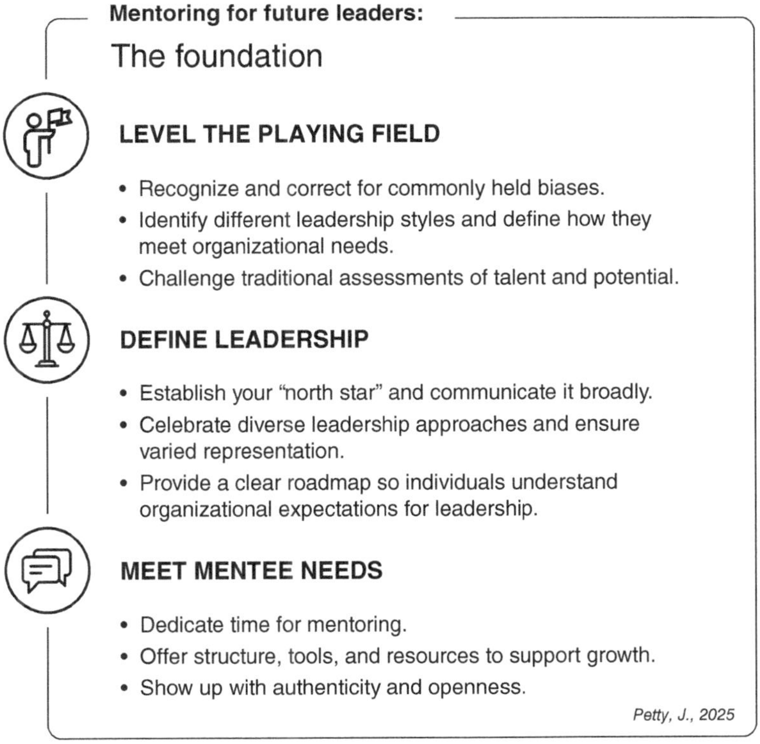
Mentoring for future leaders:
The foundation
LEVEL THE PLAYING FIELD
• Recognize and correct for commonly held biases.
• Identify different leadership styles and define how they meet organizational needs.
• Challenge traditional assessments of talent and potential.
DEFINE LEADERSHIP
• Establish your "north star" and communicate it broadly.
• Celebrate diverse leadership approaches and ensure varied representation.
• Provide a clear roadmap so individuals understand organizational expectations for leadership.
MEET MENTEE NEEDS
• Dedicate time for mentoring.
• Offer structure, tools, and resources to support growth.
• Show up with authenticity and openness.
Petty, J., 2025

FIGURE 5.1 The Foundation. *Source:* Courtesy of Jessica Petty (2025).

LEVELING THE PLAYING FIELD

A core function of mentorship is preparing individuals for increased responsibility and new skill sets. Yet research shows that mentoring experiences can differ significantly between men and women. **Men are often prepared for their next role, while women are more often coached for their *current* one** (Bohnet, 2016). This bias—rooted in longstanding norms about who is seen as a "natural" leader—can affect the nature and effectiveness of the mentoring relationship. Importantly, this imbalance persists even though women now make up the clear majority of veterinarians in the United States—nearly four out of five practicing veterinarians and the vast majority of current veterinary students (AAVMC, 2023; Vezeau and Fèvre, 2025). While development within the current role is essential, building a leadership pipeline requires a focus on stretch goals, gap-filling, and experience-building that prepares individuals to take the next step.

It's also important to acknowledge how gendered expectations can shape perceptions of career potential. Communal traits such as understanding, compassion, and care are often labeled as feminine (Gebauer et al., 2013), while agentic traits—like dominance, ambition, and competitiveness—are typically associated with men and with leadership potential (Gebauer et al., 2013; Lyness and Heilman, 2006).

These ingrained norms can create a blind spot that overlooks leadership potential in those who lean toward a communal style. While men who display communal behaviors are generally perceived as just as likable as when they are assertive (Carli and Eagly, 2016), women who adopt agentic traits—confidence, decisiveness, and independence—are often judged as less likable. This double standard complicates development and career growth for women.

The imbalance plays out in daily practice, too. Female doctors, for example, spend 10% more time with their patients and tend to share more information about symptoms, lifestyle, and mental health—yet they receive the same satisfaction ratings as their male counterparts (Roter and Hall, 2015). Even when women *don't* violate gender norms, they often must do more to be seen as equal.

Mentor training that accounts for these pitfalls is critical. We all carry assumptions—many ingrained from childhood—that can be difficult to unlearn. Creating awareness of these inequities allows more individuals to grow and succeed.

REDEFINING WHAT WE MEAN BY "LEADER"

If asked to describe a great leader, your answer would likely reflect your lived experiences. For example, someone raised in a collectivist society like those in the Asia-Pacific region may see leadership as caring for the group. In contrast, someone from an individualist culture like the United States might describe leadership as a competition, where the person who climbs to the top fastest is seen as the winner.

Your views are also shaped by family dynamics and workplace experiences. Many of us unconsciously mimic early role models—even flawed ones. For instance, if you grew up in a household where only the man worked outside the home, it may be harder to recognize leadership potential in women. One study found that men whose spouses do not work outside the home are less likely to promote women who report to them (Sandberg, 2013).

Leadership styles are also evolving as generational values reshape the workforce. The command-and-control model—"wait your turn" and "stay at one company until retirement"—resonates far less with younger generations (Gerhardt et al., 2021).

Fortunately, this shift has made room for **transformational leadership**, a style that emphasizes developing others, mentoring team members, and recognizing individual needs. It's a style more commonly associated with women—and increasingly effective in today's workplace. Importantly, this approach allows those who exhibit communal traits to succeed without violating social norms (Northouse, 2016).

By clearly defining what leadership looks like and how it shows up day-to-day, organizations can create a road map for development. Without that clarity, mentorships lack structure—and without structure, development suffers.

LISTENING TO WHAT MENTEES NEED

Research on mentorship in the animal health industry identified several recurring themes (Petty, 2020). One key finding: both mentors and mentees emphasized the need for *dedicated time* to nurture the relationship. When organizations provided time during the regular workday to meet, participants were more likely to stay engaged. When mentoring had to be squeezed into an already busy schedule, it was more likely to stall.

Another recurring theme was the need for *structure and tools*. A clear cadence of meetings, defined roles for mentor and mentee, and a system for feedback gave the relationship a strong foundation. Mentors also appreciated having a toolkit—books, podcasts, micro-learnings, and access to other mentors—to support their mentee's growth.

Finally, and perhaps unexpectedly, authenticity and vulnerability emerged as critical. **Mentees valued hearing about their mentors' successes—but they found even more value in hearing about how they handled adversity.** Navigating difficult colleagues, professional disappointments, and the struggle to balance work and life were powerful learning moments. This level of trust doesn't happen overnight, but when it's established, it creates deep, lasting impact.

Helping others avoid pitfalls and grow from shared experience is an often-overlooked benefit of strong mentorship.

An internal battle I've faced since childhood is a need for perfection. It makes me guarded at times, and in evaluating career opportunities, too cautious almost all the time.

Seared into my memory is a moment where I was offered a role that I didn't have on my radar. It was an internal move into a different area of the business and my impostor syndrome reached panic mode. I locked myself in a windowless office and sent the SOS text to a trusted colleague. She quickly joined me in the closet/office where I was nearly in tears, certain the person offering me the job was somehow fooled into thinking I was qualified when in fact, I would be an epic failure, thereby ruining my career and the company (how can one person think so little and so much of themselves—embarrassing to admit).

In that moment, that successful, calm woman looked at me and said "welcome to the club." She went on to share her own winding path to advancement and her struggle with negative internal dialogue. In just a few minutes of conversation, I felt seen, and while my confidence was not immediately restored, I knew that what I was feeling was not only normal but also surmountable.

In the years since that moment, I've openly shared this story of the path almost not taken. That one conversation changed the trajectory of my career and I'm so thankful for her life lesson; being afraid isn't the limiting factor, it's the reaction to it that matters.

THE BOTTOM LINE

For organizations and individuals alike, the return on mentorship is directly tied to the effort invested. Without a strong foundation, good intentions often fizzle out. But when we understand the biases that exist, define what talent looks like, and embrace authentic human connection, we create real opportunities for growth.

Clinics, research labs, leadership teams, and entire companies are only as strong as their people. Investing in people pays dividends—for the individual and for the collective. And investing in a structured, inclusive, and authentic mentorship program is one of the smartest investments any organization can make.

CONCLUSION

Mentorship extends beyond clinical instruction to encompass role modeling, career guidance, and professional development. Effective mentors demonstrate integrity and resilience in their daily work, challenge mentees to think critically, and provide emotional support while maintaining clear professional boundaries. They open doors through carefully curated networks, guide career development without creating dependency, and prepare mentees for the nonlinear reality of professional advancement.

Yet individual mentorship operates within larger systems. Organizations that provide dedicated time, structured programs, and clear leadership pathways amplify mentorship impact. Understanding how bias affects mentoring experiences is essential for building equitable leadership pipelines. When mentors receive training on these dynamics, when leadership is defined broadly to include diverse styles, and when mentees have access to authentic conversations about struggle and success, mentorship becomes a sustainable mechanism for developing capable, confident professionals.

BIBLIOGRAPHY

AAVMC (2023). *Annual Data Report: 2022–2023*. Washington, DC: American Association of Veterinary Medical Colleges https://www.aavmc.org/wp-content/uploads/2023/09/2023-AAVMC-Annual-Data-Report-September23.pdf.

Bohnet, I. (2016). *What works: Gender equality by design*. Cambridge, MA: Harvard University Press.

Byars-Winston, A. and Dahlberg, M.L. (ed.) (2019). *2, The Science of Mentoring Relationships: What Is Mentorship?* www.ncbi.nlm.nih.gov [online]. Washington, DC: National Academies Press (US) https://www.ncbi.nlm.nih.gov/books/NBK552775/ (accessed 11 March 2025).

Carli, L. and Eagly, A. (2016). Women face a labyrinth: an examination of metaphors for women leaders. *Gender in Management: An International Journal* 31 (8): 514–527.

Carruthers, R. (2023). 15 expert tips for first-time mentors. Together Mentoring Software. www.togetherplatform.com. https://www.togetherplatform.com/blog/how-to-mentor-someone (accessed 12 March 2025).

Coleman, K. (2019). L3 leadership transcriptions: ken coleman on the proximity principle: the proven strategy that will lead to a career you love. [online] L3Leadership.org. 13 May. https://l3leadership.org/l3-leadership-transcriptions-ken-coleman-proximity-principle-proven-strategy-will-lead-career-love/ (accessed 11 March 2025).

Ducket, T. (2023). You rent your title, but you own your character. https://www.linkedin.com/pulse/you-rent-your-title-own-character-thasunda-brown-duckett/.

Gebauer, J., Paulhus, D., and Neberich, W. (2013). Big two personality and religiosity across cultures: communals as religious conformists and agentics as religious contrarians. *Social Psychological and Personality Science* 4 (1): 21–30.

Gerhardt, M., Nachemson-Ekwall, J., and Fogel, B. (2021). *Gentelligence*. London, United Kingdom: Roman and Littlefield.

Ibarra, H., Carter, N., and Silva, C. (2010). Why men still get more promotions than women. *Harvard Business Review* 88 (9).

Lyness, K. and Heilman, M. (2006). When fit is fundamental: performance evaluations and promotions of upper-level female and male managers. *Journal of Applied Psychology* 91 (4): 777–785.

Northouse, P. (2016). *Leadership: Theory and Practice*. Thousand Oaks, CA: Sage.

O'Connell, M. and Kung, M. (2007). The cost of employee turnover. *Industrial Management* 49 (1): 14–19.

Petty, J. (2020). *Trevecca Nazarene University ProQuest Dissertations & Theses*, 71–97.

Roter, D. and Hall, J. (2015). Women doctors don't get the credit they deserve. *Journal of General Internal Medicine* 30 (3): 273–274.

Sandberg, S. (2013). *Lean In: Women, work, and the will to lead*. New York, NY: Random House.

Vezeau, N. and Fèvre, S. (2025). *Women Leaders in the Veterinary Profession*. World Organisation for Animal Health https://theanimalecho.woah.org/en/women-leaders-in-the-veterinary-profession/.

Trust

CHAPTER 6

INTRODUCTION

Dani Rabwin

Trust forms the invisible foundation upon which all effective mentorship is built, yet it's often the most overlooked element in formal mentorship programs. Without genuine trust and rapport, even the most well-structured mentorship initiatives can feel hollow and transactional, failing to create the safety that mentees need to be vulnerable about their struggles and open to growth.

Because this foundation is so critical, we devote an entire chapter to it here. Other sections of this book touch on related concepts—communication, feedback, and boundaries—but trust, rapport, and the psychological safety they create are so central that they warrant focused attention.

For this essential chapter, I've chosen two complementary voices. Dr. Sonja Olson's unique perspective bridges clinical practice with coaching and wellness education. As founder of Heartstorming Wellness and author of *A Call to Life*, Sonja has supported over 8000 veterinary associates through her work with BluePearl's veterinary social workers. Her journey from emergency veterinarian to full-time wellness educator gives her an intimate understanding of both the challenges mentees face and the skills mentors need to create truly supportive relationships.

Josh Vaisman brings the science of psychological safety to veterinary workplaces. As founder of Flourish Veterinary Consulting and author of Lead to Thrive, Josh helps veterinary teams translate evidence into practices that build thriving workplaces. His credentials include a master's in applied positive psychology & coaching psychology and accreditation as a Fearless Organization Scan Accredited Practitioner (2021). Having experienced burnout firsthand as a hospital owner and leader, Josh understands the struggle intimately and has dedicated his career to elevating veterinary teams so they can authentically flourish.

Sonja's approach emphasizes what she calls "sincere vulnerability"—the courage to share authentically while maintaining appropriate boundaries. Her framework moves beyond traditional mentor–mentee power dynamics toward relationships built on mutual respect, cultural humility, and genuine care for the whole person. She illustrates these principles through her own reflections and vignettes contributed by former mentees, offering powerful firsthand perspectives on how authentic connection can shape careers and lives.

Josh extends this foundation by exploring psychological safety—the environment where trust enables mentees to take intelligent risks, admit uncertainties, and learn openly without fear of judgment or punishment. He provides practical frameworks including the GROW model and Just Culture principles that help mentors create spaces where learning truly flourishes.

This chapter will guide you through the essential elements of building trust and rapport with your mentees, creating psychological safety, and fostering the kind of authentic connections that transform mentorship from obligation into opportunity.

BUILDING TRUST AND RAPPORT

Sonja A. Olson

> You cannot transmit wisdom and insight to another person.
> The seed is already there. A good teacher touches the seed,
> allowing it to wake up, to sprout, and to grow.
>
> —Thich Nhat Hanh (2011)

Establishing trust and rapport is the cornerstone of any successful mentorship relationship, particularly in the veterinary field. Veterinary professionals navigate demanding and emotionally charged environments, making strong, trusting relationships essential for personal and professional growth. Creating an authentic space of trust with any other person requires the essential elements of vulnerability, curiosity, and humility.

Mentorship in veterinary medicine is more than just guidance; it is about fostering an environment where growth and confidence can flourish. A lack of trust, respect, and rapport can lead to ineffective communication, hesitation in seeking guidance, and ultimately, professional stagnation. In this chapter, we will delve into the practical ways in which mentors and mentees can cocreate the conditions that establish and maintain healthy interpersonal relationships and learning.

MY PROFESSIONAL ZIG-ZAG JOURNEY: MENTORSHIP WAS NOT REALLY "A THING"

During my time in veterinary school, internship, and initial clinical role, I did not have access to a formal mentorship relationship. Nonetheless, several veterinary colleagues significantly influenced me, providing clarity on my professional development and goals.

My aspiration to become a zoo veterinarian was catalyzed by my high school senior research project experience at the National Zoo in Washington, D.C. There, I realized that a veterinary degree could be used to pursue wildlife conservation in the field, to provide care to animals in wildlife parks or zoos, or even to pursue research and education contributing to the protection of endangered species and ecosystems. Throughout college and veterinary school, I consistently volunteered at the National Zoo and worked as a veterinary assistant at local practices to build experience. One coveted position for a qualified 3rd year veterinary student was a three-month clinical externship with the zoo's veterinary team, encompassing both hospital work and teaming with keepers on wellness care.

Determined to secure this role, I cultivated supportive relationships through my volunteer activities each summer at the zoo until I had the necessary qualifications to apply for the externship. My efforts and strong academic performance were rewarded with this unique opportunity. I gained insights into zoo veterinary care dynamics, including collaboration, conflict, and the impact of politics and historical patriarchal attitudes. I also experienced informal mentorship from three exceptional zoo veterinarians, whose intelligence, creativity, grit, and dedication deeply inspired me. They provided crucial realism as well as encouragement, fostering trust through their authenticity and vulnerability.

Upon completing my veterinary training and rotating internship, I maintained communication with these mentors. Residencies in zoo medicine were, and continue to be, few in number. My efforts to build relationships were rewarded by having the National Zoo residency offered to me post-internship. However, there was no funding available as I was to start the training, and there was no clarity about when finances would be available. Reluctantly but realistically, I opted for a paid clinical role in a large GP/ER practice providing care to both companion animals and exotic patients. This ended up being a wonderful incubator of a first job where informal mentors and supportive teammates helped me build clinical competency and confidence.

The following year, I reapplied for the residency and again it was offered without compensation. **Faced with the difficult decision of sacrificing financial stability for professional dreams, the guidance from my zoo mentors was invaluable.** Discussions with them revealed fulfillment in my current emergency clinician role, leading me to embrace ER clinical medicine over zoo residency. Supported by family, colleagues, and informal mentors, I chose private practice in ER medicine with exotic patients and teaching responsibilities. This pivot taught me the value of introspection, of trusted mentorship, and of personal courage in shaping my professional identity.

Mentorship played a key role in my subsequent professional development, particularly concerning clinical skills and nonclinical support. Moving to a larger ER/Specialty hospital with robust exotics services allowed me to explore mentorship further, both receiving and providing it. The experience underscored the importance of addressing job-related distress, work–life balance, and emotional management. Observing similar struggles in colleagues and in my mentees motivated me to enhance my own self-care and offer compassionate, informed nonclinical support to my fellow veterinary professionals. This was to become the groundwork that would give me the experiential confidence and motivation to embrace the professional pivot that was essential when I identified clinical burnout in myself. All these elements have informed the person I am and the role I am in today as a full-time veterinary wellness educator, speaker, and author supporting veterinary professionals globally.

Reflecting on those early mentoring relationships, I can now identify the qualities that made them transformative—qualities I intentionally bring to my own mentoring today:

- **Genuine kindness and lifelong curiosity**—Challenging what I know and don't know with less judgment of myself and others
- **Realistic optimism**—Balancing hope with reality
- **Compassion and discerning empathy**—Creating safe space for honest conversation
- **Authenticity**—Showing up with self-respect, humility, honesty, and courage
- **Cultural humility**—Acknowledging "I don't know your experience, but I care about it" through thoughtful questions and awareness of my own biases
- **Experiential humility**—Recognizing that perfection is impossible and the best professionals are creative collaborators who work toward the best outcome for each patient

THE FOUNDATION OF TRUST IN MENTORSHIP

> Trust is the glue of life. It's the most essential ingredient in effective communication. It's the foundational principle that holds all relationships.
>
> —Stephen R. Covey (1996)

Trust is the bedrock of any mentoring relationship. In mentorship, trust is the perception that you are sincere, honest, benevolent, and credible. When we build trust, a partnership is formed. This will increase comfort, decrease anxiety, and build a relationship based on trust rather than power dynamics. It is vital to intentionally create a space of safety and a sense of mutual respect from the beginning to foster productive discussions going forward. In a trusting relationship, a sense of equality exists and both parties are able to feel understood, safe, and valued.

Without trust, communication suffers, and the effectiveness of mentorship diminishes. In veterinary mentorship, trust ensures that mentees feel more comfortable sharing their concerns and seeking guidance without fear of judgment or repercussions. Trust enables risk taking and learning through errors. New ideas can be explored and opinions expressed without criticism. This is a learning environment where the mentee can feel valued, heard, and encouraged to grow. **In veterinary medicine, where guidance can directly impact patient care, professional development, and personal confidence, establishing trust is essential**. Equally, understanding and upholding the elements that support psychological safety is essential for trust to be built in this and all other professional relationships.

Psychological safety is foundational to trust. Josh Vaisman will explore this concept in depth later in this chapter, providing practical frameworks for creating psychologically safe mentorship environments.

THE ROLE OF COMMUNICATION IN STRENGTHENING TRUST

Clear and empathetic communication is the lifeblood of a healthy mentoring relationship. Effective communication is fundamental to building trust in veterinary mentorship, creating an environment where mentees feel valued and understood. One of the most important skills is listening deeply—giving full attention without interrupting—so that the mentee feels heard. Using nonjudgmental responses, both verbal and nonverbal, fosters psychological safety, encouraging open dialogue.

Acknowledging the mentee's ideas and emotions demonstrates empathy and validation, reinforcing mutual respect. Thoughtful, open-ended questions invite mentees to contribute to their perspectives, promoting a sense of collaboration and shared learning. Minimizing distractions and maintaining focus during conversations signal genuine engagement, showing the mentee that their thoughts matter. Additionally, relating questions to specific events, situations, people, or actions helps ground discussions in real-world experiences, making the conversation more meaningful and applicable. By integrating these communication practices, mentors create a foundation of trust that supports professional growth and confidence in the veterinary field.

EFFECTIVE COMMUNICATION STRATEGIES TO BUILD TRUST

- **Clarity**—Ensure that instructions and feedback are straightforward and constructive.
- **Empathy**—Consider how messages will be received before delivering them.
- **Active engagement**—Encourage mentees to express their thoughts and feelings freely.
- **Regular check-ins**—Keep the dialogue open beyond structured meetings.

AVOIDING COMMON COMMUNICATION PITFALLS

- Speaking in overly technical terms without checking for understanding.
- Being dismissive of a mentee's concerns.
- Overloading the mentee with too much information at once.

Note: Chapter 9 goes into greater detail about understanding healthy, impactful communication in mentorship.

TRUST EXERCISE

- Ask your mentee about a challenge they are facing.
- Actively listen without interruption.
- Summarize their concern and ask how you can support them.
- Follow through on any commitments made during the discussion.

To illustrate how trust and rapport can shape the mentor–mentee relationship, I invited a few of my former mentees to reflect on their experiences. The following reflection is from a former mentee of mine, Dr. Chris Givens, who highlights the emotional nuance and long-term impact of creating a safe space for authentic vulnerability in a mentoring relationship.

STORYTELLING: DR. CHRISTOPHER GIVENS, EMERGENCY VETERINARIAN

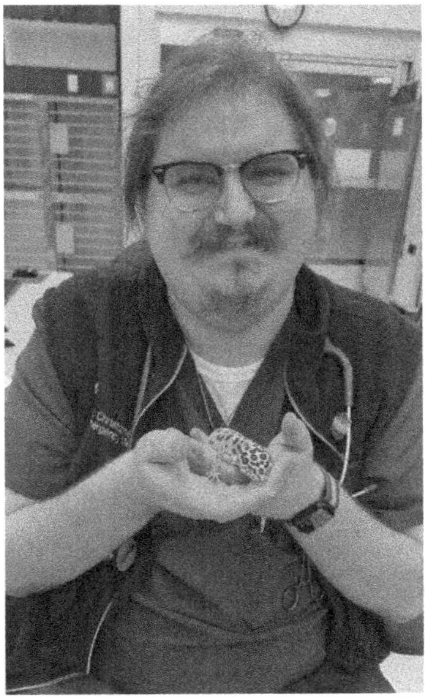

To me the most important aspects of mentorship are mutuality and openness. The ability to impart wisdom while also recognizing and appreciating the knowledge of the mentee and molding the advice to each individual. After all, we are all unique beings with unique life experiences and perspectives. And for a mentor to recognize that and incorporate that into their mentorship makes me trust them much more. I think the primary reason my mentorship relationship with Sonja was so successful is that we learned from each other and that allowed her to tailor her mentorship to me, rather than giving blanket advice from the context of a more seasoned ER veterinarian; an advocate for health and wellness; and an advocate for diversity, equity, and belonging. Rather, she got to know me, we connected, and we learned from each other. Another important aspect is a willingness to be vulnerable. Being willing and able to share your own struggles in a similar situation made it easier for me to feel okay doing the same. Hearing that someone else has slogged through the muck through which you're currently traversing and made it out alive has given me hope on more than one occasion, and I hope the same is true for people I have advised in the past. Vulnerability comes in many forms. Some examples in my field include having patients die and learning

from those experiences, dealing with burnout and compassion fatigue, and handling complicated interpersonal relationships. I also strive to be vulnerable when it comes to being a mentor as a queer individual navigating life. Sharing my coming out story with my parents, the struggle of me making the decision to come out publicly, and the decision I make every day to live authentically and make the conscious choice to come out are a few other examples of vulnerability in queerness.

BUILDING RAPPORT: THE KEY TO EFFECTIVE COMMUNICATION

In a trusting relationship, a sense of equality exists, and both parties are able to feel understood, safe, and valued. Rapport is the emotional connection between mentor and mentee that fosters comfort, engagement, and mutual respect. When this relationship is intentionally respectful and empathetic, both parties feel heard and understood. Without rapport, even the most well-intentioned mentorship efforts can fall flat—learning can feel forced, and communication barriers may arise.

Ramani et al. (2006) emphasizes that trust in relationships is built through mutual respect, recognition of each other's strengths and differences, and transparency. In stressful situations, trust helps us stay grounded and maintain higher-level thinking, rather than reverting to reactive fight-or-flight responses. While trust develops over time, rapport forms more quickly and is shaped largely by nonverbal cues—such as posture, tone, and gestures—which often carry more meaning than words alone.

CHARACTERISTICS OF STRONG RAPPORT

- Open and relaxed communication
- Mutual respect and understanding
- Shared interests and goals
- A balance of professionalism and approachability

ESSENTIAL ELEMENTS FOR CREATING RAPPORT

- **Active listening:** Show genuine interest in your mentee's thoughts and concerns. Maintain eye contact, stay present and focused, and respond thoughtfully. Demonstrating that you value your mentee's contributions and perspective builds rapport quickly.
- **Empathy:** Recognize the challenges mentees face and validate their experiences. Even if a mentor has overcome the same challenges, it is important not to diminish a mentee's struggles.
- **Shared experiences:** Bonding over similar struggles strengthens connections. Mentors should share personal anecdotes to normalize the struggles of veterinary practice.
- **Nonverbal cues:** A warm tone of voice, nodding in agreement, and an open posture can help mentees feel more at ease.
- **Adaptability:** Different mentees require different approaches. Some mentees may respond well to humor, while others may need structured guidance.
- **Encouragement:** Celebrate achievements, both big and small, as well as "a ha" moments of learning and insight.

HOW TO BUILD RAPPORT?

To build rapport, it can be helpful to share a little bit about yourself and how you are doing at the beginning of your check-in conversation. For example, something new that you learned that you are excited about, a professional challenge that you navigated and gained new skills around, and something in your life that you are grateful for or are celebrating. I personally love bringing that energy into the conversation to remind the mentee that they are more than their veterinary role and that there are positive, meaningful experiences occurring everyday. In this way, we can shift our mindset toward **growth, purpose, and possibility**.

This intentional shift toward "what is the opportunity here?" and "what can I learn from this?" supports what is called **cognitive reframing.** When we take a moment of challenge that may come with associated uncomfortable emotions and/or adverse physical sensations, we can bring awareness to this experience and utilize the reframing practice to regulate the nervous system when experiencing distress. An additional "ninja move" that efficiently and effectively moves your neurophysiology and emotional state toward one of balance and perspective is utilizing the power of **gratitude**. "Gratitude to change your attitude" can help to frame the challenging moment as a growth opportunity and bring to mind all that is in your life that is not distressing and perhaps even enjoyable. When out in the dynamic environment of the "real world," these tools help you to meet challenges and stressors as they inevitably arise.

QUICK RAPPORT BUILDERS

- Start meetings with a personal check-in. A simple "How are you doing?" at the start of each session fosters connection and trust.
- Find common ground beyond work (hobbies and interests).
- Use open-ended questions to encourage conversation, e.g. your mentee's career aspirations or check on a goal that was previously discussed.
- Use humor appropriately to ease tension.

This reflection from my former mentee, Dr. Melissa Dalton, expresses beautifully how a mentorship relationship that is founded on trust, rapport, and genuine care can be fortifying, providing a boost of self-confidence and courage when needed.

STORYTELLING—DR. MELISSA DALTON, SMALL ANIMAL ASSOCIATE

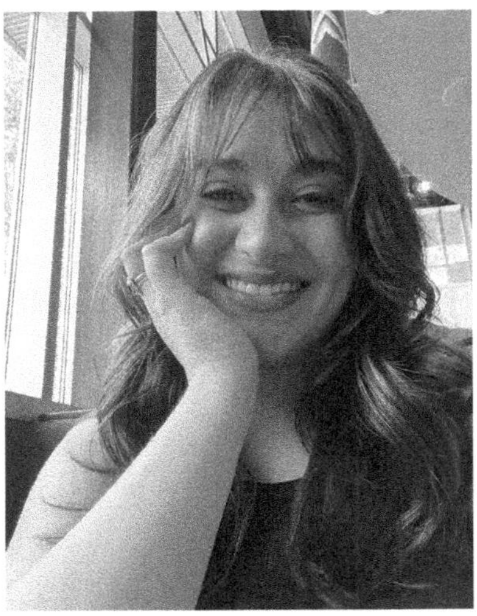

If someone were to ask me what mentorship can be, I'd tell them it's a relationship like any other, where communication, openness and willingness to be uncomfortable will help you grow. With the right person, mentorship never feels judgmental.

I white-knuckled through my first job and eventually found another (job) that fit my professional goals and personal values. And yet, I was still struggling. I couldn't understand how my senior colleagues could handle the day and not appear to be drowning—which I felt like I was. Every. Single. Day. It wasn't that I didn't have help at work, or resources outside of work, but I didn't know what I needed, how to use my resources or have any semblance of work/life balance. My days off were spent recovering and growing anxious in advance of what was to come.

It took one person (our practice manager at the time) to see me struggling and let me know it didn't have to be this way. She recommended a program called MentorVet, which is aimed at helping new grads find balance and wellbeing through mentorship. It was through this program that I met Sonja.

Our first few conversations were light, getting to know each other on a surface level, talking about our pets and backgrounds. It can be difficult to open up to a stranger over a zoom call, but Sonja has a way with people. I soon felt myself connecting with her and sharing things I hadn't verbalized to someone who understood like she did. We talked about overwhelm, chronic stress, career pivots, self-worth, moral distress, and quality of care. We even discussed personality traits like the caregiver tendency that's so common in our field and how it can be an inadvertent form of self-harm without boundaries and balance.

We've shared personal experiences, discussed difficult cases as well as how to navigate interpersonal relationships or conflict at work. I've learned that there can be strength in gentleness—because that's who she is. Through my connection with Sonja and the self-work I'd been doing in therapy, I've learned that there's power in vulnerability and how it can foster connection and create a foundation of safety and trust. I have come to understand how one person opening up about a time they struggled or a mistake they made can make you feel less alone and overwhelmed. Most importantly, I came to understand how having the right mentors—a network of people in and out of vet med—can make all the difference.

OVERCOMING BARRIERS TO TRUST AND RAPPORT

Building a strong, trusting mentorship relationship in veterinary medicine is not without its challenges. Both mentors and mentees may encounter obstacles that hinder open communication and growth. However, recognizing these barriers and proactively addressing them can make all the difference in fostering supportive and productive mentorship.

1. **Fear of Judgment**
   - **Impact:** Mentees may hold back on sharing struggles or uncertainties, fearing it will reflect poorly on their competence. This guardedness prevents open dialogue, leaving critical learning opportunities unexplored.
   - **Solution:** Create a nonjudgmental environment by modeling vulnerability. Share your own learning experiences, mistakes, and professional hurdles. This sets the tone that growth is a process and normalizes the challenges associated with it.
   - **Example:** A mentor might say, "I remember early in my career when I struggled with time management during surgical procedures. It took time and practice to build efficiency. If you're facing similar challenges, we can work through that together." This opens the door for honest conversation and reduces the fear of judgment.
2. **Time Constraints**
   - **Impact:** Busy schedules and demanding caseloads can disrupt regular mentorship engagement, leaving mentees feeling undervalued or disconnected. This inconsistency can slowly erode trust over time.

- **Solution:** Prioritize regular, brief check-ins that are structured and focused. Even short 15-minute conversations can maintain momentum and signal commitment. Scheduling these in advance ensures they are not deprioritized.
- **Example:** A mentor could implement biweekly 15-minute "coffee chats," either in person or virtually, with a set agenda: *"Let's touch base on your recent challenges, goals for the next two weeks, and any questions you have."* This regularity reassures the mentee of consistent support.

3. **Personality and Communication Mismatches**
   - **Impact:** Differences in communication styles—whether preferring detailed discussions versus quick check-ins, or written updates versus face-to-face conversations, can lead to misunderstandings and frustration.
   - **Solution:** Adapt your approach to match the mentee's communication style. Ask early on how they best receive feedback and prefer to communicate. Demonstrating flexibility reduces friction and fosters smoother interactions.
   - **Example:** If a mentee prefers written communication, a mentor might follow-up verbal discussions with a brief email summary: *"Here's a quick recap of our meeting today, along with action steps. Let me know if I missed anything!"* This bridges any gaps and reinforces clarity.
4. **Unclear Expectations and Mentorship Fatigue**
   - **Impact:** Ambiguity in roles, goals, or the structure of the mentorship can lead to frustration and burnout for both mentor and mentee. When expectations are misaligned, progress stalls, and engagement diminishes.
   - **Solution:** Cocreate a mentorship agreement that outlines scope, goals, boundaries, and expectations for communication. This serves as a living document that can be revisited and adjusted as the relationship evolves.
   - **Example:** At the start of the mentorship, a mentor and mentee might draft a simple agreement: *"We will meet biweekly for 30 minutes, focus on surgical skills development, and maintain email updates between sessions. We'll reassess our goals every three months."* This clarity prevents misunderstandings and sustains momentum.
5. **Mistrust from Past Experiences**
   - **Impact:** If a mentee has had negative experiences in previous mentorships, they may approach the relationship with guardedness, making it harder to build trust.
   - **Solution:** Acknowledge the possibility of past experiences and affirm your commitment to a supportive environment. Be patient and consistent, allowing trust to build gradually over time.
   - **Example:** A mentor might say, *"I know that past mentorship experiences aren't always positive. My goal here is to provide a safe space for growth, where questions and mistakes are part of learning."* This sets the stage for openness and reassurance.
6. **Lack of Consistent Feedback**
   - **Impact:** Sporadic or vague feedback leaves mentees uncertain about their progress, which can cause doubt in the mentor's engagement and erode trust.
   - **Solution:** Implement regular feedback loops that are specific and actionable. Make feedback a standard part of each meeting, not just when issues arise.

- **Example:** A mentor can say, *"I noticed last week's procedure went more smoothly compared to before—great job applying the new techniques. Let's keep refining that approach."* This kind of specific acknowledgment builds confidence and trust in the mentor's attentiveness.

By proactively addressing these common barriers, veterinary mentors can cultivate meaningful, lasting relationships that empower mentees to thrive in their careers (AAVMC, 2022).

SELF-REFLECTION QUESTIONS FOR MENTORS

- *Do I create a welcoming environment for open discussion?*
- *Have I shared my own challenges to make my mentee feel safe?*
- *Am I adapting my mentorship style to my mentee's needs?*

Trust and rapport flourish when both mentor and mentee show up prepared, present, and accountable. From the first meeting forward, certain shared commitments help sustain the relationship and reinforce psychological safety.

MUTUAL COMMITMENTS TO SUPPORT A HEALTHY MENTORSHIP RELATIONSHIP

- Be prepared
- Consider the proper setting and amount of time for the meeting
- Be present
- Be accountable
- Show compassion and gratitude
- Determine what follow-up will look like, e.g. what resources will be shared by the mentor and what the mentee is to prepare for the next meeting

In the 2023 AAHA Mentoring Guidelines, the section on "Managing Expectations—Laying the Foundation from The Start" provides a wide variety of helpful strategies for early relationship-building. What I found particularly valuable were the task force members' open-ended questions designed for the first meeting. These questions do more than establish logistics—they build trust by inviting vulnerability, demonstrating genuine curiosity about your mentee's needs, and creating the foundation for psychological safety. By thoughtfully asking and listening to these questions, mentors signal their commitment to a relationship built on mutual understanding and respect.

AAHA 6.2 Open-Ended Questions to Ask at the First Mentoring Meeting

Questions to Ask of Each Other

What are you looking for in this mentoring relationship? What do you hope to gain? What can I do to support the way that you work or think? How do you like to communicate and how would you like to be communicated with? What do I need to know about you that will help make this mentoring relationship successful for you? How long should we engage in this mentoring relationship? How will we know the mentoring relationship has come to an end?

Questions from Mentor to Mentee

Why is this important to you? What kind of support are you looking for specifically? How do you learn best? How do you like to be celebrated and acknowledged? How can I help you create mileposts for your goals and timelines for when to meet them? How else can I be of support to you?

Questions from Mentee to Mentor

How can you best support me in reaching my goals? How will you help me stay on track and assess whether I am achieving my goals? What resources do you have available that could be of use to me? Who can you connect me with that may help me in achieving my goals? How have you helped someone with a similar issue? (Reinhard et al., 2023).

Preparing the conditions for your regular meetings to be productive and effective requires intentionality from mentor and mentee. To support full attention being given to the conversation, minimize distractions of being in a public place, a workspace where others may overhear the mentee's contributions or have the conversation while driving. When meeting virtually, it is ideal to have cameras on, to confirm quality audio, and to each be fully focused on the conversation for an hour of time. This time should be treated as "sacred" self-care time for the mentee where they know that they are going to be receiving the mentor's full attention and that they can ask questions freely. This is an important training space where if emotions do come up for the mentee, they are supported and validated by the mentor supporting emotional regulation in the moment and the ability to do this for themselves and others outside of the mentoring meetings.

I love sharing with my mentees the analogy of doing reps at the gym to become stronger. In these skillful and authentic conversations, they are practicing articulating their questions, reflections, and concerns with a peer mentor. This helps them to be more confident and prepared for other professional circumstances where these skills are essential in interpersonal relationship building. This is rare air for veterinary professionals. The opportunity to be in a space of not-knowing-yet and to know that their full human selves are welcome strengthens their confidence and professional identity building muscles in a supportive environment.

Mentoring IS	Mentoring is NOT
Reciprocal—Both mentor and mentee learn from each other.	**A power play**—It is not about dominance or control.
Dynamic—The relationship evolves over time.	**Therapy or counseling**—It is professional support, not personal therapy.
Reflective—Encourages self-awareness and growth.	**About one person becoming knowledgeable**—It is a two-way developmental relationship.
Based on professional support—Focused on career and skill development.	**One-sided**—It is not just about the mentor giving advice, but about mutual learning.
A privilege and an opportunity—A chance for both individuals to grow.	**Rigid or fixed**—Mentoring adapts to the needs of both parties.

Source: Olson (2022).

SETTING AND RESPECTING BOUNDARIES AND COMMITMENTS

Boundaries are essential for healthy individuals and relationships, yet making, articulating, and honoring them can be challenging—both within and beyond the veterinary profession. Rooted in personal values, healthy boundaries support well-being, resilience, and the long-term sustainability of relationships, especially in high-demand caregiving environments (Olson, 2022).

As a mentor, one helpful boundary is setting limits around venting—such as time-boxing it to under five minutes—so the conversation can stay focused on identifying problems and exploring solutions. This allows space for the mentee to reflect and move forward, rather than getting stuck in frustration.

A strong mentorship relationship is built on being genuinely present and creating a safe environment for inquiry and discovery. Instead of offering quick fixes, guide mentees to ask their own questions and arrive at their own answers, using open-ended inquiry to slow down and foster deeper thinking.

CONFLICT MANAGEMENT

Conflict is anything that causes disruption in a relationship and is honestly inevitable between humans. There are so many conditions that can lead to conflict occurring between individuals such as whose perspective matters the most, power dynamics, values at play, and differing life experiences and beliefs. That said, healthy conflict is possible and can lead to strengthening personal and professional relationships. Being prepared is the key. Assessment and discussion of values, dominant conflict style(s), and personality types and tendencies early in the mentorship relationship create the space for meaningful reflection and clarification of what each person brings to the conversation. There are a wide variety of assessment tools and exercises available to support this exploration.

How mentors and mentees navigate disagreement directly impacts trust. Conflict handled with respect, curiosity, and care can actually *strengthen* rapport by demonstrating that the relationship can weather difficulty. Conversely, poorly managed conflict erodes psychological safety and damages the foundation you've built.

VALUES HELPFUL IN NAVIGATING CONFLICT

- Patience
- Curiosity
- Humility
- Compassion
- Respectfulness—not the same as agreement or compliance (dignity and unique perspectives being honored; others may have different core values)

A. Framework for Navigating Conflict

When conflict arises, use this approach:

1. **Identify and Define the Core Problem**
   - What is the actual issue at hand?
   - Is this a solvable problem (clear, immediate resolution possible) or a perpetual one (requires ongoing dialogue, compromise, or acceptance)?
2. **Assess What You Can Control**
   - What aspects of this situation are within your influence?
   - What do you need to let go of or accept?

3. **Manage Emotions First**

   Before problem-solving can happen, regulate the emotional climate:

   - Lower your voice volume and slow your pace
   - Relax your posture (hands in lap, sitting vs. standing)
   - Practice deep breathing
   - Use reflective listening: validate emotions without trying to fix them immediately

4. **Use Available Resources**

   - Draw on past experiences, trusted colleagues, or training
   - Identify barriers you cannot control and work around them

5. **Create Realistic Next Steps**

   - Use SMART goals for conflict resolution
   - Start small—incremental change is sustainable change
   - Consider: Do we need a "do-over conversation"? Should we revisit our shared values?

6. **Ensure Dignity and Respect for All**

   Both parties must feel heard and valued for resolution to last.

7. **Reflect on the Process**

   - What went well?
   - What could be improved next time?
   - Avoid perfectionism—focus on progress

When navigated skillfully, conflict becomes a catalyst for growth rather than a source of damage. Disagreements can improve the quality of decisions by surfacing perspectives that might otherwise remain hidden. They stimulate necessary discussions that move relationships and projects forward, and they increase innovation and productivity by challenging assumptions and encouraging creative problem-solving. Perhaps most importantly, successfully working through conflict builds group cohesion and cooperation—proving that the relationship can withstand tension strengthens trust. Both mentor and mentee develop stronger conflict management skills through practice, and the process itself supports individual personal and professional development by building resilience and emotional intelligence.

REFLECTION EXERCISE

Have you ever felt misunderstood by a mentor? What could have improved the situation?

TRUST AS THE FOUNDATION FOR MEANINGFUL FEEDBACK

Providing constructive, skillfully delivered feedback is both incredibly valuable in the mentorship relationship and requires preparation and practice. Creating a positive feedback environment means being specific, timely, and genuine. When combined with honest acknowledgment of success and progress, feedback becomes less challenging and more rewarding for both parties. Expressing gratitude for the mentoring relationship and the shared growth process helps regulate emotions and foster a healthier mindset.

When trust and rapport have been established, mentees receive feedback with curiosity rather than defensiveness. This openness allows for productive conversations about realistic next steps. Even with the best preparation and intentions, receiving feedback can be difficult. Be prepared to offer emotional support and connect mentees with additional resources when warning signs of mental health concerns arise. Respond with kindness, honesty, and calm presence. Leaning into the trust you've built, stay in communication and follow-up with authentic compassion.

Note: Dr. Kelly Cooper will provide more details, approaches, and resources around healthy and effective feedback in Chapter 12.

THE LONG-TERM IMPACT OF TRUST AND RAPPORT

When mentorship is built on trust and rapport, the benefits extend far beyond the immediate relationship. A successful mentorship does not just provide short-term guidance, it creates a lasting impact and possibly a long-term professional friendship. Additionally, when a mentee has a positive mentorship experience, they are more likely to embody and replicate this experience when given the opportunity to teach or to mentor a colleague. The value of collaborative problem-solving and seeking support is validated. Healthy mentorship built on trust and rapport creates long-term benefits for both parties.

BENEFITS FOR MENTEES

- Increased confidence in clinical and personal decision-making
- Greater willingness to seek help and advice
- A stronger sense of belonging in the profession

BENEFITS FOR MENTORS

- Personal fulfillment from shaping the next generation
- Improved leadership and communication skills
- Strengthened professional network

Studies show that mentorship relationships characterized by high levels of trust and psychological safety lead to greater professional satisfaction and career longevity in veterinary medicine (Carlson, 2023).

In this final personal reflection from another amazing former mentee, the immediate and long-term impacts of mentorship are brought to life. This veterinarian was able to find her way out of a toxic practice environment and into one that met her values, her professional goals, and embraced the practice culture that she had come to understand was essential for sustainable professional satisfaction and growth.

STORYTELLING—DR. AMANDA MONDT, ASSOCIATE SMALL ANIMAL VETERINARIAN, BREWERTON HOSPITAL FOR ANIMALS

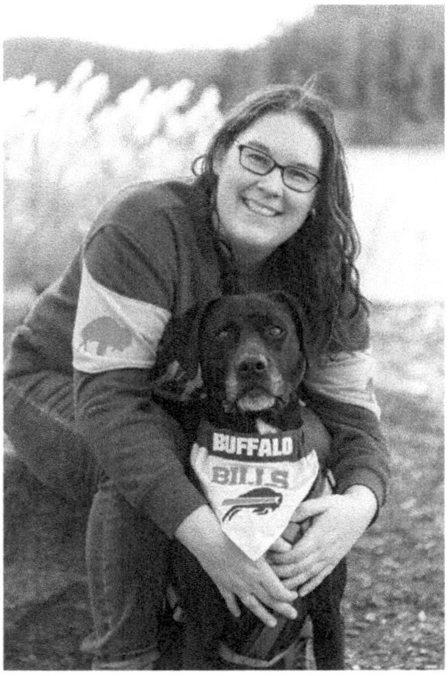

When I graduated from veterinary school in 2020, I was eager to start my first job with the hope and promise of mentorship. Due to circumstances outside of my control, that did not happen as I hoped it would. I was searching for that mentoring connection when my practice manager sent me some information about a formal veterinary mentoring program that supports early career veterinarians. The program offers mentorship and the structure to learn valuable skills to navigate the innate challenges of veterinary medicine. Over the next several months, I completed the program and, as an optional part of that, chose to be assigned a mentor. That was Dr. Sonja Olson. That mentor-mentee relationship started with a conversation about boundaries, expectations and an understanding that we would learn from each other. Through many conversations, my mentor helped me solidify my core values, as a person and as a veterinarian, and begin to outline what I wanted out of the career I had worked so hard to achieve.

After about three years at my first job, I decided to leave that position to pursue different opportunities closer to home. Because of the solid foundation I now had, I felt that during interviews for my next job, I knew what I was looking for in a practice, what I felt I could bring to the table for my clients, patients and staff and what I deserved. Conversations with my mentor continued through this transition and flowed easily into discussions about our personal lives. I finally got settled at a "unicorn practice" with an amazing owner and practice manager team who share similar core values. I am finding great job satisfaction with this team, the clients and the patients and, as a young, single career woman, I bought a house in the area because I plan to stay part of this team for a long time.

The experience I had with my own mentor/mentee relationship was, and continues to be, so vitally important to my growth as a young professional. I embraced the opportunity to become a mentor through the same program that I went through. My relationship with my own mentees has allowed me to not only find ways to connect with early career vets but also to continue to learn with them, exercise communication and active listening skills, and continue to explore ways to support veterinarians as they navigate this challenging but rewarding field. I feel strongly about changing the culture of veterinary medicine to become a field that people want to be a part of and stay a part of for a long time. With the help of my mentor and other supporting people in my life, I navigated the hurdles I was faced with early in my career and found myself in a stable place, both professionally and personally. Because of that, I now feel that I possess enough tools, resources and knowledge to be a part of positive change in the veterinary community.

THE LASTING IMPACT OF TRUST AND RAPPORT IN MENTORSHIP

Trust and rapport are the foundation upon which all meaningful veterinary mentorship is built. They transform professional guidance into deeply rewarding, lasting relationships. When trust is prioritized, both mentor and mentee thrive—not only as clinicians but also as whole people navigating growth, change, and self-discovery.

Mentorship is not just about skill development or career advancement; it is about fostering a culture of openness, humility, and mutual respect. The most powerful mentors create space for vulnerability, allowing mentees to bring their authentic selves to the relationship. It is in this space—free from judgment, rich with support—that learning is most profound.

As a mentor, your role is not to dictate, but to guide—offering honesty, encouragement, and when needed, the difficult truths that help mentees build resilience. This means knowing when to advise, when to instruct, and when to step back, allowing your mentee to take the wheel. Growth flourishes in the balance between challenge and support, between learning from mistakes and celebrating achievements (Gotian, 2024).

Ultimately, the trust cultivated in mentorship extends far beyond the individuals involved. It strengthens the veterinary profession, enhances patient care, and builds a more sustainable and supportive community—one where well-being is prioritized and the value of each professional is recognized for who they are, not just what they produce.

Mentorship, at its core, is about believing in others until they believe in themselves. It is about offering wisdom, sharing resources, and walking alongside someone as they navigate their own path. When we commit to this work with sincerity and care, we help shape a future where every veterinarian is empowered not just to succeed, but to find fulfillment, purpose, and lasting connection within this profession we all love.

Editor's Note: *Trust and rapport form the foundation of meaningful mentorship, but they serve a higher purpose: creating an environment where true learning can flourish. When mentees trust their mentors and feel genuine connection, they become more willing to engage in the vulnerable work of growth—asking difficult questions, admitting uncertainties, and learning from mistakes without fear of judgment. This psychological safety is not separate from trust and rapport but rather their natural extension into the learning environment. Josh Vaisman explores how mentors can intentionally cultivate this psychologically safe space, transforming mentorship from a supportive relationship into a truly transformational experience where both mentor and mentee can take the interpersonal risks necessary for deep professional development.*

ENSURING PSYCHOLOGICAL SAFETY—JOSH VAISMAN, MAPPCP, CCFP

Josh Vaisman

Despite the best of intentions, I was a failed leader.

In 2016, I found myself in the position of managing partner for the largest small-animal hospital in a new city. In addition to my ownership role, I was to serve as the on-site hospital director. This acquisition was oozing opportunity as the hospital had been flailing for years. Financial performance was mediocre, to be sure, but what most stood out to me was the divisive, almost toxic culture the team members had endured.

For me, this was a chance to lead a cultural turnaround and have a positive impact on nearly forty deserving lives. With vitalized enthusiasm, I dove in headfirst, certain I'd facilitate success in the fullest definition of the word. That certainty and verve blinded me to alternative possibilities. The only possible path, I felt, was forward and upward.

Eighteen months later, at the darkest depths of burnout I'd ever experienced, I left the practice burdened by a sense of defeat. Not only had I failed to revive the hospital culture, it appeared to be worse off than when I found it. Only then did I receive the feedback I needed.

After my last day on site, I reached out to a team member who I knew had insight into the perspective of most, if not all, of the team. I asked her, "what went wrong?" She told me, "Josh, at first, you made a big difference. Everyone thought we finally had a leader who cared. But over time people realized you were only open to hearing one perspective, having one type of conversation. So people stopped sharing their true thoughts, feelings, and ideas with you."

Why had no one told me this when I could have changed course? Why did it have to crash and burn for me to get this important feedback?

First popularized by Amy Edmondson (1999), psychological safety—a shared belief within a work relationship that interpersonal risk-taking will be free from fear or judgement or punishment—is an essential ingredient for learning, development, innovation, and professional success. This phenomenon is at the foundation of effective veterinary mentorship.

Veterinary professionals face emotionally intense scenarios, critical clinical decisions, and sometimes rigid hierarchies. In these environments, a psychologically safe mentorship approach isn't just beneficial—it's essential. When mentees feel psychologically safe, they're more likely to seek guidance openly, admit uncertainties, and learn continuously, dramatically improving both individual growth and overall team health (Vaisman, 2023; McKay and Vaisman, 2023).

WHY PSYCHOLOGICAL SAFETY MATTERS?

Veterinary professionals operate in uniquely stressful conditions. **Daily pressures from demanding clients, urgent medical decisions, and high expectations can quickly erode confidence, especially among new graduates. A culture of psychological safety directly combats these pressures by fostering resilience, openness, and mutual support within mentorship relationships (Edmondson, 1999, 2018; Vaisman, 2023).**

Research highlights that veterinary work-related relationships rich in psychological safety contribute to significantly lower turnover rates, greater team cohesion, and higher employee satisfaction (McKay and Vaisman, 2023; Carter, 2024). Conversely, teams lacking psychological safety often face higher burnout rates, decreased morale, and poorer patient care outcomes (St. Clair, 2023).

CREATING PSYCHOLOGICAL SAFETY IN VETERINARY MENTORSHIP

Build Trust Through Openness and Vulnerability

In mentorship, trust is foundational. One can think of psychological safety as a special form of trust. When psychological safety is present, mentees are more likely to engage in the "difficult" learning conversations they need in large part because they *trust* their mentor will respond with support, interest, and without judgement.

One way mentors can begin nurturing this type of trust is by example, openly sharing their past mistakes and professional growth experiences. This signals to mentees that vulnerability is accepted and valued, encouraging them to speak openly without hesitation. I recall a young hospital manager who sought my mentorship. After hearing about their situation (and fears), I shared the story of my first year as managing partner in a small-animal hospital, including all the stumbles and mistakes I had made. When this individual first reached out, the image of me they had was one of success and accomplishment. Hearing about my early-career shortcomings and missteps had a tangible effect, almost instantly adding comfort and connection to our conversation.

Effective mentors are also great listeners, leveraging active-listening skills such as reflection, sense-making, curiosity, and inviting nonverbals. These listening skills show empathy and interest and help mentees feel validated and heard, all variables that contribute to enhanced trust and psychological safety (Shaw and Coe, 2024). After sharing my story, this new manager began sharing similar examples from their first few months of practice. The more intently I listened, the more I showed my interest, the more they shared. This led to a deeper discovery. This manager wasn't afraid of their role so much as terrified of letting the hospital owner down. It took courage and vulnerability to admit that to me.

Finally, mentorship should be strengths-based and future-oriented. In truth, every veterinary mentee, no matter their role or phase of their career, comes to mentorship with existing strengths and a history of successes. Even in the face of challenging developmental conversations, a mentor should identify, affirm, and help a mentee see the strengths they have, the tools at their disposal, and the ways in which those strengths have and can continue to serve them. After a few questions, it became clear that the manager who approached me had many gifts. Showing those gifts to her visibly empowered her. It also helped her see that even in her darkest moments, I'd find the light within her, further strengthening the growing psychological safety between us.

VISUAL AID: MENTOR TRUST-BUILDING CHECKLIST

- Share personal learning experiences, including your own mistakes.
- Listen actively, ensuring mentees feel heard and validated.
- Regularly affirm mentees' strengths and contributions.
- Maintain confidentiality in mentorship discussions.

SET CLEAR, SUPPORTIVE EXPECTATIONS

Ambiguity breeds anxiety, so clearly communicating mentorship roles and expectations is crucial. When mentees understand precisely what's expected of them—and what they can expect from mentors—they feel more confident and supported. Clear expectations also help mentees navigate stressful veterinary scenarios effectively (Vaisman, 2023).

PROVIDE CONSTRUCTIVE, COMPASSIONATE FEEDBACK

Feedback is most effective when framed constructively and supportively. The Situation-Behavior-Impact (SBI) method allows mentors to address mistakes sensitively, focusing discussions on specific actions and impacts rather than personalities, fostering an environment focused on improvement rather than blame (Laird et al., 2024).

SBI feedback can be effective in both positive and constructive feedback. In positive feedback, a mentor might say:

> *It sounds like yesterday at the hospital (Situation) you tried the new communication approach with your technicians we had discussed last month (Behavior). From what I gather, this worked really well, bringing the team together and making you feel more confident in trusting your techs to handle treatments on their own (Impact). Bravo!*

In constructive feedback, a mentor might say:

> *What I'm hearing is that yesterday, when things got really busy at the hospital (Situation) you felt concerned about getting out on time. As a result, you focused on patient care and didn't talk to your technicians much at all (Behavior). This morning, you heard through the grapevine they all think you're mad at them (Impact). You don't want them to feel that way (Impact). What are some ideas you have to increase your communication with the team the next time it gets busy like that?*

HANDLING MISTAKES AND DIFFICULT CONVERSATIONS

Normalizing Mistakes as Learning Opportunities

Embracing a "just culture" approach in veterinary mentorship can transform mistakes into powerful learning opportunities. By distinguishing between honest errors and negligence, mentors help mentees understand that mistakes are natural parts of learning and growth. In truth, the majority (perhaps almost all) mistakes and missteps a mentee might make are of the "human" variety, not due to negligence or a lack of care, but simply due to contextual factors. Discussing mistakes openly and constructively encourages continuous learning and innovation rather than fear and avoidance (Vaisman, 2023).

Years ago, a hospital team member sheepishly entered my office to own up to a big mistake. She had accidentally undercharged a client by several hundred dollars. The client had paid the (incorrect) bill and taken their pet home. A short while later, the team member discovered her error and toiled for well over an hour, terrified to tell me. Encouraged by other team members, she mustered the bravery to face her boss.

Certain this was to be the end of her employment with us, she fessed up. I responded with this: "Well, of course I'm disappointed in the mistake but it's obvious you didn't do this on purpose. You're clearly an honest, diligent person and I can see how this is weighing on you. I'm grateful you brought this to me so together we can figure out a way to ensure no one else in the hospital ever has to feel how you feel now. Walk me through what happened. . ."

Surprised by my response, she paused. Then she began sharing all the details, and together we discovered a gap in our systems. We closed the gap, and this kind of error never happened again for her or anyone else. She remained with our hospital, a significant contributor, for many more years.

ENCOURAGING OPEN DIALOGUE IN CONFLICT SITUATIONS

Conflicts and mistakes in veterinary medicine are inevitable, but they can be managed constructively in a psychologically safe environment. Mentors should model calm, empathetic communication, emphasizing collaborative problem-solving and accountability. For instance, when a mentee incorrectly diagnoses a patient, a mentor might calmly guide them through the case review, focusing on future strategies rather than dwelling on the error.

At times, a mentee may directly disagree with a mentor or share that something a mentor has said or done offended or hurt them. In these (hopefully rare) moments of interpersonal conflict, it is essential the mentor responds with calm, contrite curiosity and openness. These are the moments in which psychological safety is tested. The mentor's response will either strengthen the trust and safety between them and their mentee or damage it significantly, perhaps permanently.

PRACTICAL FRAMEWORKS FOR MENTORSHIP CONVERSATIONS

Using Established Models

Amy Edmondson's psychological safety model (Edmondson, 2018) offers foundational insights for veterinary mentorship, highlighting the importance of creating safe spaces for interpersonal risk-taking. Additionally, the GROW model (Goal, Reality, Options, Will), championed by coaching psychology pioneer John Whitmore (2009), provides a clear, practical tool for structured mentorship discussions:

Visual Aid: GROW Model for Veterinary Mentorship

Step	Explanation	Veterinary mentorship example
Goal	Identify mentee's specific objectives or challenges.	"Improve my ability to handle difficult client discussions."
Reality	Discuss current situation and perceived obstacles.	"I feel anxious during euthanasia consultations."
Options	Collaboratively explore potential strategies	"Practice client communication scenarios; shadow experienced veterinarians."
Will	Confirm actionable steps and mentee commitment.	"Schedule biweekly meetings to reflect and assess progress."

Mentors can lean on the GROW model to help facilitate effective developmental conversations with mentees. In leveraging this coaching-informed approach, mentors are likely to enhance trust and psychological safety in the mentorship relationship. Furthermore, they will find their mentees are more creative in their problem-solving and personal development, as well as more motivated to enact the solutions discussed, as they will be "self-selected" solutions. We tend to attach more strongly and with greater perseverance, to the solutions we create on "our own." The GROW model is a time-tested, evidence-based approach mentors can use to cultivate the space in which this becomes possible.

Psychological safety transforms mentorship in veterinary practice from a transactional interaction into a transformational experience. By prioritizing openness, empathy, clear expectations, and continuous improvement, mentors empower veterinary professionals to grow confidently and collaboratively. Investing in psychological safety enhances retention, improves job satisfaction, and cultivates a resilient, engaged veterinary team prepared to deliver exceptional patient care (Vaisman, 2023; McKay and Vaisman, 2023).

CONCLUSION

Trust, rapport, and psychological safety are inseparable elements that transform mentorship from guidance into genuine partnership. When mentors create environments where vulnerability is welcomed and interpersonal risks feel safe, mentees gain the confidence to ask difficult questions, admit uncertainties, and learn from mistakes without fear of judgment.

The emphasis on sincere vulnerability and authentic connection provides the relational foundation, while frameworks for psychological safety translate these principles into actionable practices. Together, they demonstrate that effective mentorship requires both emotional intelligence and intentional structure—the courage to share authentically alongside the discipline to create consistently safe spaces for growth.

Veterinary professionals who experience this kind of mentorship don't just develop clinical skills; they build resilience, professional identity, and the capacity to extend this same transformational support to future generations, strengthening the profession as a whole.

BIBLIOGRAPHY

American Association of Veterinary Medical Colleges (AAVMC) (2022). Veterinary intern and resident wellbeing guidelines. Enhancing Mentorship. October. https://www.aavmc.org/AAVMC-Wellbeiing-InternResident-Guidelines (accessed 8 December 2024).

Carter, H. (2024). Psychological safety in veterinary practices. *Today's Veterinary Nurse* 2024 (Spring): 76–78.

Carlson, R. (2023). Mentoring our next generation of veterinarians. *Journal of the American Veterinary Medical Association* 261 (9): 1266. https://doi.org/10.2460/javma.261.9.1266.

Covey, S. (1996). *First Things First*, 203. New York, NY: Free Press.

Edmondson, A.C. (1999). Psychological safety and learning behavior in work teams. *Administrative Science Quarterly* 44 (2): 350–383.

Edmondson, A.C. (2018). *The Fearless Organization: Creating Psychological Safety in the Workplace for Learning, Innovation, and Growth.* Hoboken, NJ: John Wiley.

Gotian, R. (2024). 6 Essential traits of exceptional mentors. *Forbes* (02 June). https://www.forbes.com/sites/ruthgotian/2024/06/02/traits-of-exceptional-mentors/ (accessed 20 January 2025)

Hanh, T.N. (2011). *Planting Seeds: Practicing Mindfulness with Children*, 15. Berkeley: Parallax Press.

Laird, D., Bloom-Feshbach, K., McNamara, T. et al. (2024). Psychological safety: creating a transformative culture in a faculty group peer-mentoring intervention. *Chronicle of Mentoring & Coaching* 8 (1): 127–140.

McKay, C.H. and Vaisman, J.M. (2023). Psychological safety, purpose, path, and partnership reduce associate veterinarian desire to leave current employment. *Journal of the American Veterinary Medical Association* 261 (10): 1518–1524.

Olson, S.A. (2022). *Creating Wellbeing and Building Resiliency: A Call to Life*, 127. London: CRC Press.

Ramani, S., Gruppen, L., and Kachur, E.K. (2006). Twelve tips for developing effective mentors. *Medical Teacher* 28 (5): 404–408. https://doi.org/10.1080/01421590600825326 (accessed 5 March 2025).

Reinhard, A., Quicksall, M.S., Bourquin, B. et al. (2023). AAHA mentoring guidelines. https://www.aaha.org/resources/2023-aaha-mentoring-guidelines/ (accessed 30 November 2025).

Shaw, J.R. and Coe, J.B. (2024). *Developing Communication Skills for Veterinary Practice.* Hoboken, NJ: Wiley.

St. Clair, B. (2023). Psychological safety in the workplace: the impact of staff mentoring programs. PhD dissertation. University of Pittsburgh.

Vaisman, J. (2023). *Lead to Thrive: The Science of Crafting a Positive Veterinary Culture.* Lakewood: AAHA Press.

Whitmore, J. (2009). *Coaching for Performance: GROWing Human Potential and Purpose.* London: Nicholas Brealey Publishing.

Cultivating Emotional Intelligence

CHAPTER 7

INTRODUCTION

Dani Rabwin

Veterinary medicine is both intellectually demanding and emotionally intense. Success in the profession depends not only on sharp clinical reasoning but also on the ability to navigate stress, connect with clients, and lead teams through challenging moments. These are the domains of emotional intelligence (EI), a skill set increasingly recognized as essential for sustaining both individual well-being and healthy workplace cultures.

The challenge for mentors is that, while we intuitively know emotional skills matter, we often lack frameworks for developing them systematically. How do we teach a mentee to stay composed during a crisis? How do we help them build empathy without absorbing every client's pain? How do we model resilience in a profession where emotional labor is constant and largely invisible?

In this chapter, Dr. Gershon Alaluf draws upon more than three decades in the profession, spanning roles from kennel assistant to practice owner, and his current doctoral research at Pepperdine University on stress, emotional labor, and culture in veterinary medicine. Having personally mentored more than 20 people into veterinary school, all of whom continue to thrive in the profession, Gershon brings both lived wisdom and scholarly insight to the intersection of EI and mentorship.

This chapter explores how EI competencies such as self-awareness, self-regulation, empathy, and social skills translate into mentor behaviors that build trust, provide psychologically safe feedback, and strengthen professional resilience. Through research, clinical vignettes, and applied strategies, Gershon demonstrates how emotionally intelligent mentorship not only supports mentees but also fosters healthier, more sustainable veterinary workplaces.

Perhaps most importantly, this chapter highlights how EI transforms mentorship from an informal exchange of advice into a deliberate, measurable system that reduces emotional labor strain, improves retention, and prepares the next generation of veterinarians to thrive.

EMOTIONAL INTELLIGENCE IN MENTORSHIP

Gershon L. Alaluf

Emotional intelligence (often referred to as EQ or EI; for the purposes of this chapter, EQ will be used throughout) has emerged as a critical skill in professions that demand high interpersonal engagement, including veterinary medicine. Veterinarians must not only manage complex medical cases but also navigate emotionally charged interactions with clients, colleagues, and staff. The capacity to recognize, understand, and regulate emotions enhances communication, decision-making, and resilience in high-stress environments. In the context of veterinary mentorship, EQ is a foundational element that shapes adaptive leadership, effective teaching, and professional wellbeing. Mentors with strong EQ can model positive coping strategies and empathetic communication, thereby fostering these competencies in their mentees (Figure 7.1).

This chapter explores the fundamental components of EQ and their significance in veterinary mentorship. It reviews core EQ competencies and theoretical frameworks, then examines how mentors can apply EQ to build trustful mentor–mentee relationships, manage challenges, and support mentees' growth. The chapter also provides evidence-based strategies for developing EQ in new veterinary graduates through mentorship and training, including practical approaches for mentors. Recent research and expert insights are integrated throughout, underscoring best practices and outcomes associated with emotionally intelligent mentoring. By the end of the chapter, readers will understand how focusing on EQ within mentorship can not only enhance individual mentor–mentee dynamics but also contribute to a healthier, more resilient veterinary workplace.

CONCEPTUAL FOUNDATIONS OF EMOTIONAL INTELLIGENCE

The concept of EQ has been shaped by multiple theoretical models. Salovey and Mayer (1990) originally defined EQ as an ability-based construct with four branches: perceiving emotions, facilitating thought with emotions, understanding emotions, and managing emotions. Goleman (1995)

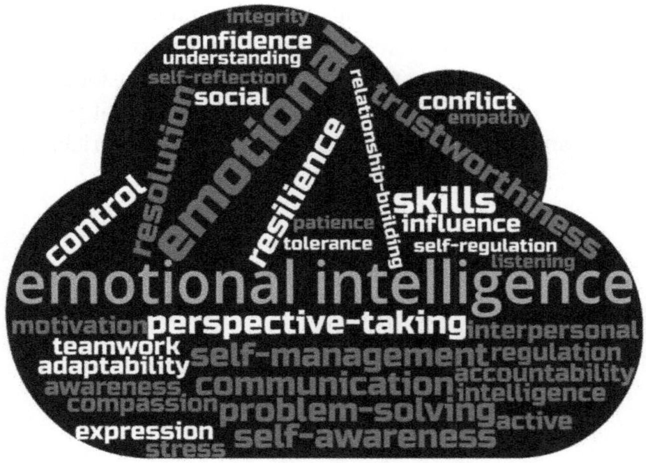

FIGURE 7.1 Word cloud illustrating the breadth of emotional intelligence competencies relevant to veterinary mentorship. *Source:* Gershon Alaluf, DVM.

Table 7.1 Four-Point Perspective of Emotional Intelligence (EI)

EI and the self	EI and others	EI and thought	EI and action
• Develops self-awareness, regulation, and motivation • Adapts during emotional moments • Learns from social interactions • Uses emotions to improve social and interpersonal effectiveness	• Possesses self-awareness and management of emotions • Exhibits intrapersonal and interpersonal EI • Gauges emotional states of others and adjusts behavior accordingly • Exhibits empathy toward others	• Able to reflect on emotions of self and others • Reasons with emotion • Perceives emotions • Understands emotions • Reflects on emotional states of self and others both during and after social interaction • Uses insights from reflection on emotions to shape future social interactions • Learns from emotional interactions	• Manages emotions • Adapts to others' emotional states • Manages stress • Controls mood • Evaluates emotional situations and identifies effective responses • Uses situational judgment • Selects best responses during conflict • Maintains calm • Offers support to others • Helps others identify emotions

Source: Clutterbuck et al. (2017) / with permission of Sage Publications.

later broadened the concept in a mixed model, highlighting five key competencies: self-awareness, self-regulation, motivation, empathy, and social skills. These competencies extend EQ into social and leadership domains, emphasizing how emotional skills translate into effective workplace behaviors. More recent work by Fiori et al. (2021) introduced emotion information processing as another component of EQ, underscoring the role of rapidly interpreting emotional cues for adaptability under pressure (Goleman, 1998). Each framework contributes to a deeper understanding of EQ, but all converge on the idea that emotional competencies can be identified and developed (Table 7.1).

For veterinary mentors, understanding these frameworks is more than theoretical—it is practical. Veterinary medicine often presents intense emotional contexts, from comforting a grieving pet owner to guiding a team through a crisis. An awareness of EQ models helps mentors recognize the range of emotional skills involved in these situations. It reinforces that effective mentorship goes beyond technical instruction—it requires attunement to both one's own emotions and those of others. In emotionally charged environments, the ability to perceive and manage emotions can significantly influence professional success and mental resilience. By grounding their mentorship approach in established EQ competencies, mentors can better prepare themselves and their mentees to handle the personal and interpersonal challenges of veterinary practice.

Model (author, year)	Core branches/competencies
Salovey and Mayer (1990)	Perceiving, facilitating, understanding, and managing emotions
Goleman (1995)	Self-awareness, self-regulation, motivation, empathy, and social skills
Fiori et al. (2021)	Emotion information processing

CORE COMPONENTS OF EMOTIONAL INTELLIGENCE

EQ is commonly described through several core components or competencies. The following core components of EQ are especially relevant to veterinary mentorship:

EQ component	What it means	Mentor strategies
Self-awareness	Recognizing one's own emotions, triggers, and their impact on others.	• Debrief after challenging cases, prompting mentee to name their emotions. • Use journaling prompts on key interactions.
Self-regulation	Managing impulses and stress responses to remain calm and constructive.	• Model deep-breathing breaks (box breathing) during high-pressure moments. • Coach mentee to pause and reframe before reacting.
Motivation	Sustaining drive, optimism, and persistence despite setbacks.	• Share personal stories of early-career challenges overcome. • Set clear, achievable goals and celebrate small wins.
Empathy	Understanding and validating others' feelings through active listening and perspective-taking.	• Role-model empathic statements in client or staff interactions. • Conduct "check-in" conversations to gauge how mentee feels.
Social skills	Communicating clearly, resolving conflicts, and fostering inclusive teamwork.	• Facilitate mock client or staff conflict scenarios and guide resolution. • Give balanced, timely feedback in private setting.

EMOTIONAL INTELLIGENCE VS. INTELLIGENCE QUOTIENT IN VETERINARY PRACTICE

Veterinary medicine is both intellectually demanding and emotionally intense. Traditional measures of intelligence, like the Intelligence Quotient (IQ), have long been valued for academic and clinical success. IQ reflects cognitive abilities such as logical reasoning, problem-solving, and analytical thinking (Wechsler, 1958), and there is no doubt that a strong IQ is important for mastering medical knowledge, diagnosing complex conditions, and making evidence-based decisions. However, research has made it clear that IQ alone does not fully predict a veterinarian's professional success or job satisfaction (Vratskikh et al., 2016; Treglown and Furnham, 2023). In many cases, EQ plays an even more critical role in day-to-day veterinary practice.

UNDERSTANDING IQ AND EQ

IQ is typically assessed through standardized tests that evaluate abilities like math, language, and spatial reasoning. It remains relatively fixed after early adulthood and is a useful predictor of academic performance. EQ, on the other hand, is the ability to perceive, understand, manage, and influence emotions—both one's own and those of others (Goleman, 1995). Unlike IQ, EQ can be developed and improved over time with conscious practice and training. Numerous studies have found positive correlations between EQ and job performance, career success, and personal well-being (Ealias and George, 2012; Vratskikh et al., 2016). The key components of EQ (self-awareness, self-regulation, social awareness/empathy, and relationship management) complement cognitive intelligence by enabling professionals to apply their knowledge more effectively in real-world situations (Goleman, 1998).

It is often said that "hard skills" (technical knowledge) get veterinarians through school, but "soft skills" like EQ distinguish outstanding practitioners in the field (Schmid and Mast, 2021). For instance, a veterinarian with a high IQ might accurately diagnose a medical condition, but if they lack empathy or communication skills, they may struggle to convey the situation to a pet owner compassionately, possibly undermining client trust. In fact, statistics indicate that raw intellectual ability contributes only a fraction to career success—some estimates suggest IQ accounts for roughly 25% of success, with the remaining influence coming from emotional and social intelligence factors (Hunter and Hunter, 1984). Notably, one analysis pointed out that 70% of the time, people with average IQ outperform those with the highest IQ, underscoring how vital EQ and related skills are in practical environments (Neisser et al., 1996).

THE EMOTIONAL CHALLENGES OF VETERINARY PRACTICE

Veterinary professionals regularly face situations that test their emotional resilience. These include delivering difficult news (such as discussing a terminal diagnosis or the need for euthanasia), managing clients' expectations and emotions (especially when outcomes are poor or uncertain), handling ethical dilemmas regarding treatment and animal welfare, and coping with workplace stressors like high caseloads, long hours, and exposure to traumatic cases. Each of these scenarios requires not just medical knowledge but also emotional savvy. For example, delivering bad news demands empathy and tact; managing client frustration requires patience and emotional control; ethical decisions call for self-awareness and sometimes moral courage; and workplace stress management benefits from self-regulation and support-seeking.

Veterinarians with high EQ are better equipped to navigate these challenges. They tend to manage stress more effectively, exhibit greater empathy toward clients and colleagues, and maintain a more positive outlook during adversity. This emotional resilience can protect against common problems in the field such as compassion, fatigue, and burnout. Research in similar caring professions (like nursing) has shown that individuals with higher EQ experience lower stress and better well-being in high-pressure roles. A study in veterinary students similarly found that those with higher EQ had significantly lower levels of stress, anxiety, and depression—indicating that building EQ could be a protective factor for mental health in the veterinary profession (Pulido-Martos et al., 2020; Schmid and Mast, 2021). Recognizing these emotional challenges and the value of EQ in addressing them is a first step for mentors who aim to prepare their mentees for the realities of practice.

IQ VS. EQ IN VETERINARY PRACTICE

Veterinary work demands both rigorous clinical reasoning and finely tuned emotional skills. Standardized IQ tests (e.g., Wechsler, 1958) predict academic success and diagnostic accuracy, but they account for only about 25% of career performance in caring professions (Vratskikh et al., 2016; Treglown and Furnham, 2023). EQ—our capacity to perceive, understand, manage, and use emotions—fills the gap by driving stronger client relationships, smoother team dynamics, and greater resilience under stress. **Critically, unlike IQ, EQ can be developed through targeted training and reflective practice** (Elias and George, 2012).

Dimension	IQ	EQ
Core focus	Logical reasoning, problem-solving, and analytical thinking	Perceiving, understanding, regulating, and leveraging emotions
Assessment	Standardized tests (Wechsler, Stanford-Binet)	Ability-based tests (MSCEIT) or mixed-model instruments (EQ-i, TEQQue)
Development	Largely fixed after early adulthood	Malleable—improves with coaching, feedback, simulations, and reflection
Predictive power	Academic grades, technical mastery, and diagnostic accuracy	Client trust, treatment adherence, team leadership, conflict resolution, and stress management
Practical impact	A high-IQ vet rapidly integrates lab data to form a differential diagnosis	A high-EQ vet senses a client's anxiety, adapts their communication, and builds rapport before treatment plans

EMOTIONAL CHALLENGES IN PRACTICE

Veterinarians regularly face emotionally taxing situations: delivering terminal diagnoses or euthanasia recommendations; managing distraught or angry clients; wrestling with ethical dilemmas around treatment choices; and coping with high caseloads, long hours, and exposure to trauma. Each scenario demands more than medical know-how—it requires emotional savvy: empathy, patience, resolve, and self-awareness.

HOW EQ MAKES THE DIFFERENCE?

Veterinarians with strong EQ navigate these challenges by:

- **Empathetic communication:** Actively listening to clients' fears and framing bad news with compassion to maintain trust.
- **Team cohesion:** Sensing staff stress and defusing conflicts before they impact patient care.
- **Resilience under pressure:** Employing stress-management techniques (mindfulness, debriefs, and peer support) to prevent burnout and compassion fatigue.

APPLYING EMOTIONAL INTELLIGENCE IN VETERINARY MENTORSHIP

ESTABLISHING TRUST THROUGH EMOTIONAL INTELLIGENCE

Mentorship is fundamentally a relationship built on trust, communication, and mutual respect. Emotional intelligence enhances these aspects by equipping mentors to perceive and manage emotions—both their own and their mentees'—in ways that build trust. Research indicates that mentors with high EQ are particularly adept at fostering trust. For example, a study by Chun et al. (2010) found that mentors' emotional intelligence was positively related to the degree of confidence and trust their mentees placed in them. When mentees perceive their mentors as emotionally stable, empathetic, and consistent, they feel safer and more willing to engage openly in the mentorship process (Berki, 2005).

There are several EQ-driven strategies mentors can use to establish and maintain trust.

Active listening: By giving mentees full attention, acknowledging their concerns, and providing thoughtful responses, mentors validate their mentees' feelings and experiences. Active listening might involve nodding, summarizing what the mentee said, and asking clarifying questions. This behavior signals to the mentee that their perspective is valued, thereby strengthening trust.

Empathetic communication: Mentors should strive to understand mentees' emotions and respond with sensitivity. If a mentee expresses anxiety about a surgical procedure, an empathetic mentor might say, "I can see why you'd feel nervous; I felt the same way when I was learning. Let's work through it together." Such responses show solidarity and understanding. High empathy in mentors has been linked to providing better psychosocial support and career guidance to mentees, which further deepens the trust in the relationship.

Consistency and reliability: Trust builds over time when mentors consistently follow through on their promises, maintain confidentiality, and offer steady support. An emotionally intelligent mentor manages their moods and stress so that they can be a dependable presence. For example, if a mentor schedules regular check-in meetings or feedback sessions, they honor those commitments and come prepared. Consistency in temperament is also important—mentees trust mentors who react to mistakes or bad news in a measured, understanding way rather than with unpredictable anger or disappointment.

Honesty with compassion: Trust doesn't mean always telling mentees what they want to hear; it means telling the truth in a constructive manner. Emotionally intelligent mentors give honest feedback or difficult news (like pointing out a clinical error) with tact and caring. They frame criticism around behaviors and improvements, not personal flaws, and balance it with reassurance about the mentee's potential to grow. This approach helps mentees trust that feedback is given for their benefit, not as personal attacks.

By consciously applying EQ principles such as empathy, active listening, and self-regulation in their interactions, mentors create a safe and supportive space. Mentees who trust their mentors are more likely to ask questions, admit uncertainties or mistakes, and seek guidance when facing challenges. This openness greatly enhances the learning process and allows the mentor to more effectively impart knowledge and advice. Over time, a strong foundation of trust can transform the mentorship into a powerful catalyst for the mentee's professional and personal development.

ENHANCING COMMUNICATION AND FEEDBACK

Effective communication is at the heart of any successful mentorship. Emotional intelligence plays a significant role in shaping how mentors convey information, provide feedback, and engage in dialogue with their mentees. An emotionally intelligent mentor is skilled at delivering feedback in a manner that encourages growth rather than causing discouragement or defensiveness. This involves being mindful of the mentee's emotional state and adapting one's communication style accordingly (Mayer and Caruso, 2002).

HOW EMOTIONAL INTELLIGENCE ENHANCES COMMUNICATION AND FEEDBACK?

Tailoring communication to mentee needs: Mentors should recognize that each mentee may have a different communication style and emotional disposition. Some mentees might prefer direct, blunt feedback; others may respond better to a gentle, roundabout approach. By being socially aware (an EQ component), mentors can gauge how a mentee reacts to feedback and adjust their delivery. For instance, if a mentee seems particularly anxious about their performance, a mentor might start feedback by acknowledging what the mentee did well before addressing areas for improvement, to avoid overwhelming them.

Encouraging self-reflection: Rather than always telling mentees what to do, emotionally intelligent mentors often pose questions that prompt mentees to reflect on their own experiences and feelings.

For example, after a challenging consultation, a mentor might ask, "How did you feel that appointment went, and why?" This invites the mentee to engage in self-assessment, reinforcing

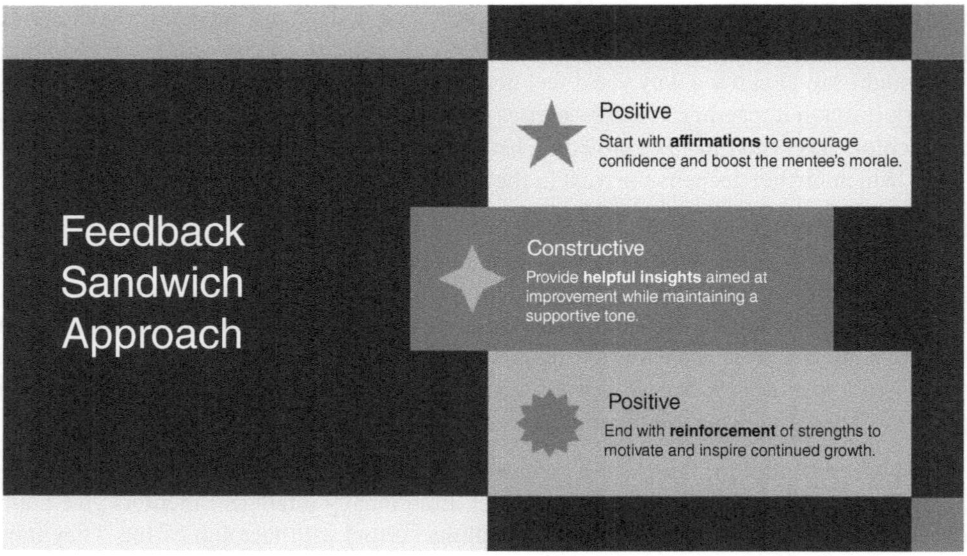

FIGURE 7.2 The Feedback Sandwich Approach. Open with positive affirmation, deliver constructive guidance in a supportive tone, then close with reinforcement of strengths to sustain the mentee's motivation. *Source:* Dr. Gershon Alaluf

self-awareness, and learning. The mentor can then guide the discussion, affirm correct insights, and gently correct any misjudgments. This Socratic method of feedback not only conveys the mentor's perspective but also helps mentees develop critical thinking and emotional insight.

Using positive reinforcement: An EQ-savvy mentor knows the importance of confidence in a mentee's development. They deliberately point out the mentee's strengths and improvements, not just the mistakes. For instance, "You communicated the treatment plan to the client very clearly—that was well done. One thing to work on for next time might be to pause a bit more to allow the client to ask questions." This kind of feedback sandwich (positive–constructive–positive) ensures the mentee hears the critique in a constructive context. Positive reinforcement of what the mentee is doing right builds their motivation and openness to learning (Figure 7.2).

Nonverbal communication and tone: A mentor's body language, facial expressions, and tone of voice can greatly influence how a message is received. Emotional intelligence helps mentors remain aware of these nonverbal cues. A supportive tone, open posture, and appropriate eye contact can convey encouragement even when the content of feedback is critical. Conversely, sighs, crossed arms, or an annoyed tone may shut down communication. By managing their emotions (self-regulation) and being aware of the mentee's, mentors can maintain a neutral or positive demeanor that keeps communication flowing.

The benefits of EQ-driven communication are clear: mentees feel more understood and less judged, which makes them more receptive to feedback and more engaged in learning. Indeed, studies have shown that when mentors communicate with empathy and clarity, mentees report greater confidence in their development and fewer misunderstandings in their interactions (Banerjee et al., 2024). Over time, this supportive communication style cultivates an environment of continuous feedback and improvement, where mentees feel comfortable discussing mistakes and successes alike.

THE ROLE OF EMOTIONAL INTELLIGENCE IN CONFLICT RESOLUTION

Conflicts or disagreements can sometimes arise in mentorship relationships, as well as in the veterinary workplace where mentor and mentee operate. These conflicts may stem from differences in expectations, communication breakdowns, or the general stress of the job. EQ is a powerful tool for navigating and resolving such conflicts constructively. A mentor high in EQ will approach conflicts with composure, empathy, and a collaborative mindset, transforming potential rifts into learning opportunities.

APPLYING EQ SKILLS TO MENTOR—MENTEE CONFLICT

Emotional regulation during conflict: When tensions flare—perhaps a mentee reacts poorly to criticism or a mentor is frustrated by a mentee's repeated mistake—strong self-regulation is crucial. A mentor who can stay calm and avoid reactive outbursts sets the tone for a more rational discussion. By keeping their own emotions in check, the mentor prevents escalation. For example, if a mentee becomes defensive at feedback, an emotionally intelligent mentor might take a deep breath and respond in a measured tone, "I see this is upsetting you. Let's talk through it," instead of snapping back. This de-escalation helps both parties focus on the problem, not the emotion.

Perspective-taking and empathy: Conflict often arises from misinterpretation of intent or lack of understanding of the other person's viewpoint. EQ allows mentors to pause and consider the mentee's perspective. They might ask themselves, "Why might my mentee be feeling this way? What concerns or stressors are influencing their reaction?" By empathizing, mentors can address the root causes of the conflict. For instance, a mentee's resistance to feedback might be rooted in feeling insecure or overwhelmed. A mentor who senses this could say, "I understand that you're feeling criticized, and that's not my intention. I'm giving this feedback because I believe in your abilities and want to help you improve. How can we work on this together?" Such empathy-driven dialogue reassures the mentee and opens the door to resolution.

Constructive framing of the conflict: EQ helps in reframing a conflict from "personal attack" to "collective problem to solve." A mentor might steer the conversation toward shared goals—"We both want you to succeed with surgical skills; how can we address what happened in a way that helps you progress?" By focusing on solving the issue (e.g., a surgical technique that needs improvement) rather than blaming the person, the mentor uses social skills to guide the interaction in a positive direction.

Collaborative problem-solving: Mentors can involve mentees in generating solutions to the issue at hand. This shows respect for the mentee's agency and often leads to better buy-in. For example, if a conflict arises because a mentee is consistently late to rounds, instead of simply scolding, the mentor could discuss, "It seems timing has been an issue. What do you think is causing it, and what strategies could help ensure you're on time?" Perhaps the mentee reveals they are struggling with another duty that overlaps. Together, they might find a work-around or schedule adjustment. This collaborative approach not only resolves the specific conflict but also empowers the mentee to take responsibility and feel heard.

Maintaining respectful communication: Even in disagreement, mentors should model respectful language and behavior. No shouting, no insults, and no dismissive gestures. By maintaining professionalism and courtesy, mentors demonstrate that disagreements can be handled without personal animosity. This is an invaluable lesson for mentees, who learn to mirror the same composure and respect in their future interactions.

When conflicts are handled with EQ, the outcomes can actually strengthen the mentor—mentee relationship. Successfully navigating a disagreement can build mutual respect and trust, as both parties see that issues can be resolved fairly and feelings can be openly discussed without jeopardizing the relationship. Moreover, mentees gain confidence and conflict-management skills of their own by observing and participating in the process. They learn that differences of opinion are natural and manageable, rather than something to fear. In the long run, these skills extend beyond the mentorship into the mentee's broader professional life, making them more capable of handling conflicts with colleagues and clients in practice (Figure 7.3).

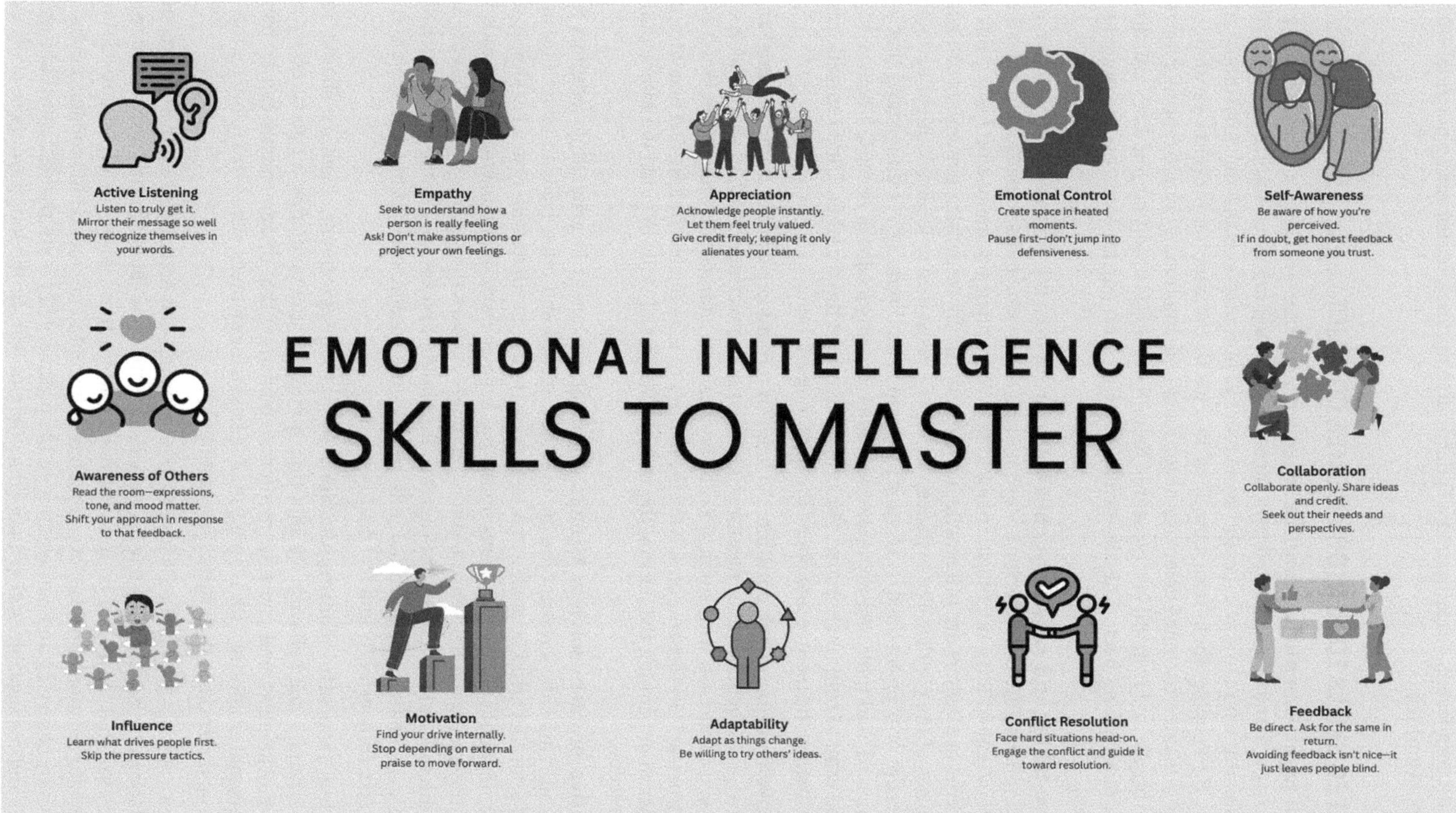

FIGURE 7.3 Emotional intelligence skills to master: active listening, awareness of others, influence, empathy, appreciation, motivation, emotional control, adaptability, collaboration, conflict resolution, and feedback. *Source:* Dr. Gershon Alaluf (2025)

VIGNETTE: A MENTORING MOMENT

Dr. Alice, an experienced veterinarian and mentor, is overseeing Dr. Ben, a new graduate, during a busy afternoon at the clinic. A tense situation arises when Dr. Ben administers an incorrect dosage of medication to a hospitalized dog. The dog is not harmed, but the pet's owner, upon hearing of the mishap, becomes very upset.

Sensing the owner's rising anger and Dr. Ben's panic, Dr. Alice immediately steps in with a calm demeanor. She gently apologizes to the owner for the confusion, empathizing, "I understand why you're upset. This is your beloved pet, and you expected the best care. I'm sorry this mistake happened. Let's discuss what it means and how we will ensure your dog is safe."

Her voice is steady and compassionate. As she speaks, Dr. Alice places herself physically at the owner's eye level, demonstrating openness and concern. The owner, seeing Dr. Alice's composed and caring response, begins to breathe more evenly and listen. Dr. Alice explains the medical implications of the dosage error in simple terms, reassuring the owner that the team has assessed the dog and found no ill effects. She outlines the additional monitoring they will do to be absolutely certain. By the end of the conversation, the owner's anger has cooled to appreciation for the transparency and care shown by Dr. Alice. They even thank her for the prompt honesty and attention.

After resolving the client's concerns, Dr. Alice turns to Dr. Ben, who is shaken and close to tears, fearing he'll be harshly reprimanded. Guiding him to a private area, Dr. Alice speaks kindly: "Ben, I know that was scary. Let's talk about what happened." Her tone is not accusatory but curious and supportive. Dr. Ben admits he was feeling overwhelmed and misread the dosage instructions. He anxiously adds, "I'm so sorry—I feel like I've failed and made a mess of everything."

Dr. Alice places a hand on his shoulder and replies, "I appreciate your honesty. Mistakes happen, especially when we're learning. I made a similar error early in my career—I was mortified, but my mentor helped me learn from it. What's important is understanding how to prevent it next time." Together, they review the clinic's medication protocols and identify that Dr. Ben missed a step in double-checking dosages due to rushing. Dr. Alice suggests practical changes: "Let's have you slow down and use a quick mental checklist before giving any drug. I'll cover the next appointment so you can collect yourself. And remember, you can always ask for a second look if you're unsure."

As they talk, Dr. Ben visibly relaxes. He expected anger, but instead he found empathy and guidance. Dr. Alice's reaction—staying calm, showing understanding, and working with him on a solution—demonstrated high emotional intelligence. Not only was a potential conflict averted, but Dr. Ben also learned how to handle errors responsibly. He feels grateful to have a mentor who supports him even when things go wrong. Walking back into the clinic, Dr. Ben is determined to be more careful and is comforted by the knowledge that Dr. Alice "has his back." The trust between them deepens, and Dr. Ben gains a powerful example of how to handle difficult situations with clients and colleagues in the future.

EMOTIONAL INTELLIGENCE AND MENTEE DEVELOPMENT

One of the ultimate goals of mentorship is to support the mentee's professional growth and personal well-being. By applying EQ, mentors can significantly enhance their mentees' development on multiple fronts. Research shows that mentees who are guided by emotionally intelligent mentors often report higher job satisfaction, better stress management, and greater self-efficacy in their careers (Bar-On, 2004). In practice, this means these mentees are more likely to thrive in their roles, take on new challenges confidently, and remain in the profession.

HOW EQ-FOCUSED MENTORSHIP BENEFITS MENTEE DEVELOPMENT?

Providing emotional support: Veterinary careers can be emotionally taxing, especially for newcomers. A mentor attuned to their mentee's emotional state can offer timely reassurance and encouragement. This might involve acknowledging the mentee's feelings ("I know dealing with that case was heartbreaking. It's okay to feel upset") and normalizing their experiences ("Many of us have felt overwhelmed in emergency situations. You're not alone, and you handled it as well as anyone could"). By addressing the mentee's emotional needs, the mentor helps them build resilience. Mentees feel they have an outlet for their stress and someone who genuinely cares about their well-being, which can buffer against burnout.

Encouraging professional autonomy: An emotionally intelligent mentor balances support with empowerment. This means gradually giving the mentee more responsibility and decision-making power, while still being available as a safety net. For example, a mentor might let the mentee take the lead in a routine client appointment or surgical procedure, stepping in only if needed. The mentor's confidence in the mentee's abilities (implicitly communicated through this trust) boosts the mentee's self-confidence. If the mentee encounters difficulty, the mentor remains calm and helps them troubleshoot rather than taking over immediately, thus sending the message "I believe you can do this." This approach fosters self-efficacy—the mentee learns by doing and gains the confidence to act independently. Over time, this autonomy, supported by empathetic oversight, produces veterinarians who are capable and assured in their skills.

Modeling emotional intelligence in action: Mentees learn a great deal by observing their mentors. When mentors consistently model EQ behaviors—such as staying composed under pressure, treating clients and staff with empathy, and handling mistakes with accountability and learning-oriented attitudes—mentees internalize these norms. They see what effective professional behavior looks like.

For instance, if a mentor navigates a difficult client interaction with patience and empathy, the mentee witnesses the positive outcome of that approach (perhaps the client calms down and the issue is resolved). This serves as a powerful lesson that might not be found in textbooks. Essentially, mentors act as role models for EQ. Over the course of the mentorship, the mentee can mimic and practice these behaviors in their own work, gradually making them part of their professional identity.

Building a growth mindset: Through emotionally intelligent mentoring, mentees learn to view challenges and setbacks as opportunities to improve rather than as insurmountable failures. A mentor who responds to a mentee's error by calmly discussing what can be learned, rather than expressing anger or disappointment, reinforces that mistakes are part of learning. This nurtures a growth mindset in the mentee—they come to believe that skills and competencies (including emotional skills) can be developed through effort and experience. Such a mindset makes mentees more resilient and proactive in seeking out learning experiences. They are more likely to volunteer for new tasks, ask questions, and engage in self-improvement activities without fear of embarrassment.

Career satisfaction and retention: By addressing both the technical and emotional aspects of the veterinary profession, mentors help mentees find deeper meaning and fulfillment in their work. Mentees feel supported not just as workers but as whole persons. This comprehensive support has been linked to higher career satisfaction (Berki, 2005) and can influence their decision to stay in the field long term. When a mentee feels valued and equipped to handle their job's challenges, they are less likely to become disillusioned or leave the profession. **In a field like veterinary medicine, where retention of talented professionals is a concern, emotionally intelligent mentorship is a critical strategy for nurturing and keeping the next generation of vets (Figure 7.4).**

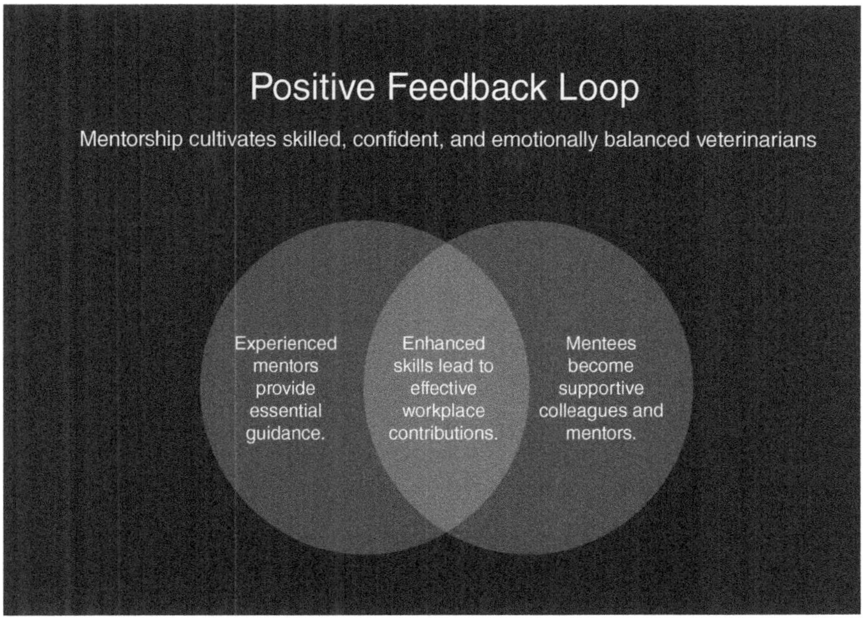

FIGURE 7.4 The positive feedback loop of mentorship: experienced mentors provide guidance, enhanced skills lead to effective workplace contributions, and mentees grow into supportive colleagues and mentors themselves. *Source:* Gershon Alaluf (2025).

STRUCTURING EQ-INTEGRATED MENTORSHIP PROGRAMS

Beyond individual mentor–mentee pairs, many veterinary schools, hospitals, and professional organizations are interested in formal mentorship programs. Integrating EQ into the design and operation of these programs can amplify their effectiveness. Institutions that have implemented EQ-focused mentorship initiatives report improvements such as increased mentor effectiveness and higher mentee retention and success rates (Joseph, 2010).

STRUCTURING AN EQ-INTEGRATED MENTORSHIP PROGRAM

1. **Training mentors in EQ competencies:** It's valuable to provide mentors with dedicated training or workshops on EQ. This could include sessions on self-awareness (perhaps using personality or EQ assessment tools for mentors to learn about their own styles), communication skills, and empathy exercises. Equipping mentors with knowledge about EQ and practical techniques (like active listening or conflict de-escalation strategies) prepares them to intentionally apply these skills in their mentoring. In some cases, organizations use role-playing during mentor training to simulate common mentorship challenges (for example, a mentee struggling with impostor syndrome) so that mentors can practice supportive, EQ-informed responses.

2. **Mentee orientation to EQ:** Similarly, introducing mentees to the concepts of EQ can be beneficial. A brief orientation might cover the importance of EQ in the profession and how they can use the mentorship to develop those skills (for example, encouraging them to seek feedback on communication or to discuss emotional challenges with their mentor). When mentees understand that EQ development is an expected part of the mentorship, they may be more open and proactive in those areas.

3. **Pairing and matching considerations:** EQ can also inform how mentors and mentees are matched. Programs might use questionnaires or interviews to gauge aspects like communication style, values, or interpersonal preferences, aiming to pair mentors and mentees who are compatible or who can have a productive rapport. For instance, a mentee who is very anxious might be paired with a mentor known for patience and empathy. While skill and interest alignment are important in matching, considering emotional dynamics is equally crucial for a harmonious mentoring relationship.
4. **Reflective practices built in:** An EQ-integrated program should encourage regular reflection for both mentors and mentees. This could take the form of structured journaling (with prompts provided), periodic check-in meetings that specifically address how the mentorship is affecting both parties, or mentor peer-group discussions to share experiences and emotions. By normalizing reflection, the program helps participants continuously apply self-awareness and adjust their behaviors. For example, a program might ask mentors to write a short reflective summary each month about what they learned or found challenging in mentoring, which fosters ongoing growth in their EQ as well.
5. **Measuring and evaluating EQ outcomes:** Just as technical competencies are often evaluated, programs can measure progress in emotional competencies too. Simple tools like mentee self-assessments (rating their comfort with client communication, stress management, etc., before and after the program) or 360° feedback processes can be employed. Some programs use validated instruments (e.g., the Emotional Quotient Inventory or other EQ scales) at the start and end of mentorship to see if there are notable changes. Tracking these metrics emphasizes that EQ development is a tangible goal. If data show improvement, it validates the approach. If not, it provides insight into where the program could strengthen its focus.
6. **Supportive community and resources:** An emotionally intelligent mentorship program recognizes that mentors also need support. Facilitate mentor support groups or a community of practice where mentors can share difficulties and advice (confidentially and without breaching mentee trust). Provide resources such as counseling services or burnout prevention workshops accessible to both mentors and mentees. By caring for the emotional health of mentors, the program ensures they are in a good position to care for their mentees' emotional development.
7. **Leadership buy-in and culture:** Finally, for such programs to succeed, organizational leadership must value and promote EQ as a core aspect of professional excellence. Leaders and senior veterinarians should champion the program, perhaps by sharing their own experiences or endorsing the importance of mentorship and EQ. When the workplace culture supports openness, learning from mistakes, and empathy (as opposed to punitive or purely results driven mentalities), mentorship efforts in EQ truly flourish. By intentionally structuring mentorship programs around EQ, veterinary organizations create an environment where both mentors and mentees are aware of and actively cultivating these skills. This structured approach can produce a generation of veterinarians who not only excel clinically but are also prepared to lead with empathy, resilience, and strong interpersonal abilities. In turn, this contributes to a more positive professional culture and better outcomes for teams, clients, and animal patients alike.

TEACHING EMOTIONAL INTELLIGENCE TO NEW GRADUATES

Mentorship of new veterinarians often extends beyond clinical skills to include helping them develop professional soft skills, including EQ. As new graduates transition from academia to the fast-paced, high-pressure environment of clinical practice, EQ becomes pivotal in navigating client interactions, teamwork, and personal wellness. This section provides evidence-based strategies for mentors and educators to teach and reinforce EQ in early-career veterinarians. These approaches are drawn from research in veterinary and other high-stress fields, and they emphasize practical, experiential learning tailored to young professionals.

Integrating EQ training into veterinary education and mentorship is essential for several reasons. First, studies in veterinary populations have linked higher EQ with positive outcomes like increased job satisfaction, lower stress, and improved client relationships (Ashton-James and McNeilage, 2022). Second, unlike IQ, EQ can be significantly developed through training and practice, especially in the supportive context of mentorship. New graduates are in a formative stage where habits and professional identities are still being shaped, so timely intervention can yield long-lasting benefits.

Approach	What it builds	Example activity
Experiential learning and reflection	Self-awareness, emotional insight	Journaling daily cases; guided case debriefs
Simulation and role-play	Empathy, conflict resolution	Bad-news conversations with actors; colleague-conflict drills
Mindfulness and stress reduction	Self-regulation, resilience	Breathing exercises; cognitive reframing coaching
Feedback and emotional coaching	Relationship management	360° feedback reviews; video-review of client consults
Program integration	Professional identity, peer support	Emotional-resilience workshops; case-based mentor storytelling

A. Experiential learning and reflection

- Journaling: Log emotional reactions to cases; identify triggers and coping patterns.
- Case discussions: Mentor-led debriefs on ethical or grief-laden scenarios; share coping strategies.

B. Simulation and role-play

- Client simulations: Enact bad-news or cost-discussion scenarios; actor and mentor give real-time feedback.
- Conflict drills: Practice de-escalation with team members and anxious clients.

C. Mindfulness and stress reduction

- Breathing breaks: Two-minute diaphragmatic breathing before a shift or after a difficult case.
- Cognitive reframing: Mentor models transforming "I failed" thoughts into growth-oriented self-talk.

D. Feedback and emotional coaching

- 360° reviews: Gather input from staff, clients, and peers; spotlight patterns (e.g., unapproachable under stress).
- Recorded consults: Watch client-interaction clips together; pause to highlight empathy cues or missed signals.

E. Integration into formal programs

- Workshops/seminars: Host quarterly resilience workshops featuring mental-health experts.
- Mentor storytelling: Mentor shares a personal high-emotion case, the missteps, and the healing lessons.
- Peer support networks: Facilitate monthly check-ins or "buddy" meetups to normalize emotional challenges.

MENTOR TIP

Match the method to the mentee. Some vets thrive on simulations, others on reflective journaling. Use your own EQ to sense which approach will stick.

ASSESSING AND MEASURING PROGRESS IN EQ DEVELOPMENT

To ensure that efforts to teach and enhance EQ are effective, it's helpful to assess progress over time. By using certain tools and feedback mechanisms, mentors and programs can identify growth in EQ competencies and adjust their approaches as needed. Monitoring development also reinforces to the mentee that EQ is a key area of professional growth, just like surgical skills or medical knowledge.

TOOLS FOR MEASURING EQ

Standardized EQ assessments: Tools like the Mayer-Salovey-Caruso Emotional Intelligence Test (MSCEIT) (Mayer et al., 2002) provide an ability-based measure of emotional intelligence. The MSCEIT involves performance tasks (such as identifying emotions in faces or suggesting how to manage an emotion in a scenario) to yield scores in areas like perception, understanding, and regulation of emotions. Administering the MSCEIT at the beginning of a mentorship and then after a significant period (say a year) can show quantifiable changes. For example, a mentee might start with a moderate score in emotion regulation and improve to a higher score later, indicating better skill in that area. These results can be motivating and can pinpoint which competencies improved and which might need more focus.

Self-report measures: The Emotional Quotient Inventory (EQ-i) or similar questionnaires ask individuals to self-rate behaviors and attitudes related to emotional competencies (Bar-On, 1997). While self-reports can be subjective, they are useful for gauging the mentee's own perception of their abilities and emotional well-being. If a mentee reports higher scores in stress tolerance or empathy after mentorship, it suggests they feel more confident and capable in those domains. Any discrepancies between a tool like the MSCEIT and the EQ-i (for instance, an ability test shows high skill but the mentee self-reports low confidence) can be rich topics for mentor–mentee discussion.

360-degree evaluations: As mentioned, gathering feedback from a variety of sources provides a comprehensive view. Periodically (perhaps every six months), mentors can solicit input from coworkers, supervisors, support staff, and even clients (through comment cards or surveys about the mentee's communication). Questions would target EQ-related behaviors: "Does Dr. X communicate clearly and compassionately?" "How does Dr. X handle pressure or setbacks?" The mentor can compile this feedback (anonymously if needed) and discuss it with the mentee. The breadth of perspectives helps validate improvements—for example, multiple team members might note that the mentee has become more approachable and patient in the last few months, highlighting progress in social skills.

Reflective self-assessments: Encourage the mentee to periodically reflect in writing specifically on their emotional growth. They might answer prompts like: "Describe a situation recently where you handled your emotions better than you might have a year ago," or "Which aspects of EQ do you feel have improved, and which remain challenging?" Comparing these self-assessments over time can reveal qualitative improvements and continuing struggles.

Mentor observations: Mentors themselves can track anecdotal evidence of growth. Perhaps initially a mentee would get flustered easily by upset clients, but now the mentor observes them remaining calm and using techniques like taking the client to a private space to talk quietly. Taking notes on such instances can be useful feedback to share: "I noticed last week with the angry owner you kept your composure and managed to de-escalate the situation. A few months ago, you looked much more anxious in that kind of scenario—this is real progress!"

Mentorship review meetings: Some programs establish formal review checkpoints where mentor and mentee jointly review all the above data and set goals for the next phase. In these meetings, they might agree on areas to continue strengthening or new strategies to try. For instance, if assessments show the mentee's self-awareness and client communication have improved but they still feel high-stress levels, the plan might include a greater focus on work–life balance or advanced stress management techniques moving forward.

By tracking changes in EQ over time, mentors and educators can celebrate successes and identify where to concentrate further support. It's important to frame assessment not as a judgment, but as a feedback mechanism for development. The goal is improvement, not a "grade." For the mentee, seeing concrete evidence of their growth (like rising assessment scores or positive feedback comments) can boost their confidence and reinforce the value of focusing on EQ. It also highlights that the sometimes intangible work of emotional growth does yield tangible results.

Conversely, if progress is slower in some areas, that's useful information too. It might indicate a need to try different techniques or involve additional resources (like counseling services if stress and anxiety remain very high, for example). In some cases, it could reveal that certain workplace factors are impeding development (perhaps the environment is too chaotic or unsupportive, undermining the mentorship efforts), which might prompt higher-level changes.

In summary, assessment in EQ development serves as a compass, keeping the mentorship journey on course. It helps ensure that the time and effort invested in building EQ are translating into real-world skills and benefits. As veterinary medicine increasingly recognizes the importance of "soft skills," the ability to measure and report on improvements in those skills will likely become a standard part of professional training programs.

EQ is not merely a "nice-to-have" in veterinary mentorship—it is a fundamental pillar of effective practice, career resilience, and professional fulfillment. By cultivating EQ, veterinary mentors set into motion a positive ripple effect. They shape mentees to become practitioners who are not only clinically competent but also emotionally resilient, empathetic, and skilled communicators.

In an era where veterinary professionals face intense emotional demands, the ability to navigate these complexities is as crucial as any medical procedure. Throughout this chapter, we have seen that mentorship enriched with EQ principles yields concrete benefits. When mentors model self-awareness and self-regulation, mentees learn how to remain composed and thoughtful under pressure. When mentors use empathy and active listening, a foundation of trust and psychological safety is built, enabling deeper learning and collaboration. By providing constructive feedback with sensitivity, mentors help mentees grow in confidence and competence rather than fear making mistakes. Importantly, emotionally intelligent mentorship also contributes to better well-being. Research links high emotional intelligence to lower stress, reduced burnout, and greater job satisfaction—outcomes that are vital for the sustainability of veterinary careers.

As the veterinary profession continues to evolve—with increasing client expectations, advancements in medical knowledge, and ongoing concerns about mental health within the field—the role of EQ becomes ever more critical. Mentors have a unique opportunity and responsibility to integrate EQ development into the training of new veterinarians. This means not only teaching medical knowledge and technical skills but also openly addressing communication strategies, coping mechanisms, and the emotional aspects of veterinary work. By doing so, mentors prepare their mentees to handle difficult client conversations, ethical dilemmas, and team conflicts with professionalism and compassion. They also instill in their mentees the importance of self-care and emotional reflexivity, which can guard against compassion fatigue and career attrition.

Moreover, embedding EQ within mentorship creates a more supportive veterinary community at large. Mentorship that prioritizes EQ helps propagate a culture where asking for help is encouraged, where mistakes are treated as learning opportunities, and where empathy is extended not just to clients and patients but also to colleagues. Veterinary institutions and organizations should recognize the power of such mentorship. Investing in mentor training on EQ, providing resources for mental well-being, and formally valuing soft skills alongside clinical skills are steps that can amplify this impact. Ultimately, the well-being of veterinarians—individually and collectively—is intertwined with the emotional health of the profession. A workforce of veterinarians who are emotionally intelligent is more likely to be resilient, collaborative, and committed, thereby elevating the quality of animal care and client service.

KEY TAKEAWAYS FOR MENTORS

Model EQ through your actions. Mentors should demonstrate self-awareness, patience, and empathy in their daily work. By managing your stress reactions and treating clients, staff, and mentees with respect and understanding, you provide a living example for your mentee to emulate. Remember, mentees learn as much from observing you as from what you explicitly teach.

Build trust with empathy and active listening. Create a safe, supportive environment by truly listening to your mentee's concerns and validating their feelings. Show that you value their perspective. Encourage open dialogue, and be consistent and reliable in your support. A mentee who trusts their mentor is more likely to ask questions, admit uncertainties, and grow from feedback.

Give constructive feedback with care. When offering critiques or suggestions, frame them in a positive, growth-oriented way. Tailor your communication to your mentee's temperament—some may need gentle encouragement while others appreciate directness. Always acknowledge what the mentee is doing well. Balanced, empathetic feedback boosts confidence and improvement, whereas harsh criticism can discourage and shut down learning.

Mentor the "whole" vet, not just the medicine. Recognize that early-career veterinarians need guidance in communication, teamwork, self-care, and handling stress—not only in clinical techniques. Incorporate discussions about work–life balance, dealing with difficult clients, and coping with grief or mistakes. Share your own experiences and coping strategies. Encouraging your mentee's emotional well-being and professional soft skills will set them up for long-term success.

Encourage autonomy and reflective growth. Gradually empower your mentee to take on challenges independently, while you act as a safety net. Let them make decisions (and occasionally mistakes), then reflect together on what went well and what could be learned. Use open-ended questions to prompt self-reflection. This approach develops your mentee's self-efficacy and critical thinking. Over time, they will become a confident, emotionally intelligent practitioner capable of handling the rigors of veterinary practice on their own.

CONCLUSION

Emotionally intelligent mentorship is a catalyst for positive change. For mentors, it is an avenue to leave a lasting legacy by shaping not just what their mentees know, but how they approach their work and life. For mentees, it provides a strong foundation to build a satisfying and enduring career. And for the veterinary profession, it nurtures practitioners who can meet the challenges of the job with both expertise and empathy. Professional mentorship programs, such as Ready, Vet, Go, emphasize that integrating EQ into every layer of mentorship can make both a chapter (and a career) truly transformative. By embracing these principles, mentors and mentees together can ensure that veterinary medicine remains a science and an art—one that cares for people and animals with equal insight and heart.

BIBLIOGRAPHY

Ashton-James, C.E. and McNeilage, A.G. (2022). A mixed methods investigation of stress and wellbeing factors contributing to burnout and job satisfaction in a specialist small animal hospital. *Frontiers in Veterinary Science* 9: 942778. https://doi.org/10.3389/fvets.2022.942778.

Banerjee, S.C., Parker, P.A., Staley, J.M. et al. (2024). Mentor communication skills training improved self-efficacy and empathic communication. *BMC Medical Education* 24: 646.

Bar-On, R. (1997). *The Emotional Quotient Inventory (EQ-i): Technical Manual*. Toronto, Ontario, Canada: Multi-Health Systems.

Bar-On, R. (2004). The Bar-On Emotional Quotient Inventory (EQ-i): rationale, description, and summary of psychometric properties. In: *Measuring Emotional Intelligence: Common Ground and Controversy* (ed. G. Geher), 115–145. Hauppauge, NY: Nova Science Publishers.

Berki, E. (2005). Mentoring as a learning process – relationships and communication. *Investigations in University Teaching and Learning* 3 (1): 41–48.

Chun, J.U., Litzky, B.E., Sosik, J.J. et al. (2010). Emotional intelligence and trust in formal mentoring programs. *Group & Organization Management* 35 (4): 421–455.

Clutterbuck, D.A., Kochan, F.K., Lunsford, L. et al. (2017). *Keeping Emotions in It: Emotionally Intelligent Mentoring*, 274–289. London, England: Sage Publications. https://doi.org/10.4135/9781526402011 https://engageforsuccess.org/engaging managers/why-managers-needemotional-intelligence-for-team-success/ Retrieved April 7, 2025.

Ealias, A. and George, J. (2012). Emotional intelligence and job satisfaction: a correlational study. *Research Journal of Commerce and Behavioral Science* 1 (4): 37–42.

Fiori, M., Udayar, S., and Maillefer, A.V. (2021). Emotion information processing as a new component of emotional intelligence: theoretical framework and empirical evidence. *European Journal of Personality* 35 (2): 223–243.

Goleman, D. (1995). *Emotional Intelligence: Why It Can Matter More Than IQ*. Bantam Books.

Goleman, D. (1998). *Working with Emotional Intelligence*. New York: Bantam Books.

Hunter, J.E. and Hunter, R.F. (1984). *Validity and utility of alternative predictors of job performance. Psychological Bulletin* 96 (1): 72–98. https://doi.org/10.1037/0033-2909.96.1.72.

Joseph, P.T. (2010). The role of emotional intelligence in mentoring and coaching. *NHRD Network Journal* 4 (10): 25–27.

Mayer, J.D. and Caruso, D. (2002). The effective leader: understanding and applying emotional intelligence. *Ivey Business Journal* 67 (2): 1–5.

Mayer, J.D., Salovey, P., and Caruso, D.R. (2002). *Mayer-Salovey-Caruso Emotional Intelligence Test (MSCEIT) User's Manual*. Toronto, Ontario, Canada: Multi-Health Systems.

Neisser, U., Boodoo, G., Bouchard, T.J. et al. (1996). *Intelligence: knowns and unknowns. American Psychologist* 51 (2): 77–101. https://doi.org/10.1037/0003-066X.51.2.77.

Pulido-Martos, M., Augusto-Landa, J.M., and López-Zafra, E. (2020). Emotional intelligence and perceived stress in healthcare professionals: a systematic review with meta-analysis. *International Journal of Environmental Research and Public Health* 17 (15): 5371. https://doi.org/10.3390/ijerph17155371.

Salovey, P. and Mayer, J.D. (1990). Emotional intelligence. *Imagination, Cognition and Personality* 9 (3): 185–211.

Schmid, K.L. and Mast, T.L. (2021). Associations among stress, anxiety, depression, and emotional intelligence among veterinary medicine students. *Journal of Veterinary Medical Education* 48 (5): 626–634. https://doi.org/10.3138/jvme-2020-0107.

Treglown, L. and Furnham, A. (2023). Are EQ and IQ negatively related? The relationship between trait emotional intelligence and fluid cognitive ability. *Psychology* 14 (1): 17–31.

Vratskikh, I., Masa'deh, R., Al-Lozi, M., and Maqableh, M. (2016). The impact of emotional intelligence on job performance via the mediating role of job satisfaction. *International Journal of Business and Management* 11 (2): 69–91.

Wechsler, D. (1958). *The Measurement and Appraisal of Adult Intelligence*, 4e. Baltimore: Williams & Wilkins.

Developing Clinical Competency

CHAPTER 8

INTRODUCTION

Dani Rabwin

When we think about mentorship programs, we often default to clinical skills checklists—and for good reason. Throughout this book, we've explored the emotional, psychological, and interpersonal dimensions of mentorship, but clinical competency remains an essential component that can't be overlooked. New graduates must be able to perform the fundamental procedures that define veterinary practice, even as they develop in all these other critical areas.

The challenge isn't that mentors avoid clinical skills development—most feel comfortable in this domain. Rather, it's that the informal, ad hoc approach we typically use often fails to address the dramatic variability in new graduates' starting points. While students master vast amounts of theoretical knowledge, their hands-on experience varies wildly—some graduate having performed only "half" a spay, while others complete twenty or more procedures. Without systematic assessment and structured progressions, even well-intentioned clinical mentorship leaves gaps that can undermine confidence and competency for years to come.

For this chapter, I've chosen Dr. Janis Shinkawa and Dr. Jill Muraoka, whose unique combination of clinical expertise and business acumen has shaped their approach to systematic competency development. Both are partners at Ohana Pet Hospital and leaders in Western Veterinary Partners' Launch Mentorship Program, having guided hundreds of early-career veterinarians through structured training pathways. Their backgrounds—Janis as a former CPA and business consultant and Jill as an educator and software developer—bring methodical precision to what is often an intuitive process.

Together, they've developed comprehensive frameworks that transform mentorship from guesswork into measurable progress. Their approach emphasizes preparation before mentees arrive, systematic skills' assessment using both self-evaluation and direct observation, and individualized learning plans with clear milestones and accountability measures.

This chapter provides the concrete tools mentors need to assess clinical competency accurately, create customized learning pathways, and track progress systematically. You'll discover how to prepare your team for mentorship success, implement structured feedback systems, and leverage technology to maintain accountability. Most importantly, you'll learn how this systematic approach not only develops confident, competent veterinarians but also creates sustainable mentorship programs that benefit entire practice teams.

DEVELOPING CLINICAL COMPETENCY THROUGH MENTORSHIP

Janis Shinkawa and Jill Muraoka

It was my first surgery day in my rotating internship. I was nervous but excited and eager to learn from one of the best boarded surgical specialists in our field, Dr. Mary Dulisch. "Dr. D," as we called her, was intimidating to say the least as she was very particular about her patients and how we managed her surgical cases. She had high expectations and made sure we clearly knew what was expected of us by providing each intern new to her rotation with a detailed handbook. Naturally, scared and intimidated by her serious demeanor and expectations, our goal was simply to "not mess up." But then, of course, on my first day on her service, I did.

I scrubbed in first and was tasked with setting up the instrument packs in the surgical suite. I felt confident upon awaiting her arrival into surgery as the technical staff and I worked efficiently to get the surgery suite ready and made sure that the patient was prepped, draped, and ready to go. Dr. D finally popped into surgery just as I had placed the last pack on the instrument stand. She paused, grabbed that last pack and looked me straight in the eye and said, "you need to open the inside drape first to make sure that the pack is sterile before placing it on the table." I said to her "oh, I'm sorry, that's not how we did it in school." And then thought to myself, what are the chances that the packs weren't sterile? Well, to my dismay, this last pack that she was now holding was revealed to be NOT sterile when the inside drape was opened. Dr. D rolled her eyes and told the technicians to redrape the patient and re-gown and re-glove both of us. I was embarrassed and felt bad that we had to spend the extra time to do everything all over again. That day I knew that I did not get off on the right foot with Dr. D because I failed to heed her instructions and expectations. By the end of the internship, I understood that these published stringent expectations and rules were created to ensure patient safety and efficiency in surgery. I learned that being prepared was the key to minimizing mistakes and ensuring that my patients receive the best possible care.

Dr. D appeared outwardly austere, but underneath that stern exterior, she was an extremely caring and compassionate person. She pushed us to foster a learning mindset and not be afraid to ask questions or question something if we were uncertain. She encouraged us to do this not only in surgery but also in tackling our medicine cases as well. Dr. D stressed preparation, and it is one of the essential skills that I have passed on when training junior associate doctors in our practice. She was an amazing mentor that has graciously continued to support me through the years. Dr. Dulisch was a true inspiration to me, and it is no surprise that I ended up loving surgery in large part because of the time spent with her.

A mentor's influence on a mentee can be profound, for better or worse. Traditionally, mentors focused on helping new graduates develop clinical competence as they transitioned from academia into practice. Today's mentors are expected to go further—coaching on communication, time management, and well-being, as discussed throughout this book. Yet clinical skill development remains a core part of helping early-career veterinarians become confident, productive members of the team.

New graduates enter practice with strong theoretical knowledge but often limited experience in primary case management and surgery. A 2017 *Journal of the American Veterinary Medical Association* article highlighted the gap between employers' expectations and new graduates' confidence and competence to perform medical and surgical procedures independently. Experience levels vary widely among students, depending on the individual and their veterinary school's clinical and surgical opportunities.

A study from the Veterinary College of Surgeons (Simons et al., 2022) suggested that the minimum number of spay and neuter procedures performed by veterinary students to feel confident is 6–10 repetitions. In the many new graduates that I've interviewed during the hiring process, the experience range is vast with some new grads only having completed "half" a spay or neuter to others that have done 20 or more. The latter group typically graduated from schools that have a robust community medicine practice or a shelter medicine program that provide students access to participate in high-volume spay and neuter clinics. For veterinary students trained with limited patient and client contact during the COVID years of 2020–2022, graduates completing their clinical years during this time were at a greater disadvantage with even more limited experience with client interaction, clinical case management, and hands-on surgical training.

The American Veterinary Medical Association's Council on Education (AVMA COE) has published a list of required knowledge and skills that veterinary students must demonstrate during the course of their veterinary education. Although the standards dictate the skills and knowledge items to be performed and signed off by faculty, they do not require assessment for competence or confidence. In addition, due to time and animal resource constraints, students are typically "signed off" after their first and only attempt at performing a skill, including surgery. Therefore, vet students have limited opportunities to perform common general practice procedures such as spays, neuters, and dentistry prior to graduation. The limited practice and exposure also apply to technical skills such as venipuncture, bandaging, and IV catheter placement, which is important as often it is assumed that veterinarians are confident and competent in these basic technician skills. Students' experience in basic hands-on clinical skills training also varies by school. This makes it difficult upon entering the workplace in private practice where the burden of hands-on training in both clinical case management, procedures, and even basic technical skills falls on the more experienced doctors in the practice.

In this chapter, we will share best practices and tips on how to assist your early career veterinarian in acquiring the essential knowledge and clinical skills to launch a successful career in small animal general practice. Training and mentoring an early-career veterinarian are a collaborative team effort, where creating a plan and preparing hospital staff prior to the start of employment of your new associate is essential. During the **preparation phase**, it is crucial to establish expectations and agreements for the new associate, mentor, and hospital staff. These expectations and agreements define each party's role and responsibilities in mentoring the new associate. Once the hospital is prepared to support the early-career doctor, the next step is to **assess their skills** and knowledge followed by the development of a customized training and learning plan. Once the learning plan is established, it is equally important to create and communicate an **implementation** plan to set up the mentorship efforts for success. Finally, the most crucial step for ensuring the clinical competency of your early-career doctor is to establish and maintain a regular **feedback** schedule, coupled with the ability to track their progress.

SETTING THE STAGE: PREPARATION, ORGANIZATION, AND CREATING EXPECTATIONS AND AGREEMENTS

Being prepared and organized is key to attaining successful outcomes. Yes, things can still go awry, but preparation can help promote a smooth transition of the early-career veterinarian into your practice. By being organized and preparing yourself and your team, you can minimize the inevitable bumps in the road in the big undertaking of mentoring a doctor in the early stages of their career. An added bonus is that this process of preparation and organization will promote improved efficiency in hospital operations. This stage of preparation should be completed prior to the start date of your early-career doctor.

PREPARATION STEPS

1. Identify the key players that will be involved in mentorship activities
2. Define the role of each key player in mentorship duties
3. Define expectations for each role in mentorship—including the mentee
4. Evaluate your hospital's protocols and processes
5. Communicate the plan to all hospital staff and allow for feedback and questions

IDENTIFY THE KEY PLAYERS

Determine who will mentor the new associate in the hospital. A mentor typically leads the mentorship efforts, providing direct training. However, if no single doctor is willing or able, multiple doctors can share the role. Also, identify other hospital team members who will be actively involved in mentorship. For instance, the hospital manager should lead by coordinating schedule changes and assisting with client communications, and an experienced Registered Veterinary Technician (RVT) can guide the new associate in the hospital's anesthetic protocols. Identify team members naturally strong in training and mentorship and be sure to acknowledge and highlight the importance of mentorship as a team effort.

DEFINING ROLES

Now that you've identified the key players in supporting mentorship activities in the hospital, you can define each key player's role. This should look like a job description. Each role should include ideal attributes of the individual taking on the role in addition to defining the specific mentorship activities they are responsible for. These attributes will also be reiterated in expectations covered next.

For example, here are some of the desirable attributes and expectations of a strong clinical skills mentor:

- Patient and compassionate
- Communicates clearly and directly
- Accurately gauges how much guidance a mentee needs
- Manages time efficiently and remains approachable for questions, even when busy
- Skilled and knowledgeable in the subject they are teaching (Table 8.1)

The mindset, motivation, resiliency, and adaptability of a mentee are key attributes for their success. They may have amazing mentors, but mentees will not succeed if they lack the motivation to learn, take feedback, and keep a growth mindset.

Here are some vital attributes and expectations of the mentee:

- **Demonstrates** willingness to be coached.
- **Pays** attention to detail, even in repetition—for example, carefully completing each skin closure instead of rushing or "going through the motions."

Table 8.1 Sample Matrix for Defining and Organizing the Roles of Each Party Involved in Mentorship Activities in the Hospital

	Mentee	Mentor	Hospital manager	Support staff
Attributes	Willing to take feedback Open communicator	Patient and compassionate Direct communicator	Patient and compassionate Direct communicator	Patient Organized
Training responsibilities	Showing up Preparing for tasks at hand Asking questions Learning from experiences (both good and bad)	Surgery and dentistry Medical case management Medical records	Managing scheduling Coaching client communication Practice management software system	Technician skills training and evaluation Surgery and anesthesia review and preparation
Assigned to	Dr. Smith	Dr. Anderson	R. Gonzalez	Allie RVT

Source: Islander Veterinary Business Consultants/with permission of Janis Shinkawa.

- **Shows** motivation to learn from others, ask questions, and take feedback from more experienced veterinarians and key staff members with decades of knowledge and experience.
- **Embraces** mistakes as learning opportunities, even when they are uncomfortable or painful.
- **Invests** in their own growth and learning—such as coming in on their day off to scrub in with another veterinarian, gaining experience at a shelter, or shadowing a local specialist.
- **Commits** to improving communication and professionalism to become an effective team player and leader in the eyes of their colleagues.

SET EXPECTATIONS

After identifying the mentorship roles and their key responsibilities, the next step is to establish clear expectations for mentors, mentees, hospital managers, and staff. **Expectations refer to the demands placed upon an individual, while an agreement constitutes a promise made by the recipient of the expectations to do their best to fulfill them**. What makes expectations so effective is that they define the types of behaviors that you want your team members to exhibit. It also provides clarity to what each person is responsible for which then makes holding individuals accountable easy. Once expectations for each role have been agreed upon and defined, they should be made available to all parties. Who is responsible for creating these expectations? Typically, it will be the mentor along with other stakeholders in hospital leadership such as the Hospital Manager and/or the Medical Director (Table 8.2).

Once roles and expectations are defined, review your hospital's protocols and processes before your new doctor's start date. This ensures consistency, safety, and quality of care, while providing a clear framework for onboarding and training. These protocols should cover everything from scheduling and patient intake on procedure days to medication refill procedures. Although establishing a full set of hospital protocols and processes can be a daunting task and will take time to develop, it is worth investing in for smoother operations and setting a foundation for future growth. If you don't have protocols or processes, start building your library with small steps. Preventative care and wellness protocols or patient intake processes are usually the easiest to start with. Small steps over time will add up!

Here are some tips for managing your hospital's processes and protocols:

- Work with your patient care team to approve medical protocols (e.g., vaccine protocols)
- Work with the appropriate team members to establish routine hospital processes (e.g., surgical patient intake process)
- Evaluate the hospital's protocols and processes periodically to ensure that they are up to date
- If new doctors have suggestions or recommendations to change a protocol or process, put it on a team meeting agenda to discuss and be receptive to ideas

Table 8.2 Examples of Expectations for the Mentor and Mentee

Mentor	Mentee
Willing to scrub in on surgeries for at least the first 2–3 months	Prepare your case questions by organizing, summarizing, and looking up information before asking your mentor
Keep to a schedule of regular meetings with the mentee	Be willing to take feedback and be open to suggestion and coaching
Be patient and compassionate always	Do not engage in gossip and negativity with other team members

- Consider protocols and processes that are missing or needed to help prevent mistakes from occurring and to increase efficiencies such as the process of having a client fill out a surgery day drop-off form to verify feeding status and the patient's medications
- Train and implement with the whole team. Team meetings are an effective way to introduce new protocols and process and gather feedback

INTERNAL COMMUNICATION PLAN

Finally, in order to prepare for the start of your new early career doctor, take the time to communicate the plan to all hospital staff and allow for feedback and questions. Although preparing expectations and establishing protocols and processes are ideally done as a collaborative effort, it isn't efficient to solicit feedback from all team members. There should be 1–2 main stakeholders that are in charge of creating the content and coordinating the gathering of feedback from other team members.

Here are tips on important information to communicate with the hospital team in preparation for the start of your early career doctor:

- Let your team know as soon as possible or even during the hiring process that an early-career doctor will be starting.
- Involve your team to create a plan as to how to onboard the new doctor and get them familiar with hospital operations.
- Managers should keep an eye on the scheduling needs so that new doctors have more experienced staff working with them in case of any questions that come up during the day.
- Check in with your team frequently once a new doctor starts to ensure things are going well; ask them for observations and confidential feedback.
- Check in with your new doctor to ensure they are integrating well into your hospital (Box 8.1).

SKILLS ASSESSMENT AND CREATE A CUSTOMIZED LEARNING PLAN

Now that the stage is set and the hospital is prepared to support your new early-career doctor, the next step is to work with them to create a customized learning plan. In this section, we'll discuss the assessment or skills' evaluation process and how to use the information gathered to then

BOX 8.1 SUMMARY OF PREPARATION FOR THE ARRIVAL OF YOUR EARLY-CAREER DOCTOR

Summary of Best Practices to Prepare for the Start of an Early-Career Doctor:

- Define the mentorship roles that include both direct training and mentorship activities as well as behavioral expectations. Publish and go over with all mentorship team members.
- Review or create hospital protocols and processes to aid in the onboarding and training process that allow for consistency.
- Communicate the plan with the team and ask for feedback. Remind the team that training of an early career doctor will benefit everyone as they become a productive, revenue-generating part of the team.

Source: Islander Veterinary Business Consultants/with permission of Janis Shinkawa.

develop an individualized and dynamic learning plan for your mentee. Evaluating the mentee's knowledge and skills will help identify gaps and training opportunities. The assessment process should be ongoing and not only used for initial evaluation. It should be regularly performed to ensure that your mentee can demonstrate true clinical competence in both hands-on skills and knowledge.

During the initial evaluation, it is important to assess both hands-on skills and knowledge, especially for the early-career doctors who have worked in practice for at least a few months or a few years. Assuming a certain level of skill based on years of experience or self-assessment by the mentee is not appropriate as it is impossible to identify where there may be deficiencies and to what degree. For a new graduate, it is safe to assume that they have minimal practical experience, so the initial evaluation will focus on foundational skills such as the physical exam and essential technician skills such as IV catheter placement and venipuncture. They've gained a lot of knowledge in school which they now need to learn to practically apply in a real-world practice setting.

EVALUATING THE MENTEE'S SKILLS AND KNOWLEDGE

For a new graduate, their initial assessment will be focused on the fundamental skills and knowledge that will be applied in the types of cases they will see in the first one to twomonths in practice. This may include details of the practice's wellness and preventative care policies, performing a physical exam, medical record writing, and dental health recommendations. During the first few months, the mentor should continue to assess the mentee's knowledge of vaccines, infectious disease control, parasiticides, as well as life stage recommendations for lab work and dentistry. See Table 8.3 for an example.

Create a proposed pathway for the new graduate to follow over the course of their first year of employment. This pathway should summarize the progression of the types of cases seen and expectations for procedures that they should be able perform at specified milestones by the end of their first year. This pathway does not need to be all encompassing and should not be overly detailed. See the example in Figure 8.1. Be sure to review the pathway with the mentee

Table 8.3 Sample of Knowledge and Hands-on Skills to Evaluate for a New Graduate

Knowledge	Skills
• Wellness and preventative care recommendations based on life stages	• Physical exam
• Vaccination protocols	• History taking and vital signs
• Annual laboratory testing	• Otoscopic Exam
• Parasite prevention and treatment	• Oral Exam with Dental Disease Evaluation
• Dental health recommendations	• Venipuncture
• Workup and treatment of otitis externa	• IV catheter placement
• Sedation protocols including fear-free premedication protocols	• Safe animal handling and restraint
	• Ear cytology
	• SOAP format medical records

Source: Islander Veterinary Business Consultants/with permission of Jill Muraoka.

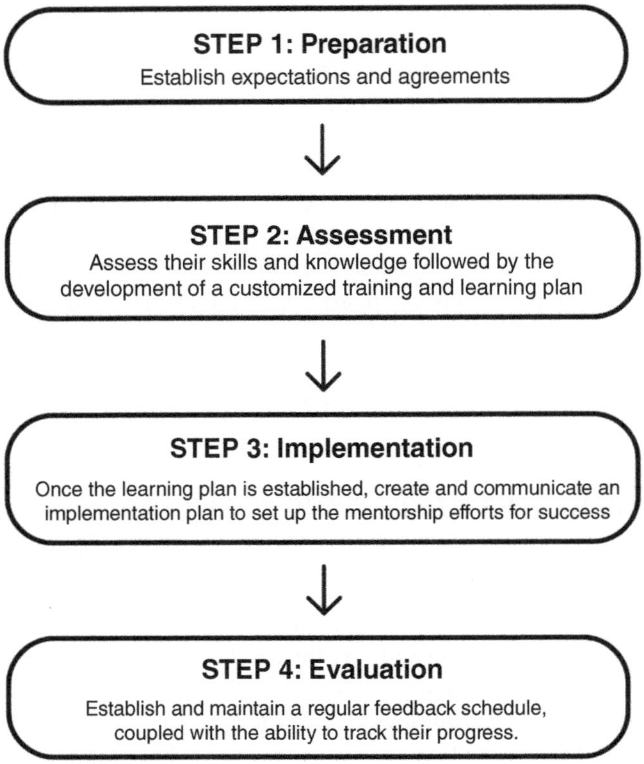

FIGURE 8.1 Early-career clinical skills' plan.

and let them know this is a suggested pathway that is flexible in both timeline and scope. It helps for them to see the path and what is expected of them, but it can also put excess pressure on them if they feel that they are unable to meet these milestones according to the pathway. It will also help keep the mentee's training focused and moving forward when working to adhere to a published timeline.

To assess the mentee's knowledge, we suggest scheduling one-on-one discussions. To avoid having them become overwhelmed with excessive direct questioning, it may help to present questions in case format. This will not only test their knowledge, but it will also show you their thought process. See Box 8.2 for an example of knowledge assessment using a case example. Mentees can be given a typed list of cases to prepare for discussion prior to meeting or you can do a more informal mix of direct questioning and case scenarios when meeting in person. Some mentees prefer the ability to think and prepare their thoughts prior to meeting while others are comfortable with impromptu discussions. This is something you should ask the mentee as it will also apply in the future when preparing to give them feedback or scheduling performance review discussions. For evaluating hands-on skills, new grads should be presented with a list where they can rate their level of confidence for each skill. Skills which they indicate confidence in should be evaluated for competency by the mentor or another qualified team member. In a further section, we will discuss how to track and manage the mentee's knowledge and hands-on skill progress. Training for skills that they are not confident with should be incorporated into the learning plan.

BOX 8.2 EXAMPLE OF A CASE-BASED KNOWLEDGE ASSESSMENT

You are presented with a 10-week-old F Labrador puppy that received 1 DHPP vaccine from the breeder at 8 weeks of age and pyrantel pamoate liquid dewormer orally at 4, 6, and 8 weeks of age. What laboratory testing, vaccination schedule, and parasite control/preventatives recommendation to give to this owner? What if the puppy was 14 weeks old instead? How would you adjust your plan?

This case will test their knowledge on puppy life stage wellness recommendations and open a discussion that will allow the new graduate to be trained on the hospital's protocols.

Source: Islander Veterinary Business Consultants/with permission of Jill Muraoka.

BOX 8.3 SETTING EXPECTATIONS FOR A SKILLS AND KNOWLEDGE ASSESSMENT

Inform your mentee that you will assess their skills and knowledge. Clarify the process, who will be involved, and encourage questions. Emphasize that the goal is to identify training needs and create a tailored learning plan, not to be punitive.

Source: Islander Veterinary Business Consultants/with permission of Jill Muraoka.

New graduate mentees should be evaluated monthly for the first three to six months, but overtime, the interval can increase but should not extend more than every three months. The learning plan will dictate the knowledge and hands-on skills that should be evaluated at the end of each period.

Again, mapping out a timeline will help the mentee be aware of the pathway and what they are expected to know and be able to do by the end of their first year. For mentees that are easily overwhelmed, dividing the pathway into smaller time increments may help to ease stress and anxiety by allowing them to stepwise build their skills and knowledge base but still see the pathway ahead (Box 8.3).

Evaluating the skills and knowledge of an early-career doctor that has been in practice for a year or more will be more challenging than doing so for a new graduate. For a non-new graduate early-career doctor, the initial assessment of their knowledge and skill level is extremely important to see where they have gaps, including "bad habits" that need to be corrected. In this situation, experienced early-career doctors should complete a more extensive self-assessment survey (see Box 8.4), but during the follow-up discussion, the mentor can use a combination of direct questioning and case scenarios to evaluate their skill and knowledge level. More experienced doctors should not be required to demonstrate all hands-on skills as mandatory for new graduates; however, competence and quality of hands-on skills such as surgical or dental procedures should be directly evaluated by the mentor. The mentor should initially shadow the mentee in different types of appointments to assess their client communication and exam room skills. In addition, the mentors should also review random medical records and shadow the mentee during initial surgery and dental procedure days during their first few months of employment. Review of medical records can be a powerful tool for the mentor to get insight on their mentee's knowledge and clinical thought process.

BOX 8.4 SELF-ASSESSMENT SURVEYS AS A TOOL TO IDENTIFY SKILL GAPS

Self-Assessment Surveys can be a very helpful tool. Mentees can rate their confidence in both skills and knowledge. The list should contain essential skills and knowledge that is reasonable for a doctor one to two years in practice. Skills or knowledge areas where the mentee lack confidence can be incorporated into their learning plan.

Example:
Please rate your confidence in the following surgical procedures:

	Not confident	Somewhat confident	Confident
Small/Med Canine OVH (<20 kg)			
Large Canine OVH (>20 kg)			
Canine Neuter			
Canine Cryptorchid Neuter			
Feline OVH			
Feline Neuter			

Source: Islander Veterinary Business Consultants/with permission of Jill Muraoka

CREATING CUSTOM LEARNING PLANS

Once you've assessed the skill and knowledge of your mentee, you can then collaborate with them to create a customized training or learning plan. It is important to have them assist in developing the learning plan for getting "buy-in" and to hold them accountable. Having skin in the game by collaborating on the learning plan greatly enhances engagement and accountability—on both the mentor and mentee sides.

The learning plan for both a new graduate and experienced early-career doctor should span their first year of employment in your practice. The plan should be broken down into, at minimum, quarterly segments and feature time-lined expectations for scheduling appointments (appointment types and duration), procedures (types and time allotted), and training objectives. See the sample learning plan overview in Figure 8.2 and detailed periodic samples in Figures 8.3 and 8.4.

For a new graduate, the learning plan should be broken down into monthly periods for the first three to six months of employment. At the end of each period, the mentee's skills and knowledge associated with their goals and training objectives should be formally assessed by the mentor. To help focus progress, encourage the mentee to create goals. Ideally, goals should be in the format of SMART goals, which are specific, measurable, achievable, reasonable, and time-bound. Utilizing SMART goal rules in goal setting will set up the mentee for success in achieving them. See Box 8.5 for samples of new graduate SMART goals. Ideally, the mentee should set no more than 1 to 2 goals per designated period, as too large a list will be overwhelming and difficult to achieve.

For more experienced early-career doctors, their assessment and learning plan should be sectioned into three month increments over the course of their first year of employment. This plan can be created after their initial skills and knowledge assessment is complete. Remember that this initial evaluation period may take the first one to two months of initial employment to complete. The learning plans for non-new graduate early-career doctors will vary depending on the individual and their experience, so it will have to be customized. Encourage the use of SMART goals to help

Aloha Animal Hospital
2025 Learning Plan Timeline for Dr. Janis Lyn (New Graduate)
Mentor: Dr. Jill Smiley
Start Date: 8/1/2025

Period	Training Items/Goals
Month 1	Appointment Times: 1.5x normal practice length Appt Types: Wellness only Procedures: None Training Objective Summary: Wellness and preventative care, discussing finances with clients, navigating the practice management software system, appropriate medical record writing, approach to working up uncomplicated illness cases (example: ear infections)
Month 2	Appointment Times: 1.5x normal practice length Appt Types: Wellness + Uncomplicated Illness Procedures: None – Start shadowing experienced DVM/Mentor Training Objective Summary: Preparing for surgery, reviewing sedation and anesthesia protocols, discharge instructions, dealing with client conflict
Month 3	Appointment Times: 1.5x normal practice length Appt Types: Wellness + Uncomplicated Illness Procedures: Shadowing +/– Canine OVH >15#<40#, Canine neuter (non-giant breed), Dentals (Mentor to assist/shadow in surgery) Training Objective Summary: Troubleshooting in anesthesia and surgery, reviewing more complicated illness cases (example renal failure, pancreatitis), teamwork and communicating with staff
Month 4	Appointment Times: Reduction to 1x normal practice length for Wellness, Uncomplicated Illness, 1.5x for complicated illness cases. No ER cases yet Appt Types: Wellness, Uncomplicated Illness + Complicated Illness Procedures: Primary surgeon on Canine OVH >15#<40#, Canine neuter (non-giant breed), Dentals (Mentor to shadow or be in hospital for help) Training Objective Summary: Review euthanasia and quality of life discussions, client education with severe and chronic illnesses, review emergency triage and CPR
Month 5…	…
Month 12	Appointment Times: Aligns with Rest of Practice DVMs Appt Types: No restrictions Procedures: Routine surgeries and dentistry matching speed and volume of DVMs in the practice. Open to performing cystotomies, GI surgery, mass removals, etc. with or without supervision based on caseload and experience. Able to manage Wellness and routine illness cases, and becoming more confident to managing complicated illness and ER cases.

FIGURE 8.2 Sample learning plan overview. *Source:* Islander Veterinary Business Consultants/with permission of Jill Muraoka.

focus their progress as well. Remember that the learning plan should include both knowledge and skills' training (Box 8.6).

IMPLEMENTATION FOR SUCCESS

Implementing a mentorship program or building a culture of mentorship in your hospital can feel daunting. However, with thoughtfulness and intention, the rewards are well worth the effort. Mentorship can improve retention rates among doctors and team members (Elce, 2021). Keep in mind that not every experienced doctor or staff member will naturally make an effective mentor—success in mentorship requires more than clinical expertise.

Now that you've started assessing your mentee's skills and knowledge, have created a learning plan, and have the team onboard and ready to launch the mentorship activities in the

Aloha Animal Hospital Learning Plan for Dr. Janis Lyn. (New Graduate)

Mentor DVM: Dr. Jill Smiley
Period: January 2025 – March 2025

Mentee Goals for this period:

1.

2.

Medical Appointment Types:

- Wellness
- Uncomplicated illness cases: ear infection, lameness, GI upset

Duration of Appointment Times:

- Wellness –30 minutes per pet./Illness – 45 minutes

Procedures:

- Canine OVH (< 40 pounds), Canine Neuter (no giant breeds)–only 1 each per procedure day
- Dentistry– surgical extractions OK–only 1 per procedure day

Training Objectives:

A. Medical Cases and Appointments:
   a. Management of recurring or complicated otitis cases
   b. Diagnostic lab work– when and what tests to run
   c. Review the orthopedic and neurologic exams

B. Procedures:
   a. Canine OVH – navigating large dog spays, review ligatures and suture selection (Dr. Quinn)
   b. Review how to determine margins needed on mass excisions and how to evaluate skin closure for appropriate tension (Dr. Quinn)

C. Communication/Administrative:
   a. Review surgery notes and discharge notes
   b. Medical records – review efficiency and completeness
   c. Discuss how to adjust treatment plans for clients that have financial constraints. (Hospital Manager)
   d. Review preparation steps for improved efficiency in getting through procedure days. (RVT Allison)

FIGURE 8.3 Sample learning plan for a new graduate. *Source:* Islander Veterinary Business Consultants/with permission of Jill Muraoka.

hospital, the next step is to put the training into action. Use the learning plan overview and periodic details and training objectives as a guide for accountability and get the training objectives done within a set timeframe.

MEETING SCHEDULE AND TRAINING PREFERENCES

Work with your mentee to create an agreed-upon schedule of meetings. Some mentees prefer structured formal meetings that are scheduled on a regular basis while others—especially more experienced early-career doctors—prefer a more informal approach. Mentees that prefer a more

Aloha Animal Hospital Learning Plan for Dr. Kate Burns
(Experienced Early Career DVM)

Mentor DVM: Dr. Jill Smiley
Period: January–March 2025

Mentee Goals for this period:

1.

2.

3.

Medical Appointment Types:

- Wellness
- All illness types
- Introducing urgent care cases

Duration of Appointment Times:

- All appointments 30 minutes per pet
- 45 min slot in AM and PM for same-day urgent care appointments

Procedures:

- OVH, Neuters, Mass removals, Dentistry–no more than 2 OVH/Neuter and 2 Dentals per procedure day
- Adding in Cystotomy, Aural Hematoma, GI surgery, Gastropexy - with Mentor approval. (Mentor to shadow procedure

Training Objectives:

A. Medical Cases and Appointments:
    a. Management of respiratory distress cases (both feline and canine)
    b. Review triage of trauma cases and CPR (Dr. Anderson)
    c. Review wound care and bandaging (RVT Allison)

B. Procedures:
    a. Review procedure for Cystotomy, Enucleation (Dr. Smith)
    b. Review Aural Hematoma repair techniques and post-op care (Dr. Smith)
    c. Review emergency GI surgery – procedure and complications (Dr. Smith)

C. Communication/Administrative:
    a. Review techniques on managing client conflict
    b. Evaluation of medical records to be concise

FIGURE 8.4 Sample learning plan for an experienced early-career doctor. *Source:* Islander Veterinary Business Consultants/with permission of Jill Muraoka.

BOX 8.5 SMART GOAL EXAMPLES

Examples of SMART Goals for New Graduate Doctors

- Within the next three months, be able to consistently complete a small-medium canine OVH within one hour from open to close.
- By the end of next month, increase the average number of patients seen per day from 15 to 18.
- By the end of the next quarter, will have exceeded $50,000 in monthly gross revenue.

BOX 8.6 SUMMARY FOR CREATING A CUSTOM LEARNING PLAN

Summary of Best Practices for Creating a Custom Learning Plan

- Skill and knowledge assessments need to be done initially and become routine throughout the active mentorship period.
- Assessing skills and knowledge for competency can be done via a combination of surveys, interviews, review of medical records, and shadowing.
- Create an overview pathway spanning one year that provides an overall view of the major milestones for types of cases seen, appointment times, and adding on procedures.
- Create detailed learning plans for each training period that includes mentee SMART goals.
- Collaborate with your mentee to create the details of the plan.

informal approach generally like to get help in the moment, do not generally have many questions, and like constructive feedback in the moment. Regardless of this preference, the mentor should meet with the mentee formally no less than once a month. We highly recommend scheduling weekly meetings with a new grad for at least the first three months.

Recommended mentee meeting agenda items:

- Follow-up on any outstanding cases, issues, etc. from the last meeting.
- Review and discuss schedule for questions or preparation for upcoming cases or procedures.
- Review learning plan to discuss or review training objective items or mentee goals.
- Provide performance feedback and comments on any assessments that may have been done since the last meeting.
- Do a mental health wellness check-in with the mentee—how are they handling stress and their workload.
- Ask the mentee for feedback and if they have questions or specific concerns.
- Confirm the next meeting time and review training goals to work on till then.

FEEDBACK AND PROGRESS TRACKING

For both new grads and experienced early-career doctors, it is imperative to create a feedback plan and stick to it. At the end of each training period, the mentee's skills and knowledge competency related to the period's training objectives should be evaluated and feedback should be provided.

BOX 8.7 FEEDBACK SUMMARY SUGGESTIONS

Suggestions for providing feedback to mentees:

- Professional behaviors—communication, attitude, and teamwork
- Time management—on time for appointments and timely record completion
- Medical records—completeness and conciseness
- Management of procedures—preparation, efficiency, and client communication

You can also ask the mentee to fill out a self-assessment survey, which gives them the opportunity to reflect on challenges and successes since the last assessment period as well as evaluate the progress on their goals. Feedback should also be solicited informally or formally, from key staff members as their perspectives, experiences, and interactions with the mentee may reveal valuable information. Once the mentee's self-assessment is complete and feedback solicited and compiled from the team, develop a concise feedback summary to review with the mentee. See Box 8.7 for a list of suggested items to include in the feedback summary.

Use the information gathered from the mentee's self-assessment and feedback summary to determine the training objectives for the next period. Work with your mentee to continue developing skills that need additional support, while also adding new objectives and updated goals for the next period.

Expectations and agreements made with the mentee should have language detailing a willingness to accept constructive feedback, but you can work with them on how they prefer to receive it. Some prefer in-the-moment feedback while others favor a private meeting away from distraction and eavesdropping team members. Mentees that are resistant to feedback should be questioned as to the reasons for their resistance. If a mentor experiences escalating resistance or hostility from the mentee, they should reach out to additional members of the hospital leadership team for assistance. The mentee's expectations should include a willingness to be honest and openly communicate in all situations, including receiving feedback.

For more detailed information about feedback, see Chapter 12.

RECOMMENDATION FOR TRAINING HANDS-ON SKILLS

Training skills should involve the whole team. An RVT competent and experienced in anesthesia would be a good trainer to help the mentee get accustomed to the anesthetic equipment and practice's anesthesia protocols. An experienced client service representative can help train a new doctor on how the practice's scheduling procedures work or how the practice handles client requests for medication refills. Another veterinarian in the practice may be more experienced in surgery than the mentor and will be the one scrubbing into surgery with the mentee. There are many ways to leverage the team to help in the training efforts. Solid communication and expectations for the team members involved in mentorship activities will ensure that the training gets done effectively and efficiently. In the example of the RVT assisting in anesthesia training, they should be informed and agree in advance that they will be the primary trainer in this area. They should be directed on the specific training objectives to cover with the mentee as well as their role in direct supervision of the mentee during the training period.

For training surgical and dental skills, the mentor or other trainer should be aware of and agree to the schedule of training days, what procedures will be scheduled, and details on what they will be doing when working with a mentee in surgery. They can work with the mentee directly to wean their active involvement with the case from scrubbing in and assisting with the procedure to eventually just being available during the time the mentee is in surgery. Mentees that are not confident even in routine spay and neuter surgeries should be encouraged to gain more experience doing volunteer surgery days at a local shelter or humane society. Encourage them to shadow other doctors doing procedures at the practice on their nonscheduled days.

KNOWLEDGE-BASED SKILLS TRAINING

Assessing and training the mentee's knowledge are done on a continual basis mainly by case discussion and review of medical records. Answering the mentee's questions when they arise may be helpful in knowing where they struggle, but pointed case discussions and feedback from medical records review should occur during formal face-to-face meetings. Some mentees need time to process the information and formulate responses. If your mentee prefers to prepare for a meeting, send them a short agenda that includes cases and topics to discuss. Feedback, especially if critical feedback, should only be delivered in person. Case discussion, knowledge assessment, and delivering feedback should occur and be documented at each official meeting, no less than once a month.

It can be helpful to ask your early-career doctor how they learn best. Understanding their learning style will help you be a more effective mentor and trainer. See Table 8.4 for examples of different learning styles and training resource options. You can also use this conversation to encourage your mentee to develop independent learning habits. They should be expected to seek out information on their own rather than relying solely on others for answers—a critical skill, especially when another doctor may not be available for immediate feedback.

Guide your mentee in identifying trusted sources of information. While Google searches can be a starting point, it's important they learn how to validate what they find. Providing access to reputable resources such as online veterinary communities (e.g., VIN.com), continuing education platforms (e.g., VetGirlOnTheRun.com), and textbooks or reference materials from the practice library can help set them up for success.

OTHER RECOMMENDATIONS FOR MENTORING

- Look ahead at the schedule to see what is coming in to prepare.
- Have the mentee read up about anything they may need to brush up on before seeing a particular case or scrubbing into any surgery.
- Train the mentee to think about necessary equipment/tools to have ready for the case at hand.
- Create a safe space for the mentee to ASK for help when needed before getting into a situation, especially if performing a medical or surgical procedure they are unfamiliar with.
- Look for alternative procedure training opportunities (e.g., scrub in with another doctor or practice on a cadaver).

Table 8.4 Learning Styles and Recommended Training Methods or Resources

Learning style	Examples of training methods or resources
Visual	Flowcharts, diagrams, images, videos, and shadowing
Auditory	Podcasts, webinars, and giving verbal step-by-step instructions
Hands-on	Have them demonstrate a technique, repetition, and cadavers
Reading/writing	Journal or web articles, books, and AI-assisted medical record platforms

Source: Islander Veterinary Business Consultants/with permission of Jill Muraoka

- Keep an open mind and search for creative ways of training if the mentee's progress is not going in the right direction.
- Train your mentee to pay attention to what is working and what is not working so that they learn from each situation or treatment plan.
- Team up more experienced staff members with your mentee so they can help guide them in items such as how to use the practice management software program, how to submit a radiograph read request, learning which ER facilities and specialists are available in local area, or working with them to improve efficiency.
- Give the mentee longer time blocks that scale down over time as they become more confident (e.g., if you normally schedule 30-minute appointments, give the mentee some 45-minute blocks till they feel comfortable).
- Consider scheduling mentees wellness and easy illness exams for the first few weeks until both the mentee and mentor are comfortable with expanding appointment types.
- Procedure scheduling (dentals, surgery, etc.) should be mutually agreed upon with the mentee and mentor.

The assessments, learning plan, and feedback notes should be documented, filed in the mentee's employee file, and shared with them as well. This is important for transparency and tracking progress. This will also be helpful information when it comes time for formal performance reviews. Tracking of knowledge and skills can also be accomplished by utilizing a digital tool such as the online training management platform, VetLevelUP.com. This platform allows you to custom build and manage training checklists without the hassle of utilizing paper-based checklists that often get lost or forgotten about. This way, as you move through assessments and training with your mentee, it is a simple and effective way to sign off on your mentee's skills and knowledge. Figure 8.5 has a screenshot of an example using the platform to track training progress on specific skills and knowledge.

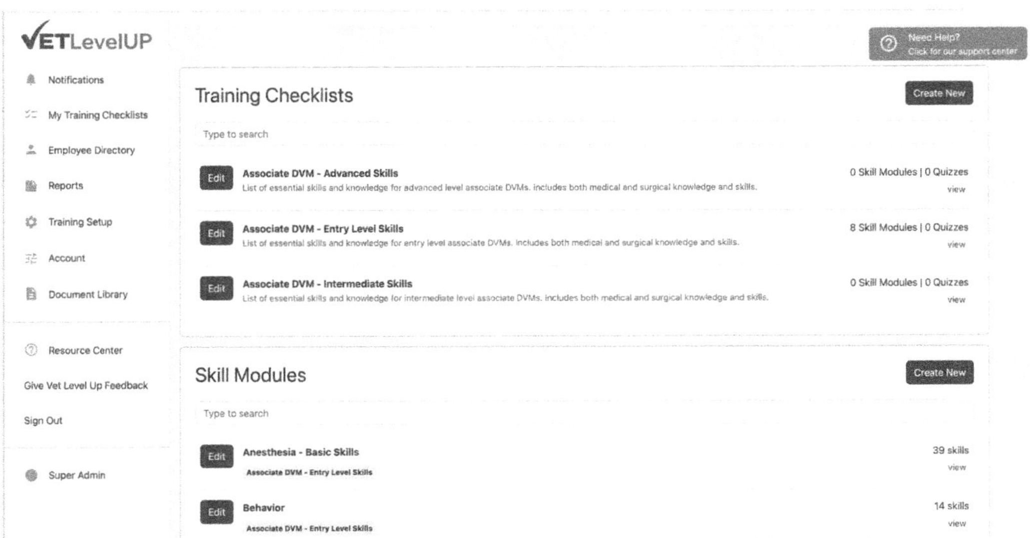

FIGURE 8.5 Vet Level UP screenshot. *Source:* with permission from vetlevelup.com

CONCLUSION

Training the next generation of our young veterinarians is imperative to the health and wellness of our animal friends, our society and to our beloved profession. Mentorship is vital to this process and can be done with each and every hospital system that embraces its value.

Remember the key steps to training your mentee for clinical competency:

- Define roles and set clear expectations for the mentor, mentee, hospital manager, and team. Set the expectations in writing and get everyone to agree to those expectations.
- Create a training plan with attainable goals and keep to a regular meeting schedule.
- Provide proper and timely feedback.

Successful mentorship programs have a strong element of team support. New veterinarians need constant support from the whole team, not just from the mentor. It doesn't take long to get a new graduate up to speed when the proper intention and guidance are put in place. There needs to be a genuine willingness, effort, and care from the entire hospital team to help make our new generation of veterinarians successful. At the end of the day, it's all about the animals. We need to remember that we are all here for the same purpose where fostering a culture of caring and mentorship helps build a strong foundation to providing our animal patients and clients with the best possible care and service.

BIBLIOGRAPHY

American Veterinary Medical Association (AVMA) (2022). Accreditation policies and procedures of the AVMA Council on Education. https://www.avma.org/education/accreditation-policies-and-procedures-avma-council-education (accessed 28 April 2022).

Cary, J.A., Farnsworth, C.H., Gay, J., and Carroll, H.S. (2017). Stakeholder expectations regarding the ability of new veterinary graduates to perform various diagnostic and surgical procedures. *Journal of the American Veterinary Medical Association* 251 (2): 172. https://doi.org/10.2460/javma.2.1.2.172.

Elce, Y. (2021). The mentor-mentee relationship, addressing challenges in veterinary medicine together. *The Veterinary Clinics of North America. Small Animal Practice* 51 (5): 1099–1109. https://doi.org/10.1016/j.cvsm.2021.04.023. (Epub 2021 Jul 6. PMID: 34238600).

Simons, M.C., Hunt, J.A., and Anderson, S.L. (2022). What's the evidence? A review of current instruction and assessment in veterinary surgical education. *Veterinary Surgery* 51 (5): 731–743. https://doi.org/10.1111/vsu.13819.

Yi, J., Adams, C., Chalhoub, S. et al. (2024). Student and clinical educator perceptions of the impacts of COVID-19 on final-year veterinary clinical training in a distributed learning model. *Journal of Veterinary Medical Education* 51 (4): 461–472. https://doi.org/10.3138/jvme-2023-0004.

Communication

CHAPTER 9

INTRODUCTION

Dani Rabwin

Communication is the cornerstone of veterinary practice, yet it is also one of the most complex skills for new graduates to master. From the exam room to the treatment area to the digital space, the way veterinarians and their teams communicate shapes trust, efficiency, well-being, and, ultimately, patient outcomes. While clinical skills may get the most attention in veterinary education, it is the quality of communication—how we listen, explain, collaborate, and connect—that determines whether care is understood and acted upon.

To address these multifaceted communication challenges, I invited three outstanding contributors to this chapter because they bring complementary expertise to the many dimensions of communication in veterinary mentorship. Amanda Donnelly, DVM, MBA, is a nationally recognized consultant and speaker. She grounds this chapter in client communication essentials—helping mentees develop the skills to build trust, strengthen relationships, and navigate difficult conversations with pet owners and their families. Alyssa Mages, BS, CVT, FVTE, draws on her deep experience in team development and education to explore communication within the veterinary team, focusing on structured tools, collaborative strategies, and inclusive dialogue that empower veterinarians and credentialed technicians alike. Finally, Caitlin DeWilde, DVM, practicing veterinarian and founder of TheSocialDVM, brings forward the rapidly evolving digital landscape of veterinary communication, showing how technology, social media, and telemedicine can be leveraged without sacrificing professionalism or wellness.

Together, their perspectives highlight that communication in veterinary medicine is not a single skill, but a continuum: it begins with the individual conversation in the exam room, extends into the collaborative language of the team, and now, more than ever, reaches into the digital channels where our clients live. Mentors play a critical role in guiding new veterinarians across all of these domains, modeling effective communication while equipping them with both practical techniques and the authentic mindset needed to connect in every setting.

EFFECTIVE CLIENT COMMUNICATION

Amanda L. Donnelly

I fell in love with veterinary medicine growing up and working at my father's small animal hospital. By the time I started veterinary school at the University of Missouri, I had a tremendous amount of real-world knowledge about practice. During my studies, I completed four, eight-week clinical rotations: two at my father's practice, one at a practice in Florida, and a surgical rotation under supervision in Las Vegas.

During my first job in Wilmington, North Carolina, I quickly discovered that I had a lot to learn, especially about client communications. It wasn't as easy as it seemed when Dad was talking to pet owners. I'll never forget seeing a small lump on a boxer and being proud of the fact that I knew to tell the clients the mass should be biopsied. I made a cavalier reference to the frequency of cancer in boxers. It wasn't until my boss called me into his office later that I found out the clients were upset with my lack of empathy and professionalism. I thought I was an expert communicator, but I wasn't.

As a new graduate and young veterinarian, it would have helped to have a mentor to guide me through client communications. I wish I knew then what I know now. Despite my interest in client communications, mastering these skills on my own required years of dedicated practice.

In this section, we'll review key communications veterinarians need to know to connect with pet owners, build client loyalty, and help pets get the care they need. You'll find specific exercises and suggestions for how to help mentees apply specific communication skills in scenarios they face in practice.

CLIENT ENGAGEMENT

The Gallup Organization defines customer engagement as making an emotional connection with people such that they become emotionally satisfied customers and feel bonded to a business. Their research shows that customers who are emotionally rather than rationally satisfied spend more, become loyal, and refer more people to the business (Fleming and Asplund, 2007). This concept applies equally in veterinary medicine with our clients and is critical to practice success as it forms the foundation for both client loyalty and compliance.

To reach higher levels of client engagement, veterinarians need to make authentic connections and appreciate the value of building a trusted relationship with clients rather than just being a healthcare provider. For busy practitioners, it's easy to focus on moving from one appointment to the next, forgetting to recognize the unique needs of each client. When this happens, clients might not feel heard or understand the value of service recommendations.

Mentors can guide mentees in developing essential communication skills that build trust and rapport with pet owners. Most importantly, mentors should emphasize that enhancing client engagement fundamentally improves patient outcomes and preserves the cherished human–animal bond.

If we don't meet the client's needs, we might not have the opportunity to meet the pet's needs.

CLIENT ENGAGEMENT SKILLS

In my work as a consultant and trainer, I've noticed veterinarians sometimes miss the opportunity to connect with pet owners using simple communication skills such as using the client's name and the pet's name, thanking owners for their trust, reassuring statements, and praising a client for how well they take care of their pet.

MENTOR TIP

Use the exercises throughout this section as discussion starters or role-play activities with your mentees to help them build confidence and skill in client communication.

EXERCISE CLIENT CONNECTION

- *What communication skills or approaches could you use to show clients you're interested in them?*
- *How could you express appreciation for your relationship with a client?*

CORE COMMUNICATION SKILLS

Research on doctor–patient communications in human medicine has served as the foundation for studies on veterinary–client communications. Communication is a core clinical skill essential to clinical competence, alongside physical examination, medical knowledge, and problem-solving (Shaw, 2006). Research in both human and veterinary medicine shows that communications can be taught and are learned skills. Using the four core communications described below can lead to better patient outcomes, more collaborative client relationships, and greater adherence to treatment recommendations. Mentors play an integral role in guiding mentees to understand and apply these core communications in specific situations to help both clients and patients.

1. **Nonverbal Communication**

   Nonverbal communication is often more powerful than verbal communication because regardless of what we say, our body language also tells a story. Veterinarians who pay attention to their own nonverbal communication as well as that of clients can build trust and develop stronger relationships.

   The Veterinarian's Nonverbal Communication

   Most people would agree that we tend to form impressions of others within seconds. Key nonverbal skills that create positive impressions:

   - Smile
   - Make eye contact
   - Raise your eyebrows
   - Keep a relaxed body posture
   - Lean in slightly (Goman, 2008)

EXERCISE NONVERBAL COMMUNICATION

- *What are some examples of when your nonverbal communication might not match your verbal communication?*
- *Encourage mentees to avoid incongruent nonverbal messages such as a forced smile that indicates impatience despite positive words or making reassuring statements while having a hand on the doorknob signaling a desire to leave.*

The Client's Nonverbal Communication

Clients' nonverbal communication provides clues about their thoughts and feelings. Signs that a client is in a hurry might include glancing at a cellphone, pacing, or standing near the door. Anger might show through a clenched jaw, lip-biting, or crossed arms. Anxious clients might clutch their pet or seem reluctant to talk, while sad clients may cry or look down. Confusion or skepticism often appears as furrowed brows or raised eyebrows.

Remind mentees to observe nonverbal messages from all of the pet's caregivers and look for any evidence of disharmony or different emotions. For example, one person might nod in agreement while their spouse shows skepticism, or one owner might be crying while another remains stoic. These contrasting reactions require attention.

Encourage young veterinarians to acknowledge clients' emotions directly: "Mr. Taylor, I noticed you looking at your watch. Are you on a tight timetable?" This gives the veterinarian an opportunity to show compassion and problem-solving rather than rushing through the appointment. An excellent response is "I'm so sorry you've had to wait. I know that is frustrating and your time is valuable. Would it work better for you to leave Jake with us and pick him up later today?"

2. Open-Ended Questions

Closed-ended questions can be answered with "yes," "no," or single-word responses, while open-ended questions invite expanded answers that help build trusted relationships. They create opportunities to learn more about the patient, the pet owner, and their special bond.

Some veterinarians might not recognize the value of using open-ended questions during an appointment simply to connect with a client. Or they might ask a question such as "How are you doing today?" which isn't engaging and often leads to a short response of "fine."

After establishing relationships with clients, asking open-ended questions become more natural. Initiating meaningful conversation with new clients, however, can be more challenging. Mentors can assist mentees with learning to apply this skill by suggesting that they have some "go-to" questions to use in the exam room to connect with clients. It's also helpful to inform them that the best open-ended questions often start with the words "how," "what," or "tell me." Here are examples:

- "How do you like living in Nashville?"
- "How did you decide to get a Golden Doodle?"
- "What kind of toys does Gidget play with?"
- "How did you decide to name him Gunny?"
- "Tell me how you spend time with Finn."

3. Empathy Statements

To become proficient in conveying empathy, mentees need to understand the difference between empathy and sympathy. Empathy is generally defined as the ability to sense another person's emotions and imagine what someone else might be thinking or feeling. Sympathy on the other hand is feeling bad for someone or identifying with their feelings. The YouTube video, Brené Brown on Empathy, offers an excellent explanation of the difference between these two communications (RSA, 2013). Expressing empathy can be more difficult because it involves being vulnerable and reaching a deeper connection with someone.

Empathy builds trust and client loyalty by making people feel heard and understood. When clients' emotional needs are addressed, they're better positioned to focus on their pet's medical needs, leading to improved compliance and outcomes.

Veterinarians who master empathy skills find that interactions with emotional pet owners become less stressful and more rewarding.

Guide mentees to approach empathy as a two-part process: first, understanding and appreciating the client's predicament or feelings, and second, supportively communicating that understanding to them. Help mentees practice both components of empathy to develop this essential skill.

Be Attentive

Appreciating someone's feelings involves being fully present with them. This doesn't mean you have to feel as the person feels or that you have to have experienced their feelings. What's important is to strive to understand what the *pet owner is feeling*. So, often in veterinary medicine, we try to fix the problem without spending enough time expressing empathy.

Think of empathy as a communication skill where "less is more" meaning less talking and more listening is the key to success. The nonverbal communications of eye contact, a caring facial expression, leaning in, and an open body posture are all part of expressing empathy.

Respond Empathetically

Veterinarians might tend to express sympathy rather than empathy. Since sympathy is feeling sorry for someone and sharing their feelings, it might come across as "glossing over" the difficult situation someone is in. Here are examples of sympathy phrases to avoid:

- "I'm so sorry you lost your job. I'm sure you'll bounce back."
- "That is awful. The same thing happened to me."
- "At least Bella doesn't have a more serious condition."

By contrast, empathy statements don't express pity, are more personal, and strive to convey a deeper level of understanding. Think about focusing on the client's feelings. Here are examples:

- "I can see by your expression that this is very upsetting."
- "Oh, I can imagine that must have been so frustrating."
- "I'm so sorry Bella isn't feeling well and I understand your concern."

4. Reflective Listening

Most veterinarians are familiar with using a reflective listening statement to summarize or repeat back to a client what they said as a way to confirm an understanding of information they communicated about their pet's clinical signs. Beyond simple confirmation, reflective listening can powerfully invite clients to share more information, helping uncover hidden feelings, emotions, or motivations. This technique is especially valuable during discussions about serious medical conditions, when assessing the client's understanding and willingness to provide care is crucial. Effective examples include:

- "I'm hearing you say you think Oliver's quality of life is not good, is that correct?"
- "I'm sensing you feel like you've done everything you could for Chloe."
- "I understand you have some budget constraints for what you can spend today."
- "It sounds like you're feeling discouraged by Tigger's response to treatment."

If veterinarians make erroneous assumptions, clients have the opportunity to clarify their thoughts and feelings or to provide additional information.

EXERCISE CORE COMMUNICATION SKILLS

1. *Identify a client's nonverbal cue (folded arms and checking phone) and have mentees interpret the potential message and formulate an appropriate response.*
2. *Practice asking each other open-ended questions to get to know each other better. Discuss which questions lead to the most information. Then discuss questions that could be used to connect with clients.*
3. *Share real-world examples of when to convey empathy. Practice saying empathy statements out loud.*
4. *Role-play scenarios where a reflective listening statement would be appropriate to learn more about a client's thoughts.*

Homework assignment: Look for the client's story.

Prompt mentees to ask clients open-ended questions to learn more about the bond they share with their pet. During the next meeting, discuss what they learned and what questions were most informative.

COMMUNICATION CHANNELS

Veterinarians routinely communicate with clients across all communication channels including text, email, phone, and video calls. Encourage mentees to apply communication skills across all communication channels. For example, nonverbal communication remains critical during video calls, just as in face-to-face interactions.

However, there are some limitations of communication skills in certain situations. Conveying empathy is appropriate in texts but may lack the power it would have when conveyed in the exam room. And of course, email exchanges limit the ability to engage in meaningful conversations.

GATHERING INFORMATION

I've observed veterinarians who don't take time to connect with pet owners at the beginning of an appointment. They tend to rush the process of gathering a patient's history and often start their physical exam while talking to a client about the pet's clinical signs. This approach risks missing critical information, fails to build trust, and misses the opportunity to communicate the value of a thorough examination.

Rather than looking at information gathering as a task to be completed, think of it as a time to be curious and get to know clients.

ATTENTIVE LISTENING

Soliciting an accurate, complete patient history is critical, which is why it's best to ask for initial information before examining the patient unless there is an urgent situation. As clients explain their pet's clinical signs, medical history, and concerns, it's important to avoid interrupting them. Unfortunately, this doesn't always happen.

Research in human medicine has shown that only 23–28% of patients participating in a study completed their opening concerns before physicians interrupted them typically within 12–23 seconds (Kurtz et al., 2005). A similar study in companion animal practice revealed that, in appointments where a veterinarian solicited the client's concerns, they interrupted the pet owner 55% of the time. The median time clients spoke before being interrupted was 11 seconds. When this happened, clients were only given the opportunity to complete their responses in 28% of appointments (Dysart et al., 2011).

Mentors can share these three reasons why attentive listening is imperative when soliciting a patient history:

- Interrupting might be perceived as a sign of disrespect and a lack of interest in what the client has to say.
- Attentive listening ensures clinicians don't miss relevant details about the patient's medical history or any client concerns.
- Concerns that aren't uncovered initially may come up at the end of appointments, which decreases efficiency and may involve the need to change a treatment plan.

When possible, mentors should observe mentees during appointments or review recordings to assess and improve their listening skills.

EXERCISE ATTENTIVE LISTENING

Ask mentees to self-reflect on their listening skills with these questions:

- *If I asked your friends if you're a good listener, what would they say?*
- *How do you think you could be a better listener?*

HISTORY TAKING

To gather a thorough history, it's best to start with one or more broad open-ended question and then funnel into close-ended questions as appropriate. Using open-ended questions encourages the client to tell the entire story of how their pet is doing. By following this approach, veterinarians can be more organized and efficient.

EXERCISE ROLE-PLAY HISTORY-TAKING PROCESS

Scenario #1
A Labrador Retriever presents with vomiting and lethargy of 36-hour duration. The first broad question might be:

- *"Tell me everything you've noticed since Jake started acting abnormally."*

Follow with focused open-ended questions:

- *"What did the vomit look like?"*
- *"Tell me about Jake's regular diet."*
- *"What do you think might be causing Jake's vomiting?"*

Conclude with targeted closed-ended questions:

- *"When was the last time Jake ate?"*
- *"Has he had a bowel movement in the last 36 hours?"*
- *"Has he done any retching like he's trying to vomit?"*

Scenario #2
When investigating nutrition-related concerns, "What diet are you feeding?" will only yield brand names. Instead, try:

- *"Tell me everything Gidget eats from the time she gets up till she goes to sleep at night."*

  If you asked me this question, I'll tell you Gidget eats 10–12 kibbles of food each night when we play fetch, a treat when she goes into her crate, small pieces of lettuce most nights, and that she licks my cereal bowl and dinner dishes. This history leads to further open-ended questions:

- *"What kind of treats do you give her?"*
- *"How much food is left on your plates?"*

Follow-up closed-ended questions might be:

- *"Have you tried cutting back on any snacks or treats?"*
- *"Have you changed Gidget's brand of food in the last six months?"*

REFLECTIVE LISTENING

As noted earlier, a reflective listening statement is a beneficial response to a client who communicates their pet's symptoms and history. A veterinarian might paraphrase what a client told them by saying:

- "So, Jake vomited once Monday night, twice yesterday, and this morning he's sluggish and doesn't want to go on a walk."

This shows the doctor was listening and interested in gaining a complete history. A client can then confirm that this is accurate or add additional details.

EXERCISE REFLECTIVE LISTENING

Let's say a pet owner brings in a dog that had a grand mal seizure at home. Ask mentees how they might respond with a reflective listening statement to demonstrate compassion.

Appropriate responses: "My gosh, he kept you up all night" or "It sounds like that was really scary for you."

CLIENT EDUCATION

When I graduated veterinary school, I felt that my primary roles were to provide the best patient care and educate clients about their pet's needs. I always wanted to share my knowledge so clients would know how to best care for their pet. Most of the time people seemed to appreciate my expertise and agreed with my proposed treatment plan. As a consultant, I've seen that the one-sided, paternalistic approach I followed still plays out in many exam room communications. Established communication habits are hard to break. Even after I learned about new models of communication, I've caught myself a few times giving a "lecture" to a friend about what food they should feed or telling a family member what treatment they should provide for their pet.

Newer models of veterinary–client communications promote a more collaborative approach. Studies have shown multiple positive outcomes when veterinarians use a relationship-centered care approach focused on developing a partnership with clients. One study found pet owners were more likely to adhere to treatment recommendations and had a greater level of satisfaction with this approach (Kanji et al., 2012). Another study showed that when veterinary teams are trained to use specific communication skills such as open-ended questions, clients felt more involved in appointments and that their veterinarian was more interested in their opinion (Shaw et al., 2016).

ASK QUESTIONS TO CREATE A CONVERSATION

Today's clients view pets as family members and come equipped with internet research. They appreciate veterinarians who ask what they want to discuss rather than dictating the agenda. Asking questions throughout appointments helps clients feel heard and enables veterinarians to provide personalized information. Clients of all ages now expect to be involved in decisions about their pet's care.

Mentors can help early career veterinarians practice communications that support forming a partnership with the client rather than talking "at" them, which might not be well received. Let's examine client education skills that help ensure veterinarians meet the needs of each client.

ASSESS CLIENT KNOWLEDGE

Open-ended questions are an excellent way to assess a client's knowledge level about their pet's preventive care so doctors can avoid making assumptions about what a pet owner does or does not know. Asking relevant questions not only helps to personalize education but can also increase efficiency if a client already has knowledge of a particular topic.

For sick pets or those with medical conditions, open-ended questions help identify what clients know and what misconceptions or misinformation they might have from their own research.

EXERCISE CLIENTS' KNOWLEDGE

Propose an exam room scenario and ask mentees what they would ask to determine a client's knowledge. Here are examples of good questions:

- *"How familiar are you with leptospirosis infections in dogs?"*
- *"How much do you know about congestive heart disease?"*
- *"What have you read about treating allergies in dogs?"*

UNCOVER CLIENT THOUGHTS AND FEELINGS

I once observed a veterinarian meet with two men whose 17-year-old cat had suffered retinal detachment and blindness from hypertension. After a brief greeting, she asked, "How do you feel about living with a blind cat?" This perfect question prompted them to share crucial information about their concerns. Without uncovering these insights, she might have missed addressing their specific worries before discussing the cat's long-term treatment plan.

Pet owners often experience emotions—anger, sadness, fear, guilt, and grief—that affect their medical decisions but remain unspoken. Direct questions help uncover these hidden thoughts and feelings. Here are examples:

- "What's most important to you about Sam's dental health and well-being?"
- "Tell me how you're feeling about what we've discussed so far?"
- "Are you feeling scared because Molly has to go under anesthesia?"

RESPONDING TO DIFFICULT CLIENT INQUIRIES AND MISINFORMATION

New graduates often struggle with "Dr. Google"—clients who arrive with internet research about their pet's condition. Sometimes clients are transparent about their Internet searches, and in other instances, they might claim knowledge that is related to misinformation they found online.

Talk with mentees about how to manage their frustration and to ideally see these situations as an opportunity to connect with pet owners. Encourage them to avoid telling clients that what they found online is inaccurate, which is likely to come across as a defensive response. Saying "Unfortunately that's erroneous information" or "That's not a good website" will sound judgmental.

Instead, encourage mentees to maintain dialogue with questions and statements that show genuine interest in the client's research and foster collaboration:

- "I love that you've been exploring information about Josie's condition"
- "It sounds like you've done some research. Tell me a little more about that."
- "I know there's quite a bit of information out there. May I share with you some of the research I'm familiar with?"

Regardless of the information's accuracy, we can always compliment clients on how much they care for their pets and invite them to explore further by providing written educational materials and/or directing them to trustworthy websites.

EXERCISE CLIENT EDUCATION

Present mentees with a specific scenario such as a dog they suspect has Cushing's disease or a cat with clinical signs of osteoarthritis. Review how to approach the exam room communications and have them answer these questions:

- *What is your goal for the appointment?*
- *What do you think the client's goals are and how would you find out?*
- *What skills would you use to educate the client about their pet's possible disease condition?*
- *What specific phrases would you use?*

PATIENT CARE RECOMMENDATIONS

Today's clients want to partner with the veterinary team and be fully empowered to make decisions for their pet. They want to be an active participant in their pet's care rather than a passive listener of recommendations. Specific communication skills can be used to form a collaborative relationship that empowers pet parents and helps them see the veterinarian as their trusted advisor.

CHUNK AND CHECK

One of the clinical communication skills that doesn't get much attention is that of chunking and checking when talking to pet owners. The process involves giving clients small amounts of information and then checking for their understanding before proceeding with a question such as "What questions do you have about what I've covered so far?" This technique is valuable because it ensures that veterinarians don't overwhelm clients with more information than they can reasonably process. Likewise, it gives clients an opportunity to ask questions about the information that is presented.

Using chunking and checking also allows veterinarians to assess how much information a client would like to know about their pet's health and possible treatment plans. I recall listening to a veterinarian interact with a couple who presented their cat for examination of a skin lesion that had been present for six months. The doctor gave a detailed, lengthy explanation of all the possible underlying causes of the skin lesion as well as multiple treatment options. I could see the clients were confused; due to the information overload, they weren't sure what was the most likely diagnosis or which treatment plan was being recommended.

EXERCISE CHUNK AND CHECK

Discuss how to present information in various scenarios. For example, here are ways to check in with a client who is hearing for the first time that their pet has heart disease:

Veterinarian:	*"How much do you know about managing congestive heart failure?"*
Client:	*"I've never had a dog with heart problems, so I don't know much."*
Veterinarian:	*"There's quite a lot of information that I can share about CHF in dogs and all the medications we might use for treatment. Some of my clients want to know as much as possible and others prefer to just focus on what's most important right now. How much information would you like me to share?"*

Client:	*"Well, I'd like to know what treatment you recommend right now, how long you think Hannah will live and what her quality of life will be like."*
Veterinarian:	*"I know we covered a lot today. Are there any other questions you'd like to ask or additional concerns that you'd like to address?"*
Client:	*"Is it OK if she still goes for walks?"*

SHARED DECISION-MAKING

Shared decision-making involves collaborating with clients to help them choose the best treatment plan for their pet and family. Instead of dictating "This is what I recommend," veterinarians guide clients through options. This approach builds deeper trust and understanding. It also avoids assumptions about client preferences or financial constraints. Instead, veterinarians transparently present options while explaining the potential consequences and benefits of each choice.

For example, in the case of a vomiting dog, the veterinarian could say "Based on Max's clinical signs and physical exam, the most likely causes of his vomiting are non-specific gastroenteritis or pancreatitis. However, we can't rule out the possibility of an obstruction, liver disease or other endocrine diseases. Since his vomiting could be associated with an upset stomach or a more serious medical condition, let's discuss the pros and cons of two different approaches. How does that sound?"

The veterinarian would then compare conservative care (bland diet and medication) with diagnostic testing to rule out serious conditions. This approach centers on the client and pet's needs while still allowing the veterinarian to indicate which plan might yield the best outcome.

SPECTRUM OF CARE

In 2021, the American Association of Veterinary Medical Colleges established the Spectrum of Care Initiative to provide guidance and enhance SOC training in veterinary education. A key aspect of spectrum of care practice is to consider all the factors that might influence a care plan including the pet owner's financial constraints. Some clients might elect care even if it means going into debt while others have limited ability to pay even with credit. When speaking about spectrum of care options, the goal is to identify a client's barriers to providing care and to clearly communicate the risks and benefits of different treatment plans (Brown et al., 2021).

The idea isn't to immediately recommend the least expensive option when a client complains about fees but rather to engage in transparent, caring conversations about the continuum of care options and to be responsive to any financial limitations. Discussing various treatment approaches and finances allows veterinarians to provide some level of care for more pets. For example, foregoing diagnostics and performing outpatient treatment might be an option for some patients. We don't want someone to feel guilty or judged because they can't adhere to the gold standard of care. Likewise, we need to be realistic about what care clients can provide for their pets.

EXERCISE SHARED DECISION-MAKING

Ask: What would you ask or say to support a collaborative approach to client decision-making. Here are examples:

- *"Tell me about your budget for today's visit."*
- *"How do you think Max will do with treatment at home?"*
- *"What questions do you have about Tigger's treatment options?"*

CONVEY CLEAR RECOMMENDATIONS

When I listen to veterinarian—client communications, at times I hear a lack of clarity which can be confusing for pet owners. Being transparent about different treatment options doesn't mean we avoid making clear recommendations. Here are examples of unclear recommendations to avoid:

- "If you decide to have him neutered, we can do that."
- "You should probably consider scheduling a dental"
- "We can schedule the dentistry procedure when you have time."

Since this language doesn't express a sense of urgency or the need to provide care within a specific time period, a client is not likely to make an appointment.

I've also heard veterinarians give clients a list of all possible rule outs for the pet's medical condition followed by a list of multiple options for treatment. They might sound like this:

- "You could take antibiotics. . ..."
- "We can try medication and see if that helps"
- "I'm thinking doing X-rays and lab testing would be helpful."

EXERCISE CLEAR RECOMMENDATIONS

Ask: How can you convey clear recommendations? To ensure clarity, mentees can practice making recommendations such as these:

- *"I recommend we schedule the dentistry procedure for Chooli now. My team will help you with scheduling."*
- *"In my experience, the best approach to treatment is. . ..."*
- *"I recommend doing both abdominal X-rays and comprehensive lab testing so we can find out what's causing Scooter's vomiting."*

COMMUNICATE VALUE

Before clients embrace the value of veterinary services, they must fully appreciate the need for care. Expressing a patient's needs is fairly easy when a patient is injured, sick, or uncomfortable, but it is often more difficult to articulate the need for preventive care when a pet is healthy. Clients might question the need for annual laboratory testing, for example, if their pet doesn't have any signs of illness.

After establishing needs, veterinarians must clearly communicate treatment benefits—an area where many fall short. When recommending dental care, practitioners often explain the process (preanesthetic testing, radiographs, anesthesia, cleaning, extractions, and medications) but fail to emphasize the benefits. While clients want quality care, they approve treatment plans based on perceived value.

Mentors can assist mentees with a "needs and benefits" exercise. Name a treatment, test, procedure or surgery and ask the mentee to describe the patient's needs and at least one benefit for the service or product. The chart below gives examples (Table 9.1).

Table 9.1 Patient Needs and Benefits of Services

Service	Needs	Benefits
Intravenous fluids	Correct dehydration	Better prognosis
	Improve perfusion	Quicker recovery
		Home sooner; feel better
Dentistry procedures	Eliminate plaque, infection	Eliminate pain
	Remove loose teeth	Slow progression of disease
		Improved quality of life
		Longer
Annual wellness laboratory testing	Early disease detection	Trends data
	Early intervention	Live longer, healthier life
		Peace of mind

For role-playing exercises, here are examples of how to effectively communicate the benefits (value) of oral healthcare to clients:

- "Mrs. Jones, the dental radiographs help us fully evaluate the health of Bella's teeth and reveal conditions such as bone loss, tooth root tip infections, and other abnormalities below the gumline. The benefit is that I can then perform any necessary treatments to make sure she stays healthy."
- "I'll remove Sophie's infected tooth and suture the gums after the extraction. Then I'll look for evidence of other teeth that may need to be extracted. The benefit of this procedure is to eliminate any pain and prevent progression of disease."

Mentors should help mentees learn to clearly articulate the unique benefits of recommended treatments. If pet owners are left to believe two or three treatment options are equally beneficial, they might gravitate toward the least expensive and least scary plan. Since clients generally don't have the medical knowledge to decide which treatment or products are best, they need the veterinarian to provide guidance.

Rather than simply saying "I recommend laboratory testing" here are phrases that bring the client into shared decision-making and communicate a clear recommendation:

- "The benefit of laboratory testing is that we will gain valuable information that will help us know how to best treat Sophie. The risk of not doing the testing is that we may not uncover whether she is dehydrated or has evidence of pancreatitis. What are your thoughts?"
- "My exam of Luna indicates she is experiencing some pain in her hips. I recommend we X-ray her hips and legs. The benefit of an X-ray is that it shows us whether she has osteoarthritis and the severity of it. It would help me tailor her treatment plan. How does that sound?"

RESPONDING POSITIVELY TO ANGRY CLIENTS

Veterinarians inevitably face angry clients, whether during appointments, over the phone, or when escalated from staff. Mentors should prepare mentees with specific techniques to de-escalate these situations and reduce stress for everyone involved.

COMMUNICATIONS TO FOSTER PARTNERSHIP AND PATIENCE

To defuse anger, first remain calm and remember that most upset clients are motivated by concern for their pet. Signal a desire to help with phrases such as:

- "I want to help you. Tell me a little more about what's upsetting you."
- "Let me see what I can do to get you some more information."

Thank clients for their understanding at the earliest sign of frustration or impatience. A doctor might say:

- "I appreciate your understanding and thank you for your patience."

VALIDATE FEELINGS AND EXPRESS EMPATHY

When facing upset clients, veterinarians need a structured approach to de-escalate the situation. The following flowchart illustrates key response techniques that help acknowledge client emotions while moving toward constructive conversation. Train mentees to recognize when to apply each technique and practice using these specific phrases in role-playing scenarios (Figure 9.1).

NONVIOLENT COMMUNICATION TECHNIQUES

A client's emotions can become heightened despite everyone's best efforts to calm them. This might lead to unacceptable behavior such as continued verbal assaults or other threatening actions. When this happens, veterinarians can respond with the following de-escalation communication technique using parts of the framework for nonviolent communication (Rosenberg, 2003):

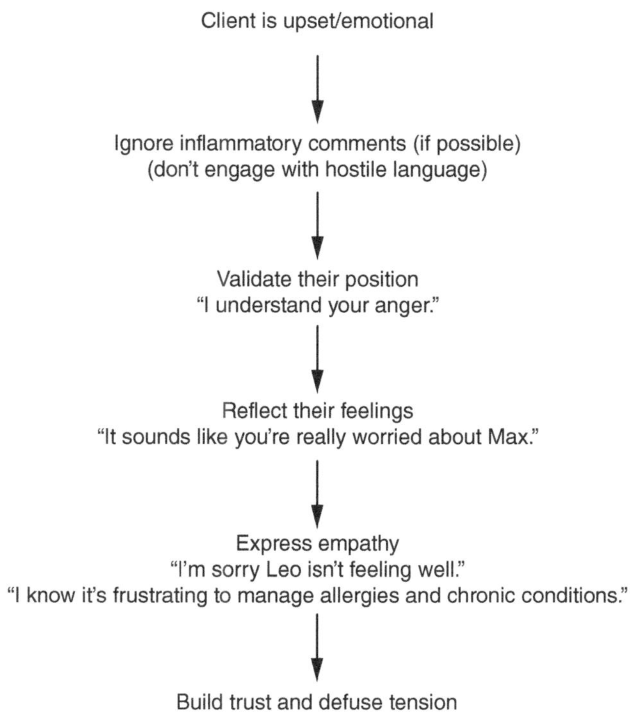

FIGURE 9.1 Flow chart: responding to client emotions. *Source:* Courtesy of Amanda Donnelly.

The two-step process starts with the doctor stating their feelings to signal to the client that the behavior is unacceptable. They might say, “Mr. Jones, I’m feeling uncomfortable with your yelling and profanity” or “Ms. Smith, I’m feeling intimidated by your behavior.”

The next step is to request the client’s cooperation. They might say, “Mr. Jones, my request is that you lower your voice and refrain from cursing” or “Ms. Smith, I need for you to step back and stop throwing anything.”

If a client doesn’t calm down, the next step is to politely fire the pet owner. If this happens, be succinct and clear, stating, for example, “Mr. Jones, it’s evident that despite our best efforts, our hospital is not a good fit for you. We won’t be able to continue to see Max and are happy to send his medical records to whatever veterinary practice you choose.”

DELIVERING BAD NEWS

Communicating a pet’s serious illness, poor prognosis, or death is challenging but inevitable in practice. Mentors should conduct role-playing exercises to prepare mentees for these difficult conversations. Emphasize appropriate nonverbal communication: position yourself at the client’s level and, when seated, at an angle that creates comfortable distance rather than directly adjacent or across from them.

The first communication skill is to signpost the bad news. This is often called a “warning shot” which alerts the client the veterinarian does not have good news and gives them a brief moment to prepare. Here are examples:

- “I’m sorry that I have some bad news.”
- “I’m afraid Chloe’s condition is more serious than we thought.”

Prepare for a client to express a range of emotions and give them time to respond to the news. Advise mentees to validate a client’s feelings and express empathy by saying:

- “I can see this is upsetting and makes you very sad.”
- “I know how much you care about Jake and I appreciate this is worrisome.”
- “I’m so sorry about Davie’s diagnosis.”

Since people might need time to process bad news, remind mentees to use the skill of chunk and check to avoid overwhelming a client with too much detail about treatment or prognosis before they’re ready to hear it. This process gives the client an opportunity to participate in the conversation. It’s also appropriate to see if clients need time to think about how they want to proceed. A doctor can ask “Would you like some time to think about your options or to call someone?”

Veterinarians should be compassionate and realistic about outcomes. Unless the pet has already died, we want to strive to maintain hope and optimism. Even if the outcome looks bleak, this gives a client time to come to terms with their pet’s prognosis and treatment plan. Talk to mentees about how to create a realistic outcome, so a client knows what to expect with statements such as:

- “In my experience, treatment can help Tigger live comfortably for some time.”
- “It can be a challenge treating dogs with congestive heart failure and we’re here to help you manage her medications and care.”

Another difficult scenario involves mistakes or accidents, such as a pet escaping from the practice or medication errors (see Chapter 11 for more on communicating about adverse medical outcomes). These situations require specific communication approaches (Table 9.2).

Table 9.2 Communications to Deliver Bad News When Mistakes Happen

Immediately convey heartfelt sentiments about the clients' feelings and avoid making excuses or giving reasons why the mistake happened.
Next, signpost the bad news.
Then be direct, clear, and transparent that something bad has happened at the practice. State the facts.
Let the client know what is being done to correct the problem or help the patient as well as what will be done to avoid future problems or errors.

Advise mentees to document information about the incident including their client communications in the pet's medical record and that the best way to handle these situations is to apologize and express empathy with phrases like this:

- "I'm so terribly sorry this happened. Please know we're doing everything we can to find Kylie."
- "I can imagine how difficult this is to hear and that you're worried about Max."
- "I understand this is extremely upsetting and we're looking at our protocols to see how we can prevent future mistakes."

TALKING ABOUT MONEY

Veterinary care costs can cause anxiety for pet owners who want the best for their pets while managing their finances responsibly. Mentors should help mentees develop confidence when discussing treatment costs with clients.

We don't want to assume money is the reason for reluctance to accept treatment recommendations. Sometimes spending money is an obstacle because clients don't understand the value of recommended care. The right questions can help clients achieve peace of mind and make decisions that are right for them. Here are appropriate questions to ask when presenting treatment plans:

- "What concerns do you have about Sophie's treatment plan?"
- "What questions do you have about the procedure?"
- "I sense you're frustrated by Tigger's response to treatment. Tell me your thoughts."
- "How can I help you make this decision?"

As patient advocates, veterinarians must emphasize care benefits. Even after initial discussions, clients often need time to process information, so reinforcing how treatments will benefit their pet is important.

The shared decision-making process often reveals clients' financial concerns. When this happens, transparent, supportive conversations about payment options are appreciated. While veterinarians aren't responsible for discussing payment details, they should know what options their practice offers. Make financial conversations more comfortable with statements like:

- "We know veterinary care is expensive and that trying to make decisions about treatment options can be stressful. However, we can discuss a few options and work with you to find what's best for your budget."
- "We have several payment options we can talk about to make care as affordable as possible."

Mentors are instrumental in guiding early-career veterinarians to refine their client communication skills so they can foster stronger client relationships and enhance patient outcomes. Using the practical strategies and interactive exercises in this chapter, you can help mentees master effective communication techniques, ensuring they can educate clients more effectively and engage them in meaningful discussions about patient care.

Editor's Note: *While strong client communication skills form the foundation of veterinary success, they do not exist in isolation. A veterinarian's ability to connect with pet owners is closely tied to how effectively they communicate with their colleagues. Misunderstandings between veterinarians and technicians can quickly spill over into the client experience, while strong collaboration behind the scenes reinforces trust in the exam room. To explore how new graduates can build confidence and competence in team-based communication, Alyssa Mages highlights structured strategies and inclusive practices that strengthen the veterinarian–technician partnership and foster a culture of psychological safety.*

A COLLABORATIVE APPROACH

Alyssa C. Mages

Effective communication is the lifeblood of veterinary medicine and a critical skill for new graduates to develop as they integrate into clinical teams. From patient care to workflow, collaboration to conflict resolution, communication shapes every aspect of practice life. Yet, despite its importance, many new veterinarians enter the workforce with limited formal training in how to communicate within a team: when to speak up, how to delegate, how to build trust with technicians, or what to do when information falls through the cracks.

This section focuses on the **collaborative nature of communication**, especially between new veterinarians and credentialed veterinary technicians (CrVTs). These relationships can either bolster a young veterinarian's confidence or erode it. Strong communication builds mutual respect, supports clinical learning, and ultimately benefits the patient. Poor communication can lead to medical errors, confusion, and team friction.

Veterinary practice presents natural communication challenges—time pressure, hierarchical structures, emotional fatigue, and generational differences, to name a few. Rather than unpacking each of these in depth here, this section zooms in on **practical tools and relationship-based strategies** to help new graduates become not just better communicators, but better teammates.

COLLABORATIVE COMMUNICATION BETWEEN VETERINARY TECHNICIANS AND VETERINARIANS

CrVTs play a crucial role in supporting newly graduated veterinarians (NGVs). NGVs bring fresh clinical knowledge but often lack confidence in real-world application, whereas experienced veterinary technicians offer practical expertise and case management insights. Beyond this relationship, when you pair a CrVT with a veterinarian in the OR, in the exam room, and while doing treatments, they both learn from one another while establishing a relationship built on mutual respect and trust that can at times even result in a dynamic that doesn't require verbal communication; they are that in sync.

STRATEGIES FOR STRENGTHENING THE VETERINARIAN–TECHNICIAN DYNAMIC

- Conduct regular case debriefs to ensure mutual understanding.
- Encourage two-way feedback to enhance learning.
- Define clear expectations regarding roles and responsibilities.
- Practice open, respectful dialogue to facilitate knowledge exchange.
- Utilize mentorship opportunities to develop clinical decision-making skills.

STRUCTURED COMMUNICATION DURING PATIENT ROUNDS

Effective patient rounds enhance case continuity and promote interdisciplinary collaboration in veterinary medicine. Implementing a standardized structure for rounds can improve efficiency, reduce miscommunication, and enhance information retention. According to O'Connell et al. (2018), structured rounds in human health care settings improve patient safety, and similar benefits apply in veterinary practice. The use of checklists, standardized handoff protocols, and active team participation ensures that critical patient information is consistently conveyed (Haig et al., 2006).

STANDARDIZATION AND EFFICIENCY

Structured rounds, such as those utilizing the SOAP (Subjective, Objective, Assessment, Plan) format or checklists, facilitate organized and efficient information sharing. Research in human medical education has shown that structured rounding reduces information loss and enhances teamwork (Starmer et al., 2014). Adopting similar strategies in veterinary settings, including predefined categories such as patient history, treatment updates, and next steps, ensures comprehensive case management.

ENHANCING TEAM COLLABORATION

Interdisciplinary rounds encourage input from veterinarians, veterinary technicians, and support staff, fostering a culture of shared decision-making. Evidence from human medical teams suggests that structured communication methods, such as **SBAR** (**Si**tuation, **B**ackground, **A**ssessment, **R**ecommendation), reduce errors and improve patient outcomes (Muller et al., 2020).

THE SBAR COMMUNICATION METHOD IN VETERINARY PRACTICE WORKFLOWS

This method is a structured framework designed to enhance communication in high-stakes environments, such as health care and veterinary medicine. Originally developed by the US Navy for nuclear submarine communication, SBAR was later adapted for medical settings to reduce miscommunication and improve patient safety (Haig et al., 2006). This model provides a standardized way for veterinary professionals to convey critical information clearly and efficiently, particularly during patient handoffs, rounds, and emergencies.

BREAKDOWN OF THE SBAR MODEL

1. **Situation (S):** Clearly state the immediate issue or reason for communication.
2. **Background (B):** Provide relevant patient history and context.
3. **Assessment (A):** Share the status or clinical interpretation of the situation.
4. **Recommendation (R):** Suggest next steps or required actions.

PATIENT HANDOFFS

Veterinary hospitals often require seamless communication between shifts to ensure continuity of care. SBAR helps structure patient handoff reports so that essential information is not overlooked.

Example—CrVT to Veterinarian

By following SBAR, the CrVT presents the case in a concise, logical order, ensuring the veterinarian has all necessary details to make an informed decision.

- **S:** "Fluffy, a 10-year-old feline, is experiencing increased respiratory effort."
- **B:** "She was admitted yesterday for dyspnea, has a history of asthma, and received oxygen therapy overnight."
- **A:** "This morning, her respiratory rate increased from 28 to 45 breaths per minute, and she seems more lethargic."
- **R:** "Would you like to recheck thoracic radiographs and adjust her oxygen flow rate?"

EMERGENCY SITUATIONS

Veterinary emergency teams rely on quick and clear communication to triage critical patients. SBAR ensures rapid information exchange. SBAR allows emergency teams to communicate high-priority information efficiently, reducing the risk of miscommunication in time-sensitive cases.

Example—Emergency Presentation to a Veterinarian

- **S:** "We have a 4 y/o, FS, GSD presenting for suspected GDV."
- **B:** "The owners report non-productive retching for two hours. The abdomen appears distended, and initial vitals show tachycardia (150 bpm) and pale mucous membranes."
- **A:** "Abdominal radiographs confirm a classic 'Popeye arm', and lactate is elevated at 8.0 mmol/L."
- **R:** "We should proceed with decompression and prepare for emergency surgery."

Remember, we're all human in this profession, regardless of position or years of experience. These conversations can sometimes feel intimidating or challenging, especially when communication styles or experience levels differ. What matters most is maintaining empathy and perspective—seeing the situation through the eyes of both the new graduate and the seasoned team member, as well as the doctor, technician, and support staff. Timing also matters. Avoid trying to have reflective or teaching conversations about communication during an emergency. Save those insights for a calm moment afterward, like a debriefing session once the patient is stable.

COMMUNICATION BETWEEN TEAM MEMBERS

SBAR fosters effective communication between the veterinary team, ensuring CrVTs, veterinary assistants, and veterinarians align on patient care. This structured approach minimizes misunderstandings and promotes decisive action.

Example—Lab Result Reporting

- **S:** "I have an important update regarding Max, the Golden Retriever in ICU."
- **B:** "He was admitted with suspected pancreatitis. Initial bloodwork showed mild elevations in amylase and lipase."
- **A:** "His repeat bloodwork shows a significant increase in lipase, and his white blood cell count has also risen."
- **R:** "Should we start IV fluids and consider an ultrasound to rule out complications like peritonitis?"

CLIENT COMMUNICATION

Veterinary professionals can also use SBAR to improve clarity in conversations with clients, particularly when explaining diagnoses, treatment plans, or financial considerations. This helps veterinary professionals explain complex information in a logical, client-friendly manner.

Example—Discussing a Treatment Plan with a Pet Owner

- **S:** "Milo has been diagnosed with diabetes."
- **B:** "He has been losing weight despite a normal appetite, and his blood glucose today was 410 mg/dL."

- **A:** "This indicates that his body is not properly processing sugar, which requires management through insulin therapy."
- **R:** "We recommend starting insulin injections twice daily and adjusting his diet to a prescription low-carb formula. Would you like a demonstration on how to administer insulin?"

WHY SBAR IS ESSENTIAL IN VETERINARY MEDICINE?

Used consistently, SBAR reduces miscommunication. In busy clinical environments—especially during emergencies or handoffs—verbal updates can be rushed or incomplete. SBAR minimizes these gaps by prompting team members to deliver information in a consistent, organized format. This is especially valuable during high-stakes scenarios such as anesthetic monitoring, postoperative transfers, or sudden patient declines, where unclear instructions can lead to critical errors.

In addition to improving accuracy, SBAR also enhances efficiency. Rather than sifting through lengthy narratives or disorganized updates, team members receive concise, relevant details that support swift decision-making. This efficiency allows veterinarians, technicians, and support staff to focus more time and attention on clinical tasks while still maintaining a high level of communication fidelity.

SBAR also plays a crucial role in enhancing patient care. By facilitating clear and consistent exchanges of clinical information, it ensures that all caregivers are aligned on treatment plans, monitoring requirements, and next steps. This alignment promotes timely interventions and continuity of care, essential elements in achieving optimal patient outcomes, particularly for those with complex or rapidly changing conditions.

Furthermore, the use of SBAR contributes to stronger team collaboration. A shared communication model fosters a sense of collective responsibility and mutual respect, as each team member learns to communicate in a language that is both professional and universally understood across roles. This shared framework encourages transparency, reduces friction, and reinforces a culture of psychological safety.

Finally, effective internal communication has external benefits, particularly when it comes to building client trust and compliance. When veterinary professionals communicate clearly among themselves, they are better prepared to deliver cohesive, confident updates to pet owners. Clients are more likely to trust recommendations and adhere to treatment plans when they perceive the team as organized, knowledgeable, and aligned.

Incorporating SBAR into veterinary practice is not simply a matter of protocol—it is an investment in clinical excellence, team cohesion, and client satisfaction. As the demands of veterinary care grow more complex, structured communication tools like SBAR offer a reliable foundation for navigating those challenges with clarity and confidence.

VETERINARY SBAR COMMUNICATION TEMPLATE

Patient Sticker/Label Here

Presenting Complaint: ______________________________

S—Situation *(What is the immediate issue? Why are you communicating this?)*

□ **Current concern:** ______________________________

□ **Urgency level (Routine / Urgent / Emergency):** ______________________________

□ **Who needs to be informed or involved?** ______________________________

B—Background *(What relevant history or context is needed?)*

□ **Relevant medical history:** ______________________________

□ **Recent diagnostics/lab work results:** ______________________________

□ **Current treatments/medications:** ______________________________

A—Assessment *(What is your evaluation of the patient's current status?)*

□ **Vital signs (TPR, BP, CRT, etc.):** ______________________________

□ **Changes since last evaluation:** ______________________________

□ **Current response to treatment (circle one: improving, stable, and deteriorating):**

R—Recommendation *(What are the next steps? What do you need?)*

□ **Proposed treatment adjustments:** ______________________________

□ **Further diagnostics needed:** ______________________________

□ **Client communication updates needed:** ______________________________

□ **Who is responsible for next steps?** ______________________________

Notes/Additional Information:

____

____

____

____

____

Put it into Practice

Two people or In a circle of 3 participants…
Speaker-The first person that begins the conversation or selects who they will speak to about a pre-determined topic.
The **Active Listener reflects what they are hearing** until the speaker feels heard and understood to their satisfaction (paraphrase or verbatim)
Then it is the **Active Listener's turn to become the Speaker**. They will then ask one of the **Silent Listeners** to become active, and the **new (Silent) listener will now reflect** what they heard
Everyone else (**Silent Listeners**) helps to hold the circle process by monitoring & sticking to the steps. The dialog continues around the circle like this for the time allotted

INFORMATION RETENTION AND CASE CONTINUITY

A structured approach to rounds improves information retention by reducing cognitive overload and ensuring consistency across shifts. Studies in both human and veterinary medicine highlight that frequent, structured communication improves knowledge retention and enhances patient care transitions (Tariq and Chavez, 2022). Regularly scheduled rounds that follow a standardized template help prevent gaps in treatment planning and ensure smooth case handoffs.

Structured communication during veterinary patient rounds is essential for optimizing case continuity, interdisciplinary collaboration, and patient safety. Implementing evidence-based strategies, such as checklists, SOAP formats, and SBAR-style reporting, enhances efficiency and information retention. By adopting structured rounds, veterinary teams can improve workflow, reduce miscommunication, and ultimately provide higher-quality patient care.

Below is an example to utilize when rounding on a patient:

VETERINARY ROUNDS TEMPLATE

Veterinarian: ____________________

Patient Sticker/Label Here

Technician(s): ____________________

Date/Time: ____________________

1. **Patient Overview**

   □ **Brief History:** (Summary of medical history, preexisting conditions, etc.)

   □ **Presenting Complaint:** (Why the patient is in the hospital today?)

   □ **Diagnostics Performed:** (Labs, imaging, physical exam findings, etc.)

   Notes: ____

   ____

   ____

2. **Current Treatment Plan**

□ **Medications (name, dose, route of administration, and frequency)**

□ **Ongoing Procedures:** (Fluid therapy, wound care, and monitoring needs)

□ **Care Priorities:** (Pain management, infection control, stabilization, etc.)

Notes: ____

____

____

3. **Discussion**

□ **Progress Observations:** (□ Improving □ Stable □ Deteriorating)

□ **Concerns from Team:** (Changes in vitals, unexpected reactions, and behavior concerns)

□ **Alternative Approaches/Adjustments Needed:**

Notes: ____

____

____

4. **Next Steps**

□ **Action Items:** (List specific tasks and who is responsible)

□ **Follow-Up Diagnostics or Procedures Needed?**

□ **Discharge Timeline or Continued Hospitalization Plan?**

Notes: ____

____

____

5. **Client Communication Plan**

□ **Key Updates for the Pet Owner:**

□ **Any Consent Needed for Additional Procedures?**

□ **Expected Follow-Up Call/Visit:**

Notes: ____

____

____

Additional Notes:

____

____

____

____

THE SBI MODEL FOR CONSTRUCTIVE FEEDBACK

Just as structured tools like SBAR support clear patient communication, structured feedback frameworks help strengthen team dynamics and professional growth, especially for early-career veterinarians still building confidence. One such model is SBI (Situation–Behavior–Impact).

Developed by the Center for Creative Leadership (CCL, 2021), SBI helps make feedback more objective, specific, and actionable (Gentry et al., 2025). It breaks feedback into three essential components:

- Situation (S): Describe the specific context where the event occurred.
- Behavior (B): Identify the observable action or behavior, without judgment.
- Impact (I): Explain the effect of the behavior on others, the team, or outcomes.

VETERINARY TEAM INTERACTIONS

Within a veterinary practice, clear, constructive feedback is essential for maintaining efficiency, professionalism, and collaboration. The SBI model helps veterinary professionals provide direct, actionable feedback that promotes learning rather than defensiveness.

Example 1: Feedback Among Team Members

If a veterinary technician forgets to complete a patient's medication administration, a supervisor can address it using SBI:

- **Situation:** "During rounds this morning, we reviewed all patient treatments."
- **Behavior:** "I noticed that the antibiotic for Bella hadn't been given as scheduled."
- **Impact:** "This delayed treatment could impact her recovery, and it required us to adjust the schedule to ensure she received it later."

This approach focuses on facts rather than blame, creating an opportunity for problem-solving and professional growth.

MENTOR SPEAKING TIPS AND CONVERSATION EXAMPLES

What a mentor might say to open the conversation?
"Hey [Name], do you have a minute to talk about something that came up during rounds this morning? I think it's a great chance for us to work through a system check together." Remember to use a neutral tone and body language that reflects curiosity rather than criticism. Sit or stand at the same level to reduce power distance.

What a mentor might say to guide reflection?
"I noticed Bella's antibiotic was delayed—can you walk me through what happened from your side?" After presenting the SBI, invite the team member into the discussion. Active listening is key—resist the urge to jump straight to a solution.

What a mentor might say to encourage learning and collaboration?
"Thanks for explaining that. What do you think we could adjust to prevent this from happening again, especially on busy mornings?" Frame the conversation around shared improvement, not individual fault. This promotes trust and growth.

What a mentor might say to affirm and reinforce progress?
"I appreciate you being open about it and helping find a solution. I know you care deeply about patient care, and that comes through." Always end feedback sessions with a positive reinforcement or recognition of strengths. This balances accountability with encouragement.

By modeling and teaching this feedback method, mentors help foster a culture of accountability and continuous improvement. The SBI model becomes not just a feedback tool, but a shared language for learning within the team.

Example 2: Reinforcing Positive Behavior

Veterinary teams should also use SBI to reinforce and encourage good workflow practices.

- **Situation:** "Yesterday afternoon, during a busy appointment block. . ."
- **Behavior:** "You stepped in to assist another technician with a difficult blood draw without being asked."
- **Impact:** "This helped reduce patient stress and allowed us to stay on schedule. It was a great example of teamwork!"

This kind of feedback boosts morale and fosters a culture of mutual support.

WHY SBI IS NECESSARY IN VETERINARY MEDICINE?

- **Reduces Miscommunication:**
  - Veterinary teams operate in fast-paced environments where misunderstandings can affect patient care.
  - SBI ensures clarity in feedback.
- **Enhances Teamwork:**
  - Constructive feedback strengthens collaboration and prevents conflicts from escalating.
- **Improves Client Relationships:**
  - Clients who feel respected and heard are more likely to trust their veterinary team, comply with treatment plans, and return for future care.
- **Promotes Professional Growth:**
  - Encouraging open, structured feedback helps individuals learn from mistakes and reinforces positive behaviors.

By implementing the SBI model in daily veterinary practice, teams can foster a culture of respectful communication, continuous improvement, and enhanced client service, ultimately leading to better patient outcomes and workplace satisfaction.

ENHANCING CLIENT-FACING COMMUNICATION

ESTABLISHING TRUST AND RAPPORT

Veterinary teams must communicate complex medical information in a way that fosters client trust and adherence. Studies indicate that clients who understand their pet's condition and treatment plan are 40% more likely to follow veterinary recommendations (Shaw et al., 2019).

Techniques for Effective Client Communication

- Use **open-ended questions** to gauge understanding.
  - "What other concerns do you have about your pet's condition?"
- Avoid medical jargon and provide clear, concise explanations.
- Confirm understanding through reflective listening.
- Utilize **written and visual aids.**
  - Discharge instructions, diagrams.

NAVIGATING DIFFICULT CONVERSATIONS

Delivering bad news or discussing financial constraints requires empathy and structure. The **SPIKES protocol** developed by Baile et al. (2000) provides a framework for these conversations. The goal is to enable the clinician, and in turn the medical team, to relay bad news in a way that the patient, and in veterinary medicine, the client, is more apt to receive it. The six steps are outlined below (FIGURE 9.2):

1. **S**etting: Choose a private, quiet space.
2. **P**erception: Assess the client's understanding of the situation.
3. **I**nvitation: Ask if they are ready for details.
4. **K**nowledge: Deliver information clearly and compassionately.
5. **E**motion: Acknowledge emotions and offer support.
6. **S**ummary: Confirm understanding and outline next steps.

FOSTERING AN INCLUSIVE WORK ENVIRONMENT: ENCOURAGING DIVERSE PERSPECTIVES

An inclusive veterinary practice values diverse viewpoints and creates an environment where all team members feel heard. Research by the American Veterinary Medical Association (AVMA) (2022) found that clinics fostering inclusivity experience higher team satisfaction and lower turnover rates.

Veterinary medicine is experiencing a turning point. Historically, our profession has been impactful in providing exceptional medical and surgical care for our patients, and yet, in doing so, we have overlooked a critical component—its people. The veterinary profession also continues to be one of the least diverse professions in the United States and has therefore NOT prioritized diversity, equity,

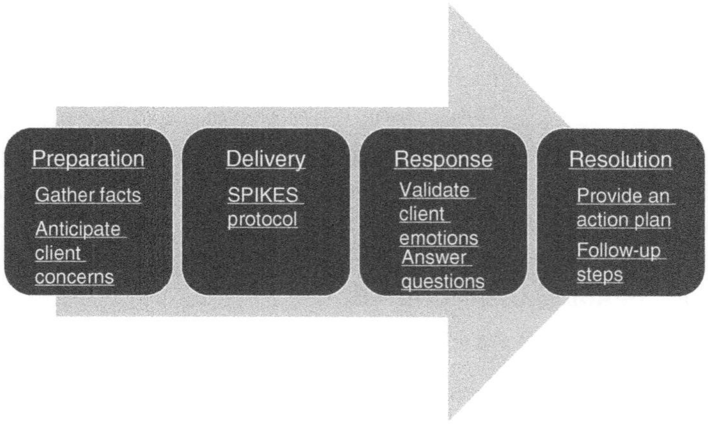

FIGURE 9.2 Flowchart utilizing the SPIKE protocol

inclusion, or belonging (DEIB) in our daily practice. This issue has directly influenced our work norms and culture, so we must acknowledge that it also leaves us culturally inept to diagnose and treat our patients when barriers such as these are left unchallenged (Ervin-Smith and Mages, 2024).

A focus on well-being without the coexistence of DEIB is a farce: DEIB is so intricately intertwined into well-being that suppressing any aspect of an individual's inherent need to express their diversity, pursue equity, search for inclusivity, or feel a sense of belongingness is a direct impact on their well-being.

One of the most primal (an early stage of evolutionary development) feelings human beings experience is the desire to BELONG, to be connected to other beings, and to be accepted as part of a "tribe." Research shows that brain scans of those individuals with social rejection create virtually identical activity to that of a physical assault. Therefore, the aspect of DEIB is not only important for a homogeneous profession such as veterinary medicine but also important for any profession across the world (Ervin-Smith et al., 2024).

STRATEGIES FOR INCLUSIVE DIALOGUE

Empathy is a critical tool in all aspects of veterinary medicine, but particularly in matters of DEIB, as it helps to establish an emotional connection, creates a safe space, aids in identifying needs, and opens the door for collaboration. This practice involves putting yourself in the "shoes of the other person" and understanding their pain or concerns as they feel them. It is also a journey of discovery and understanding to "WHY" someone may have those feelings.

This is where we engage our Emotional Intelligence (EQ) instead of our IQ by:

- Encouraging team members to voice concerns and ideas.
- Practicing active listening without interruption.
- Implementing regular team meetings focused on improvement and growth.
- Establishing a psychologically safe work environment where learning from mistakes is supported.

ADDRESSING WORKPLACE CONFLICTS

Conflict is inevitable in high-stress environments, but handling disputes professionally prevents escalation. It doesn't have to be scary or stressful. Creating—and maintaining—open channels of communication along with familiarity among team members, disagreements can often develop into more considerate conversations, which ultimately lead to mutually beneficial solutions. Is it easy? No. Will it be comfortable? Likely not. But if handled correctly, conflict, when addressed and managed appropriately, may even bring your team closer together. Start by creating a short checklist to prep yourself.

Conflict Resolution Checklist

- Identify the root cause of the disagreement.
- Listen to all perspectives with neutrality.
- Find common ground and develop a solution.
- Follow-up to ensure resolution effectiveness.

It may also be helpful to know your team members' conflict management styles. According to Thomas (1992), there are five main styles:

- **Competing:**
  - Assertive and uncooperative, focusing on achieving one's own goals at the expense of others.
- **Collaborating:**
  - Both assertive and cooperative, aiming to find a solution that satisfies all parties involved.

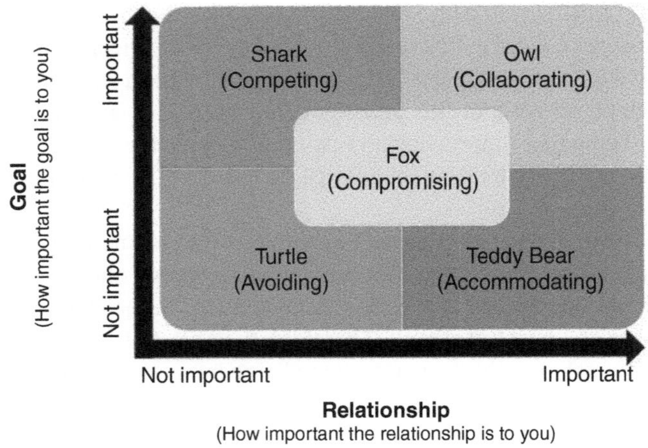

FIGURE 9.3 Online assessments are readily available, and one that the team at MentorVet utilizes is the Blake Conflict Management styles assessment, which can be found here: http://www.blake-group.com/sites/default/files/assessments/Conflict_Management_Styles_Assessment.pdf

- **Compromising:**
  - Moderate level of assertiveness and cooperativeness, seeking a mutually acceptable solution that involves some concessions from all parties.
- **Avoiding:**
  - Unassertive and uncooperative, individuals try to avoid the conflict altogether.
- **Accommodating:**
  - Unassertive and cooperative, individuals prioritize the needs of others over their own.

This was further developed by The Blake Group (2006) and then again by Stuart (2023) who took the material and created more of a matrix (Figure 9.3) based on how important the goal of the conflict is and how important the relationship is with whom the conflict is while also incorporating animal metaphors for relatability.

Enhanced communication within veterinary teams directly improves patient outcomes, client satisfaction, team morale, and workplace culture. By implementing structured communication strategies—such as SBAR for communication within teams, the SBI model for feedback, and inclusive dialogue practices—mentors can foster a collaborative and supportive environment. Strengthening relationships between team members, particularly those between veterinarians and CrVTs, prioritizing clear client communication, and resolving conflicts proactively will ensure long-term success in veterinary medicine.

KEY TAKEAWAYS

Strong communication reduces medical errors and enhances patient care.

A focus on structured feedback and collaborative learning enhances mentorship.

Client communication strategies improve adherence and trust.

Inclusive dialogue creates a trusting relationship, fosters a positive work culture, and reduces turnover.

Editor's Note: *Even the most skilled in-person communicators must now extend their reach into a digital-first world. Clients increasingly expect updates, resources, and results to be delivered through technology, and veterinary teams must adapt without becoming overwhelmed or losing personal connection. Building on the foundation of client-facing skills and collaborative team communication, Dr. Caitlin DeWilde turns our attention to the digital tools that are reshaping practice—email, text, social media, telemedicine, and AI—and shows how mentors can help early-career veterinarians use them wisely and sustainably.*

UTILIZING TECHNOLOGY

Caitlin DeWilde

Effective communication has always been the cornerstone of veterinary medicine, but in a digital world our conversations don't end at the conclusion of the exam. They continue in inboxes, apps, portals, texts, videos, social channels and even through telemedicine. For early-career veterinarians, mastering these channels is not optional; it's essential to practicing medicine efficiently, documenting properly, and building durable client trust. As mentors, our role is to demystify the tools, model sound workflows, and create guardrails that keep communications compliant, professional, and sustainable for the whole team.

TECHNOLOGY AROUND THE VISIT: BEFORE, DURING, AND AFTER

THE BEFORE

Pre-visit Touchpoints That Set You Up for Success

Most clients have already interacted with your practice digitally before they meet the doctor: online booking, automated confirmations, digital intake/history forms, senior pet, or Fear Free questionnaires. These steps set expectations and save time; they also prime clients to accept digital communication for everything that follows.

> **MENTOR TIP**
>
> Make sure your mentee knows the full cycle of service and how clients might interact (and prefer to communicate) with the practice not only in the exam room, but before they come to your practice. Discuss the importance of knowing the modalities, workflow, and client preferences for client communication based on your practice's specifics.

THE DURING

Scribing and Templates: How Mentees Win Back Time

AI-assisted scribing tools can reduce documentation time and improve completeness, especially for new graduates still finding their rhythm. Whether your practice uses an AI scribe or not, templates, shorthand/glossaries, and text-expansion tools (e.g. TextExpander and TypeDesk) keep records thorough and consistent while accelerating client-facing communication.

> **MENTOR TIP**
>
> Share your favorite or cocreate condition-based templates with default client-friendly language and customizable sections for: visit summary, what to watch for, medication instructions, home care, recheck timing, and trusted links/handouts (see "Resource Bank," below). Pilot them together for a week and refine.

THE AFTER

The Case for Written (Digital) Discharge Summaries

Client recall after veterinary visits is notoriously poor; in human medicine, patients can forget upward of half of what's discussed, particularly when anxious or older (Kessels, 2003). Providing concise, clear after-visit summaries improves recall, supports plan adherence, and enhances the perceived value of the visit.

Even for healthy pets, a "medical report card" can be brief (e.g., "continue monthly preventives; VOHC-approved dental chews; recheck in 12 months").

Emailing these post-visit summaries is not only recommended but also is now a built in functionality of many PiMS and scribing softwares, making it easy to integrate with the medical record.

> **MENTOR TIP**
>
> Share examples. Give your mentees 3–5 model discharge summaries (healthy adult, senior with OA, dentistry follow-up, GI upset with home care, and a chronic disease update). Encourage them to use discharge templates within your PIMS or build a cloud-based template library for common conditions, so summaries are consistent and quick to produce.

Sharing Resources the Smart Way

Clients value short, credible resources tied to exactly what their veterinarian just discussed—ideally delivered in their preferred format. In the room, encourage mentees to ask: "Would you like a handout or an email/text after the visit?" Matching format to preference increases the chance they'll read and act.

> **MENTOR TIP**
>
> Build a "Resource Bank" with your go-to, evidence-based links and tools so mentees aren't reinventing the wheel: AAHA/AVMA client guides, national organization resources, hospital-approved product materials, and even your favorite personal online tools (e.g. online calculators, etc.).

When you share a link, include the "why." For example, "I like the American Heartworm Society calculator because it creates a clear plan we can email to the client and download into the record."

Diagnostics: Choosing the Right Channel and Documenting Once

Post-visit communication often peaks when test results return. Efficiency in these moments depends on two things: using the client's preferred channel and ensuring the information is documented once in the medical record, rather than duplicated across multiple platforms. Post-visit communication often peaks when results return—CBC/chemistry, cytology, imaging, or specialist interpretations. Efficiency here depends on two things: honoring the client's communication preference and documenting once (not three times).

- **Simple normals/minor changes:** Brief text or email with one actionable sentence and next steps.

- **Nuanced/visual results:** A short screen-recorded video (e.g., Loom) where the veterinarian appears picture-in-picture to point to out-of-range values or show radiographic findings; clients can rewatch and share with family.
- **Complex results/decisions:** Schedule a call or telemedicine visit for shared decision-making.

MENTOR TIP

Map your practice's workflow. Which labs allow client-shareable summaries from the portal? How do you attach PDFs/links to the PIMS? If you use an AI scribe or recorder, decide when to transcribe calls so the record is complete without extra work.

Proactive Prescriptions and Refills

Clients often "think about it" before buying preventives, diets, or starting chronic meds. Sending a proactive, authorized e-prescription or product link (via your online pharmacy or approved vendor) lets them act later—without calling back or defaulting to third-party sellers. This workflow is convenient for the client, efficient for the team, keeps more revenue in-house, and—most importantly—gets pets what they need sooner.

MENTOR TIP

Teach mentees your "refill cadence" and explain where their responsibility (or delegation) lies (e.g., seven-day supply remaining → auto-text plus link; three-day remaining → staff call). Pair each trigger with the client's preferred channel and templated language.

COMMUNICATION BETWEEN VISITS: STAYING PRESENT ALL YEAR

A healthy adult pet might visit once or twice a year, and yet client questions and needs persist year-round. Practices can nurture trust and prompt timely care with a mix of channels: social media, email, website/blog posts, SMS/app notifications, and online review/reputation site engagement. For new veterinarians—especially those joining a practice where clients are used to "their" longtime doctor—these touchpoints also accelerate familiarity and rapport.

THOUGHTFUL PARTICIPATION ON SOCIAL MEDIA

New grads don't need to run the page, but their *contributions* are invaluable. Short, educational videos (seasonal hazards, home dental care basics, and OA home hacks) allow clients to meet the new doctor's face and voice before they ever see them in an exam room.

MENTOR TIP

- Keep logistics off the doctor's plate. Provide a point person for editing, approvals, and scheduling.
- Calibrate boundaries: Who posts, who replies, expected response windows, out-of-office coverage, and what escalates to clinical staff.
- Track what resonates (saves/shares/comments), not just likes, and iterate.

PERSONAL VS. PRACTICE PRESENCE

Help mentees navigate "personal" social media in a professional world: whether to accept client friend requests; how to engage (if at all) in neighborhood groups; what to set as public vs. private; and when *not* to offer medical advice online because there is no valid VCPR.

MENTOR TIP

Encourage simple reputation monitoring. Even clinics without an aggressive social media/online strategy should keep an eye on what's said about the practice and staff; AVMA outlines light-lift monitoring tools (including free options), so problems don't snowball. Set up Google Alerts for the hospital name *and* doctor names.

CONSENT, PHOTOS, AND NEGATIVE COMMENTS

Codify consent for patient photos, team photos, and video usage—and follow it. Your policy should also spell out how the practice responds to negative comments: who drafts replies, who approves them, what gets handled privately, and when you disengage. AVMA's "best practices to manage your online reputation" is a strong starting point (AVMA, 2025).

EMAIL, TONE, AND TEMPLATES

If your mentee has a clinic email (e.g., dr.lastname@practice.com), help them create reusable, professional templates for common scenarios: new-client welcome, normal results, "mildly abnormal but not urgent," chronic recheck due, and grief/condolence. Tools like Grammarly can help maintain clarity and tone consistently.

MENTOR TIP

Pair every template with a "humanizing sentence" at the top (e.g., "I know you've been worried about Bella's cough—thanks for your patience while we reviewed her X-rays."). Small empathy signals go a long way to build relationships and reduce client anxiety.

TELEMEDICINE: AN EVIDENCE-INFORMED, REGULATION-AWARE APPROACH

Veterinary telemedicine is maturing quickly, but it is still governed by state practice acts and the profession's stance on the VCPR. The AVMA advises that telemedicine be conducted only within an established Veterinarian–Client–Patient Relationship (VCPR), with only limited exceptions for emergency guidance. While some states have considered loosening these rules, most still require an in-person examination to establish a VCPR. The AVMA generally does not recommend creating a VCPR virtually because of regulatory constraints and the potential for compromised clinical care.

Translation for Mentees

- Know your state's current rules; they change.
- If your practice offers telemedicine, understand *exactly* which visit types qualify, what you can and cannot do, and how to document.

TELEMEDICINE BEST PRACTICES (WHAT TO TEACH MENTEES?)

1. **Practice with your mentor first:** Shadow or co-conduct a few virtual visits to learn cadence, exam limitations, and documentation steps.
2. **Prepare like it's in-person:** Review the chart and recent diagnostics; list differential questions you'll ask; preload client education links you might send afterward.
3. **Optimize tech basics:** Quiet, private space; eye-level camera; stable connection; clear lighting and audio. Test before the session. (Avoid over-specifying tech specs in training; prioritize outcomes: clients can see and hear you clearly.)
4. **Document once:** If the practice allows recording or transcribing (with informed consent), do it—then summarize the plan in the record and send a lay summary to the client.
5. **End with clarity:** "Did I answer all your questions?" followed by explicit next steps, expected timelines, and recheck triggers.
6. **Have a backup plan:** Get the client's phone number before you begin in case the connection drops.

MENTOR TIP

Create a telemedicine "starter kit" for mentees:

a. Eligibility matrix (what's OK, what's not)
b. Pre-visit checklist
c. Consent language for recording/transcription
d. "Post-visit plan" template you can email or text

AI AS A COMMUNICATION COPILOT (WITH GUARDRAILS)

Used thoughtfully, AI can accelerate administrative tasks and improve client-facing clarity: summarizing multiyear charts, translating plans into plain language (or another language), drafting sensitive messages (with a human final pass), or even organizing a complicated, multistep treatment path into a readable summary. There are two cautions that mentors must echo: respect privacy/security and follow practice policy; and remember that clients themselves may already be consulting AI ("Dr. ChatGPT"), so we need to be ready to contextualize or correct what they bring us.

On the professional side, emerging veterinary literature discusses responsible AI deployment—calling out owner consent, data governance, documentation of AI use in care, and transparency about limitations. Use these as teaching touchpoints when you introduce AI to mentees.

MENTOR TIP

Verify and share a brief "AI Use Policy" for your clinic:

- Approved tools and *approved* use cases (e.g., de-identified chart summaries, rewriting discharge instructions at a 6th-grade reading level, and template drafts).
- Disallowed uses (uploading identifiable client/financial data into tools or data agreement).
- Required human review and documentation ("Discharge instructions generated from template and reviewed by Dr. Smith").
- Client-facing transparency when appropriate ("We used a software assistant to draft these instructions; I reviewed and customized them for your pet.").

TEACHING THE COMMUNICATION MINDSET

Technology is the vehicle, not the outcome. What we're really mentoring is a mindset: meet clients where they are, reduce friction, document well, and close loops. Several evidence-backed points your mentees should internalize:

- **People forget:** That's normal—and why short, clear, post-visit recaps work. https://pubmed.ncbi.nlm.nih.gov/12724430/?utm_source=chatgpt.com.
- **Written summaries and open notes help:** Patients report better understanding and engagement when they can revisit the plan.
- **Digital nudges work:** Simple, timely notifications (SMS/email) improve attendance and adherence; translate that into refill and recheck workflows.
- **Regulations matter:** Telemedicine lives inside your state's practice act and the AVMA's VCPR stance; teach mentees to check before they promise.

CONCLUSION

Communication in veterinary medicine extends far beyond the exam room conversation. It encompasses the trust-building empathy shared with clients, the structured collaboration practiced within teams, and the intentional use of digital tools that connect practices to the communities they serve. Each domain reinforces the others: strong client relationships depend on cohesive team communication, efficient documentation enables better follow-through, and clear internal dialogue translates into more confident external messaging.

Mentors play a critical role in helping new graduates see communication not as separate skills to master, but as an integrated system that shapes every aspect of care. By modeling effective communication across all channels—face-to-face, team-based, and digital—mentors equip their mentees to build lasting client relationships, contribute meaningfully to collaborative teams, and adapt to the evolving technological landscape. When communication flows clearly in all directions, patients, clients, and veterinary professionals all benefit.

BIBLIOGRAPHY

Ackerman, L. (2021). *Pet-Specific Care for the Veterinary Team*. Hoboken, NJ: Wiley Blackwell.

American Veterinary Medical Association (AVMA) (2022). Diversity, equity, and inclusion in veterinary medicine. AVMA Reports.

AVMA (2025). *Best Practices to Manage Your Online Reputation*. American Veterinary Medical Association https://www.avma.org/resources-tools/practice-management/reputationnn (accessed 20 September 2025).

Baile, W., Buckman, R., Lenzi, R. et al. (2000). SPIKES – a six-step protocol for delivering bad news: application to the patient with cancer. *The Oncologist* 5: 302–311.

Blake, O. E. (2006). Adkins' conflict management styles assessment. http://www.blake-group.com/sites/default/files/assessments/Conflict_Management_Styles_Assessment.pdf.

Brown, C.R., Garrett, L.D., Gilles, W.K. et al. (2021). Spectrum of care: more than treatment options. *Journal of the American Veterinary Medical Association* 259 (7): 712–716.

Center for Creative Leadership (2021). Talking across generations at work. https://www.ccl.org.

Coe, J.B., Adams, C.L., and Bonnett, B.N. (2018). A focus group study of veterinarians' and pet owners' perceptions of the monetary aspects of veterinary care. *Journal of the American Veterinary Medical Association* 231 (10): 1510–1518.

Dysart, L.M., Coe, J.B., and Adams, C.L. (2011). Analysis of solicitation of client concerns in companion animal practice. *Journal of the American Veterinary Medical Association* 238 (12): 1612.

Edmondson, A. (1999). *Psychological safety and learning behavior in work teams. Administrative Science Quarterly* 44 (2): 350–383.

Ervin-Smith, Genine and Mages, Alyssa C (2024). What's the 411? Breaking down barriers & finding common ground – the culture of communication. Presentation at VMX 2024.

Fleming, J.H. and Asplund, J. (2007). *Human Sigma.* New York, NY: Gallup Press.

Gentry, Bill, and Stephen Young (2025). Using situation-behavior-impact (SBI)TM to understand intent. CCL.Org/Articles, www.ccl.org/articles/leading-effectively-articles/closing-the-gap-between-intent-vs-impact-sbii/

Goman, C.K. (2008). *The Non Verbal Advantage.* San Francisco, CA: Berrett Koehler.

Haig, K.M., Sutton, S., and Whittington, J. (2006). SBAR: a shared mental model for improving communication between clinicians. *Joint Commission Journal on Quality and Patient Safety 32* (3): 167–175.

Joint Commission (2020). Communication failures: a root cause of sentinel events. *Journal on Quality and Patient Safety* 47 (4): 242–249.

Kanji, N., Coe, J.B., Adams, C.L., and Shaw, J.R. (2012). Effect of veterinarian-client-patient interactions on client adherence to dentistry and surgery recommendation in companion-animal practice. *Journal of the American Veterinary Medical Association* 240 (4): 432–433.

Kessels, R.P. (2003). Patients' memory for medical information. *Journal of the Royal Society of Medicine* 96 (5): 219–222. https://doi.org/10.1177/014107680309600504 PMID: 12724430; PMCID: PMC539473.

Kurtz, S.M., Silverman, J., and Draper, J. (2005). *Teaching and Learning Communication Skills in Medicine.* Abingdon, UK: Radcliffe Medical Press.

Muller, M., Jurgens, J., Redaelli, M. et al. (2020). Impact of the communication and patient hand-off tool SBAR on patient safety: a systematic review. *BMJ Open 8* (8): e022202.

Not One More Vet (NOMV) (n.d.). Mental health support and peer assistance for veterinary professionals. https://www.nomv.org.

O'Connell, R.G., Gajewski, B.J., and Windish, D.M. (2018). Structured interdisciplinary rounds improve teamwork, communication, and patient outcomes. *Academic Medicine 93* (7): 1032–1039.

RSA (2013). Brene Brown on empathy [video] https://www.youtube.com/watch?v=1Evwgu369Jw (accessed 12 March 2025).

Rosenberg, M.B. (2003). *Non-violent Communication.* Encinitas, CA: PuddleDancer Press.

Shaw, J.R. (2006). Four Core Communication skills for highly effective practitioners. *Veterinary Clinics of North America: Small Animal Practice* 36 (2) Elsevier Saunders: 386.

Shaw, J.R., Barley, G.E., Broadfoot, K. et al. (2016). Outcomes assessment of on-site communication skills education in a companion animal practice. *Journal of the American Veterinary Medical Association* 249 (4): 428.

Shaw, J.R., Bonnett, B.N., and Adams, C.L. (2019). Effectiveness of veterinarian communication on client adherence. *Veterinary Clinics of North America: Small Animal Practice* 49 (3): 377–391.

Silverman, J., Kurtz, S.A., and Draper, J. (2005). *Skills for Communicating with Patients.* Arbingdon, UK: Radcliffe Medical Press.

Starmer, A.J., Spector, N.D., Srivastava, R. et al. (2014). Changes in medical errors after implementation of a handoff program. *New England Journal of Medicine 371* (19): 1803–1812.

Stuart, G (2023). What Are the 5 Styles of Conflict Management? Resources for Students and Practitioners, Sustaining Community, 15 Feb. 2023, sustainingcommunity.wordpress.com/2022/11/16/what-are-the-5-styles-of-conflict-management/

Tariq, R.A. and Chavez, B. (2022). Patient handoffs and transitions. In: *StatPearls* [Internet]. StatPearls Publishing.

Thomas, K.W. (1992). Conflict and conflict management: reflections and update. *Journal of Organizational Behavior 13* (3): 265–274.

CHAPTER 10

Promoting Resiliency and Adaptability

INTRODUCTION

Dani Rabwin

Resilience and adaptability are two of the most important skills for early-career veterinarians. The transition from school into practice is filled with challenges—low confidence, impostor thoughts, perfectionism, and the weight of responsibility that comes faster than expected. I wanted this chapter to offer practical, evidence-based strategies for building resilience while also sharing lived experiences that mentees and mentors alike can relate to.

To bring this conversation to life, I invited Dr. Addie Reinhard, Mariel Hendricks, and Dr. Daniel Stillwell to collaborate. Addie, the founder of MentorVet and a researcher on the Merck Animal Health Veterinary Wellbeing Study, grounds this chapter in her research on early-career stress and innovative well-being interventions. Her own journey through burnout—from that breaking point in a Meijer parking lot to founding a national mentorship program—provides both personal authenticity and scientific rigor to the discussion of resilience.

Mariel, a credentialed technician and educator, contributes the perspective of a veterinary nurse who has walked through burnout and growth and now develops training and learning systems for veterinary teams. Her transition from specialty surgery to leadership in veterinary education illustrates how prioritizing well-being isn't a luxury—it's essential for career longevity. Daniel, a licensed marriage and family therapist, adds clinical expertise in mental health, coaching, and suicide prevention, weaving in tools that help mentors support mentees through perfectionism and the challenges of adapting to change.

Together, they illustrate how resilience and adaptability are not innate traits but skills that can be nurtured through mentorship, self-care, and supportive workplace culture. This chapter will provide you with evidence-based strategies, reflective questions, and real-world stories to guide your mentees toward sustainable wellbeing. Perhaps, most importantly, it will remind you that resilience is not about avoiding hardship but about helping new veterinarians adapt, recover, and continue thriving in a demanding yet deeply rewarding profession.

IDENTIFYING STRESSORS AND UNDERSTANDING RESILIENCY

Addie Reinhard

The transition to veterinary practice is challenging. In my early veterinary career, I experienced pretty severe burnout a few different times—once at about eight months into practice and again at about three years into practice. As someone who had always excelled in academic settings, burnout felt like I was failing. Sometimes it felt like I was not meant to be a veterinarian.

Fortunately, with the support of some incredible mentors inside my practice and in my external support network, I successfully overcame burnout twice. As I started talking more openly about my experiences, I quickly learned that I was not alone in these feelings. Many of my classmates were also struggling in the transition to practice.

After getting through burnout the second time, I felt a calling to dig deeper into this issue. I was driven forward by two major questions:

- *Why are so many early-career veterinarians struggling in the transition to practice?*
- *What can we do about it?*

In 2019, I decided to go back to school to get my master's degree in Community and Leadership Development at the University of Kentucky, and I spent two years researching early-career veterinary well-being and interventions to support early-career veterinarians. In 2020, I performed a qualitative focus group study and piloted an intervention to support the mental health of veterinary professionals.

That intervention has since transitioned into a national mentorship program where I have now worked alongside thousands of early-career veterinarians in the transition to practice to reduce and prevent early-career burnout. In the work that I do everyday, I want to ensure that I am providing early-career veterinarians with tools, resources, and community so that hopefully they won't have to experience burnout in the same way that I did.

In this section, I will discuss some of the key findings of my research during my master's program as well as experiences working with thousands of early-career veterinarians including some of the key stressors in the early career. Later in this section, I will introduce the concept of resilience. In the following two sections, two of my team members will discuss strategies for fostering resilience to provide you with tools to better support those around you.

EARLY-CAREER VETERINARY WELL-BEING

Often, for those who have experienced severe burnout, we can pinpoint the exact moment we realized that we had an issue.

This is my story. I had been in practice for around three years, and my mentor was taking a much needed vacation. I was practicing as the only veterinarian in the practice for one week. I felt confident being left alone in the practice, yet I still would have higher levels of stress when practicing without my mentor in the building (Figure 10.1).

It was a Wednesday, and my schedule got a little out of hand with walk-ins and emergencies. I had several rude clients throughout the morning and several cases that I had no clue what I was dealing with. I was running around trying to provide the best care that I could for my patients, but being spread thin, I felt that each patient was not receiving the care that they deserved.

Working through my lunch, I examined a very sick, adorable little kitten that was dropped off for evaluation. After examination and some preliminary testing, I felt the need for stabilization and an exploratory surgery. At this stage, I lacked confidence in surgery, but I was willing to try the surgery if the owner could not afford referral. After communicating my recommendations to the pet owner to

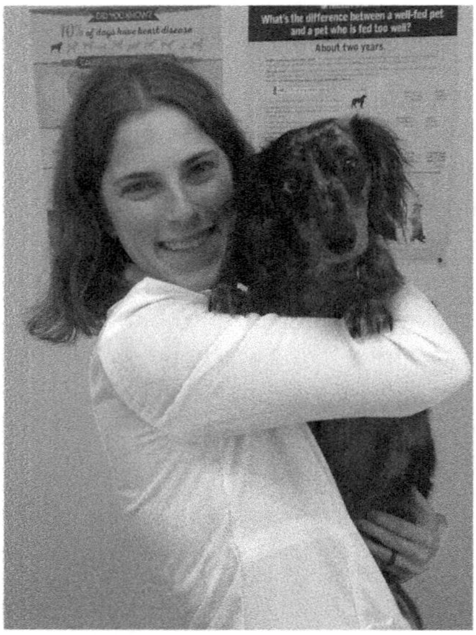

FIGURE 10.1 My early career in small animal practice.

either refer to an emergency clinic for better care or stabilizing and trying the surgery myself, they explained that they had almost no money to put toward this kitten and opted instead for euthanasia.

At the end of my shift and having stayed hours past closing time to catch up, I euthanized this sweet kitten that had likely a treatable condition.

After I left the clinic that evening and about three minutes after hitting the road, all of the stress of the day and the cumulative stress that I had been feeling over the past several months began to spill over onto my face. I couldn't see the road anymore with all of the tears, so I opted to pull into the Meijer parking lot.

That was my breaking point.

From the Meijer parking lot, I reached out to my mom on the phone telling her that I was feeling extreme burnout. That was the first step in overcoming my burnout—realizing that I had an issue and taking a step to reach out for help.

Slowly, I began taking instrumental steps to overcome my burnout. I spoke with my mentors about what I was feeling, I started setting better boundaries, and I learned skills to be more prepared to navigate the challenges that I was experiencing.

Going through this experience, I also did what any good veterinarian would do—turn to the research and literature. I quickly learned that stress in the early veterinary career was common, but very few studies assessed what we could do about it, so I set off on a path to learn more.

For two years during my master's program, I did a deep dive into early-career veterinary mental health and well-being, and for the past three years, I have served as a researcher on the Merck Animal Health Veterinary Wellbeing Study. Consistently, we find that early-career veterinarians have higher levels of serious psychological distress and lower levels of well-being compared to veterinarians who have been in practice longer (Volk et al., 2022).

This finding is not new and is not limited to veterinarians in the United States. Studies dating back to the 2000s in New Zealand and the United Kingdom suggest that, among all veterinarians, younger veterinarians experience the highest levels of stress (Gardner and Hini, 2006; Bartram et al., 2009).

Burnout, in particular, seems to be quite prevalent among early-career veterinarians, and it is estimated that around 75% of all veterinarians under the age of 35 are experiencing moderate to severe burnout (Merck Animal Health, 2022). This term, *burnout*, gets used frequently within our profession, so it is vital that we have a clear definition of this term and conceptualize the causes and symptoms of burnout.

Burnout can be defined as "a psychological syndrome emerging as a prolonged response to chronic interpersonal stressors on the job" (Maslach and Leiter, 2016, p. 103). Essentially, stress at work left unchecked (e.g. not reducing the amount of stressors you are experiencing or not coping with your stressors in a healthy way) can lead to a psychological syndrome called burnout. This syndrome is typically characterized by three main symptoms:

- **Exhaustion:** Feeling emotionally, mentally, or physically drained by your work
- **Cynicism:** Feeling angry or cynical toward clients, coworkers, or patients
- **Inefficacy:** Feeling a lack of accomplishment or feeling like the work you are doing does not matter

When I was experiencing burnout in my early career, I remember telling others that I felt mentally, physically, and emotionally exhausted. Often, I would start the day feeling tired. Feelings of cynicism would creep in when pet owners did not accept my treatment recommendations. Finally, I felt like I was not contributing to making the world a better place.

Burnout occurs on a range (e.g. mild to severe symptoms), and because burnout is caused by chronic stress at work, anything that causes stress in the workplace can contribute to burnout in early-career veterinarians. I performed a literature review for my master's thesis (Reinhard, 2021) and identified key sources of stress for veterinary professionals including:

- Ethical dilemmas
- Client expectations
- Client complaints
- Client interactions
- Unexpected outcomes
- Conflict with team members
- Identity dissonance
- Professional mistakes
- Demands of practice
- Lack of support
- Student debt
- Surgery
- On-call responsibilities

To further explore stressors among early-career veterinarians, I performed a qualitative focus group study with six early-career veterinarians (Reinhard et al., 2021). In this study, our research team identified five key themes that can affect stress in the early career.

1. **Setbacks and adaptation:** Many new and recent graduates experienced setbacks and had to adapt to the challenges they were facing. Many reported sleepless nights at the start of the career, and several veterinarians mentioned experiencing discrimination based on age, gender, or other factors.
2. **Self-sufficiency and self-doubt:** Some early-career veterinarians mentioned that there was an expectation that, on their first day of practice, they needed to be self-sufficient,

which for some was a jarring transition after being in a supportive veterinary school environment. This sense of responsibility was also coupled with a sense of self-doubt, imposter syndrome, and fear of making mistakes.

3. **Changing clientele and ethical dilemmas:** The clientele of a veterinary teaching hospital is inherently different than that of many private practices. Many recent graduates reported stress when navigating the gray areas of veterinary medicine and felt unprepared for navigating the ethical dilemmas and moral stress that ensued.
4. **Leadership and conflict:** Many recently graduated veterinarians reported challenges in navigating team dynamics. As veterinarians often have to delegate and lead a team, many were unprepared for this role and the inherent conflict that resulted especially when team members did not trust their decision-making.
5. **Good mentorship vs. bad mentorship:** Mentorship has the potential to either positively or negatively contribute to stress in the transition to practice. Most veterinarians in the focus group received positive mentorship. Good mentorship helped veterinarians feel more supported, but poor mentorship was reported by one individual in the focus group, which resulted in increased stress.

While there are many challenges and stressors inherent to the veterinary profession, there is a lot we can do as mentors to support early-career veterinarians in the transition to practice. Next, we will discuss resilience.

WHAT IS RESILIENCE?

When I first started mentoring early-career veterinarians, I met a veterinarian who was only six months into practice and already feeling severe symptoms of burnout. She set up a meeting with me to talk about resources that might help her. She shared with me that she had been struggling with imposter syndrome. She told me that she didn't feel like she was meant to do small animal clinical practice because she felt like she wasn't good enough. She was also experiencing quite a bit of conflict with coworkers and clients, and she was having trouble navigating this on her own. Only six months after graduation, she was considering switching to a nonclinical role in veterinary medicine.

I listened actively to her concerns, reflected back what I was hearing, and tried not to immediately fix or offer any suggestions or advice. Instead, I validated what she was experiencing. I empathized with her challenges and shared that I had also experienced similar feelings when I first started my career. I asked her how I could better support her.

She mentioned that she was looking for more resources and support including connection with other early-career professionals who might be experiencing similar challenges as well as education and training in how to navigate the challenges she was facing. I referred her to one of our mentorship programs that offered these resources.

Over the course of the five month program, this mentee learned about how to navigate conflict with clients and team members as well as strategies for navigating her stress and coping with moral stress. She shared her challenges in a supportive environment with other early-career professionals. By the end of the program, she stated that she not only wanted to stay in clinical practice but also wanted to stay in her current practice.

This story demonstrates the incredible resilience of early-career practitioners given the right tools and resources.

Resilience can be defined as "the process and outcome of successfully adapting to difficult or challenging life experiences, especially through mental, emotional, and behavioral flexibility and adjustment to external and internal demands" (American Psychological Association, 2025).

In this instance, this veterinarian successfully navigated a challenging experience by overcoming burnout in her early career. This was done through her ability to adapt and adjust

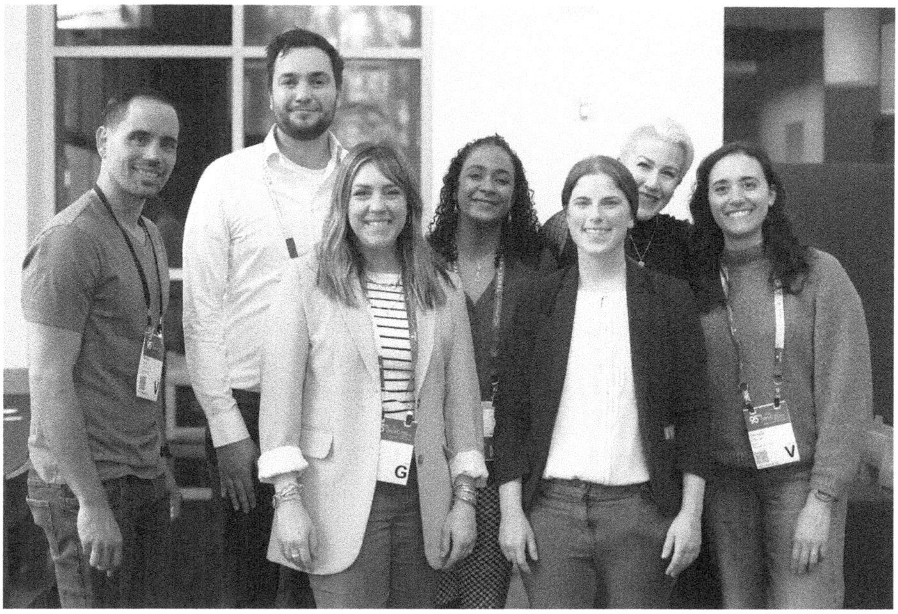

FIGURE 10.2 A support network of mentors.

to the external demands being placed on her (e.g. conflict with team members and clients) as well as her internal demands (e.g. feeling not good enough). She did this through seeking resources to support herself in navigating these challenging experiences. By seeking peer support and professional skills training, she learned strategies to cope with her stress in a healthy way. This veterinarian embodied the very definition of resilience in her early career (Figure 10.2).

Resilience is multidimensional. In one study (Cake et al., 2017), several key components of resiliency in veterinary professionals were discussed including:

- **Emotional competence:** Emotional competence or emotional intelligence (EI) may contribute to high levels of resilience. Giving veterinary professionals the tools that they need to process the emotions that they are experiencing as they are transitioning into the profession is vital.
- **Motivation:** This component of resilience included the ability to find a sense of purpose and meaning in your work. As mentors, we can help support our mentees in discovering their purpose in veterinary medicine.
- **Personal resources:** Personal resources include the ability to have autonomy, self-confidence, proactive and reflective behavior, and optimism. One of the best ways to help our mentees build personal resources is to encourage self-reflection and self-awareness through quality open-ended questions and debriefing.
- **Social support:** Seeking resources and support from those around you is one of the most powerful contributors to resilience. As mentors, we can encourage our mentees to create their own support network as well as encourage them to ask for help when needed.
- **Life balance:** Maintaining an identity and life outside of work is key in promoting resilience. I often encourage mentees to set healthy boundaries, better manage their time, and prioritize their personal life. This can lead to a more sustainable career.

- **Well-being strategies:** Certain well-being strategies can help veterinarians solve problem, process challenging thoughts and emotions, and foster well-being. This may include encouraging your mentees to seek support from a licensed mental health professional if needed or making your mentee aware of evidence-based mental health programming and resources to improve physical, mental, and emotional health.

When I was navigating my own feelings of burnout, I can recall how my mentors, friends, and loved ones supported me in each of these areas. I believe that resilience can be nurtured by those around us including within our mentoring relationships.

As I continued my career, I have always tried to model vulnerability and resilience. I think if we can be more open about discussing our challenges and how we successfully navigated them, we can show our mentees that it is okay to experience times of stress and self-doubt. As mentors, our role is to support our mentees in coming up with their own solutions to their unique challenges and stressors.

In my early career, I received a thank you card from a veterinary assistant that I mentored in my practice. In this thank you card, my mentee expressed gratitude for my vulnerability and compassion even in times of stress. I sometimes refer to it in times of doubt because it reminds me that asking for help is not a sign of weakness; rather, it can inspire others to push forward despite setbacks in this challenging career (Figure 10.3).

In the next section, Dr. Daniel Stillwell will dive deeper into more strategies to build resilience in your mentees. We will also discuss how to best support your mentee through adapting to change in their early career.

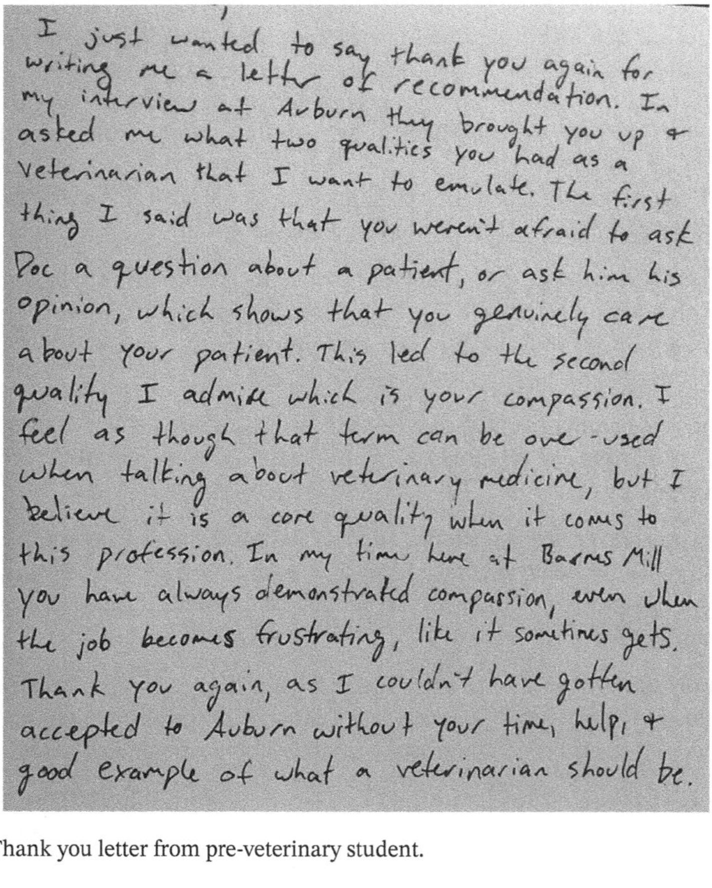
I just wanted to say thank you again for writing me a letter of recommendation. In my interview at Auburn they brought you up & asked me what two qualities you had as a veterinarian that I want to emulate. The first thing I said was that you weren't afraid to ask Doc a question about a patient, or ask him his opinion, which shows that you genuinely care about your patient. This led to the second quality I admire which is your compassion. I feel as though that term can be over-used when talking about veterinary medicine, but I believe it is a core quality when it comes to this profession. In my time here at Barnes Mill you have always demonstrated compassion, even when the job becomes frustrating, like it sometimes gets. Thank you again, as I couldn't have gotten accepted to Auburn without your time, help, & good example of what a veterinarian should be.

FIGURE 10.3 Thank you letter from pre-veterinary student.

FOSTERING ADAPTABILITY TO CHANGE

Daniel Stillwell

Fostering adaptability to change starts with understanding the nature of change and the barriers to it. Change is notoriously difficult to pin down since it is both a moment and constant, both developmental and instantaneous. Some professionals I work with in veterinary medicine seem to fixate on rigid concepts of how things "ought to be" and that stuckness seems to limit their ability to adapt to new situations, people, or moments.

Change-work is built on the *both/and* sense of reality. It emphasizes that when we stop being open to change, we stop adapting to it. Since change is inevitable and ubiquitous, we tend to be at our most functional and resilient as professionals (and people!) when we have a healthy relationship with change.

As a doctoral level relational therapist, I have been working with complex and interesting cases for over 15 years. I have been a professor, presenter, supervisor, and clinical director. I have also been fortunate enough to bring that experience to mental health coaching sessions with veterinary professionals for the past five years. Common themes have emerged in the sessions:

- Feeling like they haven't earned their professional status and could be fired if discovered to be unworthy (imposter syndrome)
- Navigating power dynamics related to clinical decisions and perceived effectiveness
- Struggling to maintain a healthy work–life balance
- Seeking the right book, therapist, or resource to help address a specific issue

What all of these have in common is the underlying issue of perfectionism or the person's relationship with how things "ought to be."

UNDERSTANDING PERFECTIONISM

The general definition of perfectionism is a combination of excessively rigid standards with excessively harsh evaluations. While most people think about these as only applying to oneself, there are actually three types of perfectionism: self-oriented, socially prescribed, and other-oriented.

Self-oriented perfectionism is the most common kind and occurs when "individuals attach irrational importance to being perfect, hold unrealistic expectations of themselves, and are punitive in their self-evaluations" (Curran and Hill, 2019). Put in another way, it is a pattern or paradigm of being hard on oneself because of an internalized belief that the person "has to be" a certain way.

My most common starter question I ask someone wrestling with the *have to's* of life is "Do you have to?" This typically gets them to pause and question an alternate reality. This simple question usually prompts a pause—and opens the door to imagining an alternate reality. Over time, they begin to recognize these moments of perceived obligation more easily, which helps reduce feelings of passivity or helplessness.

The second question I often ask is "Who told you that you had to?" This usually prompts them to reflect on the authoritative voices that have shaped their beliefs. From there, we can begin to untangle the message itself from the people or institutions behind it. **A great way to become more comfortable with change is by beginning to believe you have the authority to create it yourself.**

These authorities (God, parents, coaches, teachers, celebrities, society, etc.) are not consciously trying to control people or push them toward self-critical thoughts and behaviors. In most cases, they're not aiming to manipulate, but rather expressing their own preferences for how people should behave—often as an attempt to bring the world more in line with their own values or sense of order. Generally, these people and institutions have very good reasons for their preferences.

In veterinary medicine, many of these expectations are rooted in science and best practices for patient care and business management. I don't raise this to disparage or reject authority for its own sake, but to create space for mentees to critically examine whether these standards are fully understood and still useful to them in each context or case.

New veterinarians and technicians often struggle to feel comfortable offering care options that fall below the "gold standard." This difficulty is often rooted in the training environment of veterinary school, where aggressive diagnostics and treatment plans are emphasized, and anything less than the gold standard is often implicitly or explicitly discouraged. Yet, regardless of how well-intentioned or widely accepted an authority may be, it's ultimately up to the professional in the moment to decide whether following that standard aligns with their own clinical judgment and the specific needs of the case in front of them.

When people adopt externally given standards as their own, they also inherit a built-in framework for ethics (how to make the right decisions) and morality (what is good or bad). This can be efficient—it saves the effort of constructing a personal framework from scratch. Many children are raised with parents who say, "Because I said so" from time to time. Depending on the age and developmental level of the child, this might be very appropriate to ensure the child does not hurt themselves or someone else, especially since children often don't need to know all the reasons behind a rule. The insidious nature of these internalized messages is that, as adults, we often end up policing ourselves with inherited standards—rarely pausing to question whether these ideas of right and wrong still serve us. Holding space to check in with oneself is one of the first steps of the mindfulness practice of **self-compassion**.

SELF-COMPASSION

Self-compassion is a concept pioneered by Neff (2011). Her work helped articulate that people can't simply will themselves into feeling better. In fact, willpower or grit as a forced experience typically worsens self-esteem and quality of work. Instead of doing something because we "have to," self-compassion teaches us to pause and check in with ourselves before taking action. It teaches we are worthy of grace and compassion, not because we are successful, but because we have autonomy and agency. When we cultivate this internally, we become our best as caregivers.

This practice helps us be better at change because it improves our base level of identity and functioning. Instead of being high-strung and brittle, we are more agile. When a veterinary professional finds their schedule has just been overbooked for the fourth day in a row, a practice of self-compassion reminds them that neither the circumstances nor their performance define their worth. They can choose to pause, continue to put one foot in front of the other, and calmly communicate their needs and resources to those around them.

According to Neff, there are three components of self-compassion you can nurture in your mentees:

1. **Self-kindness** consists of responding to personal challenges with warmth and understanding, rather than criticism or harsh judgment. As a mentor, you can model self-kindness by validating your mentee's struggles and encouraging them to speak to themselves with the same care they'd offer a close friend.

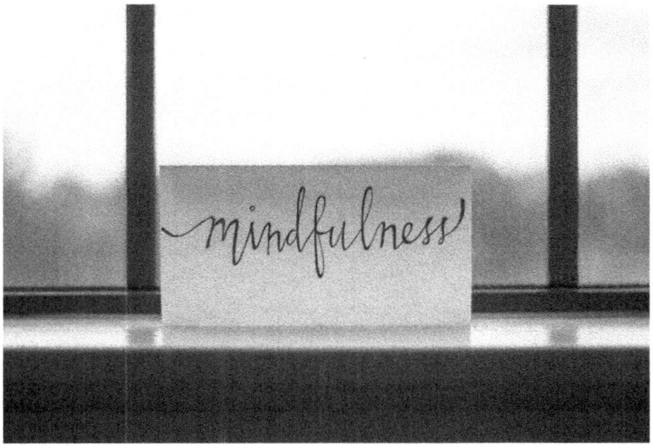

FIGURE 10.4 *Source:* Lesly Juarez/https://unsplash.com/photos/mindfulness-printed-paper-near-window-DFtjXYd5Pto/Last accessed on Jan 29, 2026.

Table 10.1 Types of Perfectionism

Self-oriented	Socially prescribed	Other-oriented
Being hard on oneself because of an internalized belief that the person "has to be" a certain way.	A form of people-pleasing where one's sense of worth is tied to meeting perceived external expectations.	A tendency to micromanage or dictate how others "should" be; being hard on others.

2. **Common humanity** is recognizing that struggles and imperfections are part of the shared human experience. Remind your mentees that they are not alone in their challenges—sharing your own stories of missteps or doubts can help normalize imperfection and foster connection.

3. **Mindfulness** includes being present with difficult thoughts and emotions without suppressing or exaggerating them, allowing for clarity and acceptance in the moment. Help your mentees build mindfulness by encouraging them to slow down, name what they're feeling, and notice their inner experience without immediately jumping to problem-solving (Figure 10.4).

By encouraging these elements in your mentorship relationships, you can help mentees develop a more grounded and resilient sense of self—one that thrives even in the high-stress environments of veterinary medicine (Table 10.1).

SOCIALLY PRESCRIBED PERFECTIONISM

The next type of perfectionism is socially prescribed perfectionism and occurs when "individuals believe their social context is excessively demanding, that others judge them harshly, and that they must display perfection to secure approval" (Curran and Hill, 2019). In many ways, this reflects a compulsive form of people-pleasing—where one's sense of worth is tied to meeting perceived external expectations.

Many high achievers have been raised in families or contexts where the approval of others mattered more than whatever the particular behavior was. The veterinary profession is full of high-achieving people pleasers, and one of the most impossible expectations they seem to internalize is that "I have to make sure everyone is okay."

Extreme standards like this are technically possible to achieve from time to time. For veterinary professionals, it is true that they can occasionally see every patient on time that needs to be seen and have every client satisfied without running over budget. Another example is that it is possible to get off work on time, get home smoothly, make dinner, and serve it hot to a family in a good mood and then get a great night's sleep so you can get up early and workout.

But are those things likely?

Can they be expected to happen literally everyday?

Of course not. So let's explore some ways to address this type of perfectionism.

THE 80% RULE

I suggest high achievers follow the 80% rule: whatever the ideal metric is, lower it by 20% and you will not only meet it more often but also be less burnt out in the process since reserves are built in for the ebbs and flows of stress. Unfortunately, those 100% metrics are the types of narratives most professionals convince themselves they need to meet each and every time. For socially prescribed perfectionists, this drive is often rooted in a desire to make others feel satisfied, valued, or reassured, even at the expense of their own well-being.

LESS IS MORE

An incredibly vital lesson I teach over and over in veterinary coaching is this: you are not responsible for other people's emotions or reactions. Typically, I am working with over-functioning people who are used to picking up the slack for those around them. When this pattern becomes the norm, then these people tend to also become the enablers of those around them. Enabling others almost always begins with good intentions—offering help, support, or care. But over time, it can evolve into an unspoken expectation: to continually rescue others from their own discomforts, challenges, or even incompetence. The path forward for socially prescribed perfectionists often starts with realizing that the change they need most isn't doing more—it's doing less for others, especially when it's rooted in seeking validation or approval.

Doing less for those around us (notably the ones we are "trying to make happy") is likely counterintuitive for most and will almost certainly cause some friction at the beginning. This highlights another crucial element of fostering adaptability to change: embrace the discomfort. People gravitate toward the familiar or the path of least resistance, instead of deciding to try something uncomfortable or different. And when people-pleasing is involved, this can be very difficult.

One tactic I give in coaching sessions is to move from "do for" someone to "do with" someone. This creates connection and shared experience, and if the other will benefit from starting to do the task on their own, the "do with" can be gradually pulled back. This is how we move from enabling to empowering.

I encourage people to ask themselves, "what am I actually responsible for?" and slowly let go of or hand off the rest.

CULTURAL AWARENESS

People are raised in communities, families, and cultures where virtues such as respect, submission, deference, and assertiveness can dictate how one is expected to relate to others. Cultural norms can be laden with power dynamics that can uplift or suppress individuals. This chapter is ultimately about regaining one's own sense of autonomy and agency over making choices with intention and not because one *has to*. True growth begins when the individual realizes they have a *choice* in how they respond. As long as someone believes they *must* conform without question, they remain stuck in a pattern that undermines their sense of freedom and self-trust (Table 10.2).

True freedom comes from making choices rooted in your own values—whether they align with your upbringing or not—and navigating life with clarity, confidence, and integrity.

Table 10.2 Tactics for Perfectionism

Mentoring tactics for perfectionism		
Self-oriented	**Socially prescribed**	**Other-oriented**
Encourage self-compassion Self-kindness Common humanity Mindfulness	80% Rule Whatever their ideal metric is, encourage them to lower it by 20%. Less is More Consider "do with" someone instead of "do for" someone.	The paradigm of choice Help mentees shift from "I should" to "I choose". Reduce all-or-nothing statements towards others.
Open-ended questions to explore Do I have to? Who told me, "you have to?"	Open ended questions to explore What am I actually responsible for? Am I seeking someone else's approval?	Open ended questions to explore What are realistic expectations? What is this feeling trying to tell me?

OTHER-ORIENTED PERFECTIONISM

The last form of perfectionism is other-oriented perfectionism. With this form of perfectionism, "individuals impose unrealistic standards on those around them and evaluate others critically" (Curran and Hill, 2019). I think this type of perfectionism is best understood as a tendency to micromanage or dictate how others "should" be—often because the individual cannot see another way to bring reality in line with their expectations. If self-oriented perfectionism is about being hard on oneself, other-oriented perfectionism is about being hard on others.

A major factor in reducing other-oriented perfectionism is to shift the anger to another emotion in moments when others are not "doing what they should." Anger is activated by unmet expectations, but many veterinarians I work with are able to eventually acknowledge their anger is covering up fear, sadness, or guilt. They might be scared about a botched surgery getting reported to the board. On days when they don't show up as their best selves, they may carry a heavy sense of guilt. By acknowledging that those other emotions are acceptable to feel, this helps change how they relate to having feelings in the first place.

EMOTIONAL INTELLIGENCE

EI can foster adaptability to change. Change means something different has occurred, and something different will almost always trigger an emotion.

An emotion can be thought of as the body talking to the mind, saying, "Hi! I have some information for you so you can take care of us." When we take our emotions out on those around us, we forget that the feeling is ours, not theirs to deal with. By pausing and asking, "What is this feeling trying to tell me?" we get better at not projecting onto others and instead focus on managing the one thing we can control—US!

Becoming more emotionally fluent not only helps you stay grounded but also creates a calming ripple effect on those around you.

This topic is explored further in Chapter 7 on Cultivating Emotional Intelligence.

THE PARADIGM OF CHOICE

By breaking down the patterns of how things "should be" and reducing the power of rigid expectations and harsh judgments, I coach people to break the cycles of shame and blame they regularly find themselves in. This helps them foster the ability to change by moving from the paradigm of *have to's* to the paradigm of choice. Below you will see the chart I walk people through to help map out how the paradigms work.

Should's are usually shorthand ways to get people to motivate themselves. In the workplace, should's have institutional weight in the form of policies and procedures. And to be functional in the workplace, most of the time, it is wise and healthy to comply with those standards. But not because you *have to*, instead because you *choose to*.

I also help individuals not overcorrect. They still have expectations and evaluations, and now they can change the patterns around requirements and judgment. I help them emphasize and empower the things and values that matter to them, thus also breaking the cycles of shame and blame that keep them believing they are not good enough.

And as self-compassion literature has demonstrated, people flourish and are adaptable to change when they have worth in their own autonomy and agency. Not doing things because you *have to*, but because you *choose to* (Figure 10.5).

FOSTERING ADAPTABILITY TO CHANGE AS A VETERINARY MENTOR

As a mentor, your role is not to fix or rescue your mentee, but to walk alongside them as they explore their own patterns, values, and choices. The goal is to create a space where they feel both challenged and supported as they grow. Below are some simple but powerful ways you can help mentees build adaptability to change while confronting perfectionism with compassion and clarity:

1. **Ask open-ended values-based questions**—Help mentees shift from "I should" to "I choose" by asking what truly matters to them. Questions like "What's important to you in this situation?" invite reflection and ownership.

2. **Normalize imperfection**—Share your own missteps or moments of uncertainty. This not only builds trust but also helps mentees understand that growth comes through imperfection, not the absence of it. In addition, discuss the gray areas and nuances of practicing veterinary medicine.

Choose	Should
Expectations	Requirement
Evaluations	Judgment
Empowerment of values	Shame/Blame

FIGURE 10.5 People flourish when "choosing to" rather than "having to". *Source:* Daniel Stillwell (2025).

3. **Model self-compassion**—When a mentee is hard on themselves, model how to pause and respond with kindness. A simple, "That sounds really tough—how are you taking care of yourself in this?" can shift the conversation toward self-kindness.
4. **Shift from "do for" to "do with"**—As a mentor, aim to do with your mentee rather than do for them. Walk alongside them through challenges instead of taking over. This approach models collaboration, supports autonomy, and helps mentees build confidence and capability without fostering dependence.
5. **Foster emotional awareness**—When mentees express frustration or anxiety, ask what might be underneath those feelings. Helping them recognize underlying emotions like fear, sadness, or guilt builds EI.
6. **Emphasize choice and agency**—Remind your mentees that they have the right to question standards and make intentional choices. Whether they follow traditional paths or forge new ones, it matters that the decision is theirs.

Fostering adaptability to change and addressing perfectionism are foundational steps in helping veterinary professionals thrive—but they don't exist in a vacuum. True growth and sustainability come when these internal shifts are supported by strong external systems and intentional self-care. Mentorship, community, and workplace culture all play critical roles in shaping well-being. In the next section, Mariel Hendricks will explore how support systems, well-being practices, and self-care strategies can reinforce the inner work mentees are doing—and help them navigate the demands of veterinary medicine with greater clarity, balance, and resilience.

SUPPORT SYSTEMS, WELL-BEING AND SELF-CARE STRATEGIES

Mariel Hendricks

When I graduated from Purdue's Veterinary Technology program in 2010, I was eager to take on the world. My plan was simple: start in small animal general practice to sharpen my nursing skills before stepping into my dream job in a specialty surgery department. I had great coworkers, a lead technician I could go to with questions, and incredible veterinarians by my side. But despite all of that, I often felt alone. I didn't realize then how much I needed a mentor—someone who truly understood my perfectionism, my introverted nature, and the weight of the expectations I placed on myself.

At that time, the culture in veterinary medicine was very much "sink or swim." After two years in general practice, I transitioned into specialty surgery, a role that came with on-call shifts and long, emotionally and physically demanding days. I worked 12-hour shifts, overnights, weekends, and holidays, pouring everything I had into my patients' healing process. Then, I would come home to my personal responsibilities, including the demands of motherhood. I was fortunate to find a surgical mentor who helped me grow in my role, but even then, I never prioritized my own well-being.

A decade into my career as a surgical veterinary technician, burnout hit me—hard. My body was screaming for relief. Chronic back pain became my constant companion, I underwent hip surgery for a labral tear, and I found myself relying on antidepressants just to keep going. Then came the COVID pandemic, bringing with it an overwhelming sense of isolation. In the midst of it all, I became a single mom and lost my own mother to brain cancer. The weight of it all became too much.

By 2021, I reached my breaking point. I looked at my life and told myself, *Enough is enough. It's time to take care of me.*

My self-care journey started with one crucial realization: I couldn't keep pushing my body past its limits. The physical demands of working on a clinic floor were no longer sustainable, and I knew something had to change. Rather than waiting for things to get worse, I took a proactive step and enrolled in a master's program in veterinary education. It wasn't easy—balancing school, work, and motherhood meant sacrificing a lot of my free time—but I knew it would be worth it in the long run.

In 2024, I earned my master's degree, and with it came a new path—one that allowed me to continue making an impact in veterinary medicine without sacrificing my health. Transitioning to a work-from-home role with MentorVet not only eased the physical strain on my body but also gave me the flexibility I needed as a single mother. More importantly, it gave me the opportunity to focus on something that had become a true passion: mentorship.

Aside from work, I started focusing on hobbies—hiking, outdoor obstacle course racing, and puzzling. This helped my brain focus on Mariel (the person), rather than Mariel (the veterinary technician). I watched what I ate, became more intentional about personal relationships with close friends and family, and made sure to put down my phone at night to get an hour or two more of sleep. I embraced meditation and breathing exercises, started a gym membership, and increased self-care activities like massages, facials, and aromatherapy. After two years of these lifestyle changes, I was 30 pounds lighter, happier than I had ever been in my life, and off of my antidepressants.

This career shift lifted both the physical and mental weight I had been carrying for years. It showed me that I could prioritize my well-being, stay in the profession I love, and still be successful—as a veterinary technician, as a mentor, and as a mother. It was a long, difficult journey to get here, but now, I know I'm exactly where I'm meant to be—helping others navigate their own paths in veterinary medicine and well-being.

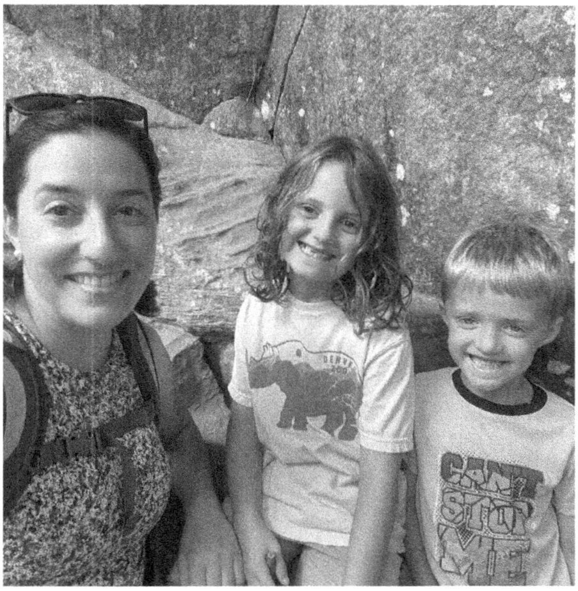

FIGURE 10.6 Mariel and her kids hiking at Turkey Run State Park in Indiana.

In this section, we'll explore how you care for yourself and your mentees. As mentors, we can't effectively support others unless we first prioritize our own well-being. By modeling healthy self-care practices, we show our mentees that a sustainable career in veterinary medicine is not only possible—it's essential. We will also give you strategies on how you can support others in developing their own self-care practices (Figure 10.6).

STRESS MANAGEMENT PLANS

Self-care isn't just about taking a break when you feel overwhelmed—it's about creating a sustainable plan that prioritizes your well-being everyday. In veterinary medicine, where long hours, emotional strain, and physical demands are the norm, having a structured stress management plan can be the difference between surviving and thriving. A self-care plan ensures that caring for yourself isn't an afterthought, but rather, a lifestyle. As veterinary mentors, it's crucial that we encourage our mentees to build these self-care habits early so our mentees can build a sustainable career.

WHAT IS SELF-CARE?

Self-care is the practice of taking intentional actions to maintain and improve one's physical, mental, and emotional well-being. It involves recognizing personal needs, setting healthy boundaries, and incorporating habits that promote overall health and resilience. In veterinary medicine, where professionals often prioritize the needs of patients and clients over their own, self-care is vital for keeping us in the profession long term.

Veterinary medicine is a deeply rewarding profession, but it also comes with significant challenges, particularly in the transition to practice. Long hours, physically demanding work, and emotional stressors—such as conflict, ethical dilemmas, and the pressure to provide the best possible care—can take a toll on us. Without intentional self-care, these challenges can lead to burnout, compassion fatigue, and even serious mental health struggles.

Prioritizing self-care is not just about feeling better in the moment; it's about building a sustainable and fulfilling career. Here's why self-care is essential in veterinary medicine:

- **Prevents burnout and compassion fatigue**—Chronic stress and emotional exhaustion can make it difficult to find joy in the profession. Self-care helps manage stress before it becomes overwhelming.
- **Supports mental and physical health**—Veterinary professionals experience higher-than-average rates of serious psychological distress and suicide risk (Tomasi et al., 2019; Merck Animal Health, 2022). Prioritizing self-care can help improve emotional resilience and overall mental well-being as well as physical health.
- **Promotes job satisfaction, team morale, and better patient care**—When veterinary professionals prioritize self-care, they feel more fulfilled in their roles, contribute to a healthier workplace culture, and deliver higher-quality patient care.

BASIC SELF-CARE

Establishing healthy habits in sleep, exercise, and nutrition has the potential to improve overall energy levels, resilience, and job performance. Helping your mentee build these sustainable self-care habits is one of the most practical ways to support their long-term well-being. Here are some key areas you can explore together:

1. Prioritizing Quality Sleep

   Adequate sleep is essential for physical recovery, mental clarity, and emotional stability. However, irregular schedules, on-call shifts, and stress can make it difficult for veterinary professionals to get the rest they need.

   - Aim for seven to nine hours of sleep per night whenever possible.
   - Establish a consistent bedtime routine to signal to your body that it's time to wind down.
   - Reduce screen time before bed to avoid blue light disruption.
   - Use relaxation techniques, such as deep breathing or meditation, to improve sleep quality.
   - If working night shifts, create a dark, quiet sleep environment during the day.

2. Incorporating Regular Exercise

   Physical activity can reduce stress, improve mood, and prevent injuries caused by the physical demands of veterinary work. It doesn't require a rigorous workout routine—small, intentional movements throughout the day can make a big difference.

   - Stretch before and after shifts to prevent stiffness and reduce injury risk.
   - Engage in low-impact exercises like walking, yoga, or swimming to build strength and flexibility. You can even include your pet to make it fun!
   - Consider resistance training to improve endurance and support proper lifting techniques.
   - Even on busy days, incorporate movement breaks—a quick walk, a few stretches, or deep breathing exercises can help reset the body and mind.

3. Fueling the Body with Proper Nutrition

   Veterinary professionals often work long shifts without regular meal breaks, leading to reliance on fast food, sugary snacks, or skipping meals altogether. Proper nutrition plays a key role in maintaining energy levels and overall well-being.

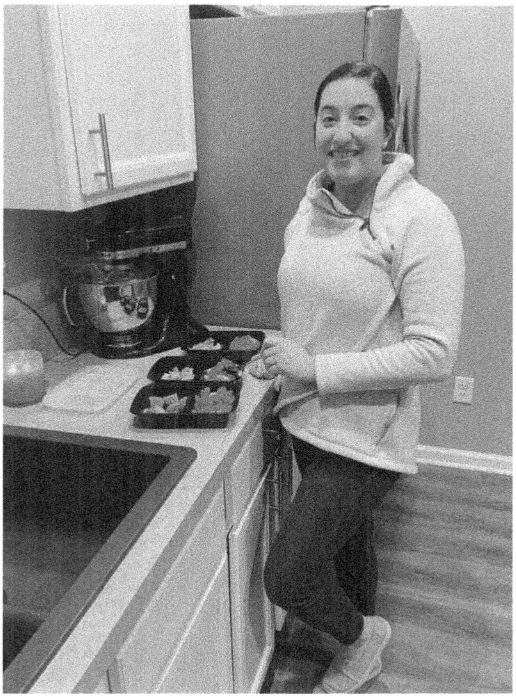

FIGURE 10.7 Mariel meal prepping to save time during the week with chicken, rice, and veggies.

- Start the day with a balanced breakfast to stabilize blood sugar and energy levels.
- Keep healthy snacks on hand, such as nuts, fruit, protein bars, or yogurt, to prevent energy crashes.
- Stay hydrated—dehydration can contribute to fatigue and brain fog. I use a water bottle with each hour of the day printed on the outside to keep me on track!
- Plan and pack nutrient-dense meals to avoid reliance on unhealthy fast-food options.
- Avoid excessive caffeine and high-sugar energy drinks; instead, incorporate hydrating beverages like water or herbal tea (Figure 10.7).

These foundational self-care practices help create a strong baseline for managing stress, preventing burnout, and maintaining long-term well-being in the profession.

ADVANCED SELF-CARE

Beyond the basics of sleep, exercise, and nutrition, self-care extends into more advanced areas of well-being that contribute to a sustainable and fulfilling career in veterinary medicine. A holistic self-care approach includes **physical, intellectual, emotional, occupational, and social well-being.** Encouraging your mentee to integrate these advanced practices can help them build resilience, improve job satisfaction, and create a long-term career that supports both personal and professional goals. The following five dimensions of well-being offer mentors a framework to help mentees reflect on their current habits and explore areas for growth.

1. **Physical Well-Being: Protecting Your Body for Longevity**

   Veterinary professionals perform physically demanding tasks daily, from lifting patients to standing for long hours. Prioritizing physical well-being can help prevent injuries and maintain long-term health.

- Ergonomic Awareness—Use proper body mechanics when lifting and adjusting tables and equipment to reduce strain.
- Preventative Care—Prioritize regular medical checkups, physical therapy, or chiropractic care to address early signs of injury or physical stress.
- Workplace Modifications—Utilize tools like anti-fatigue mats, supportive footwear, and adjustable stools to reduce discomfort.

2. **Intellectual Well-Being: Lifelong Learning and Professional Growth**

   Engaging in intellectual self-care fosters curiosity, keeps the mind sharp, and enhances job satisfaction by continuously growing within the field.

   - Continuing Education—Stay engaged with CE opportunities, workshops, and conferences to enhance skills and confidence.
   - Reading and Research—Stay updated on emerging trends, research, and best practices in veterinary medicine.
   - Teaching and Mentorship—Share knowledge with colleagues, students, or interns to strengthen leadership skills and inspire the next generation.

3. **Emotional Well-Being: Managing Stress and Compassion Fatigue**

   Veterinary professionals often experience emotional strain from client interactions, euthanasia, and high caseloads. Actively managing emotional health helps build resilience and maintain passion for the field.

   - Self-Reflection Practices—Journaling or mindfulness exercises can help process emotions and prevent emotional exhaustion, like compassion fatigue.
   - Healthy Coping Mechanisms—Develop strategies like deep breathing, meditation, or hobbies that provide a mental reset.
   - Seeking Support—Regularly connect with mentors, therapists, or peer support groups to discuss challenges in a safe space.

4. **Occupational Well-Being: Thriving in the Workplace**

   A fulfilling work environment plays a significant role in overall well-being. Occupational self-care includes creating a healthy workplace culture, clarifying job roles, and advocating for professional growth.

   - Define Clear Roles—Ensure all professionals are utilized to their full potential with defined responsibilities that match their training.
   - Encourage Collaboration—Work closely with management, leaders, and colleagues to create a team-centered environment where everyone's contributions are valued.
   - Set Boundaries—Communicate workload expectations and ensure a balance between responsibility and capacity.

5. **Social Well-Being: Building a Strong Support System**

   Building a strong support system—both personally and professionally—is essential for long-term success and well-being in the veterinary field.

   - Cultivate Meaningful Relationships—Stay connected with friends and family, prioritize quality relationships, and make time for social activities (Figure 10.8).

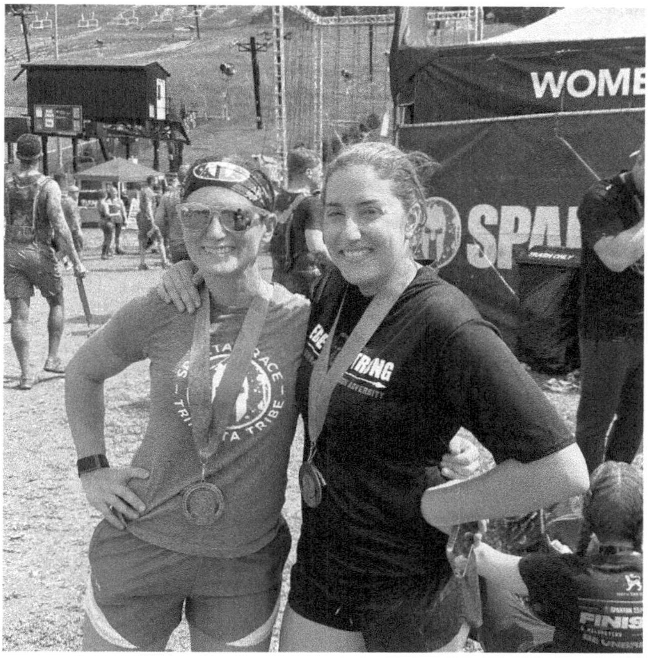

FIGURE 10.8 Mariel and a friend celebrating their Spartan finish.

- Seek Quality Mentorship—Surround yourself with a diverse group of mentors, including those with more experience and trusted peers who can offer valuable support.
- Expand Your Professional Network—Join veterinary organizations and attend conferences to connect with like-minded professionals.

CREATING A STRESS MANAGEMENT PLAN

I highly recommend all mentors and mentees complete a stress management plan to help put ideas on paper as a quick-reference guide to their personal self-care strategies. While creating this plan, be sure to make SMART goals that are Specific, Measurable, Achievable, Realistic, and Time-Limited. For example, if I know I wasn't exercising enough and wanted to start exercising more, I wouldn't just write down on my self-care plan "exercise more." I would write, "Run 2 miles on Mondays, Wednesdays, and Fridays" (Figure 10.9).

As you and your mentee are creating self-care plans, think about the following questions and comments:

1. What is your main concern? Narrow down concerns to the most important.
2. What processes will allow you to focus on the most important concerns? This will allow you to prioritize processes that will target concerns that will give you immediate results, which is encouraging.
3. How can you make your self-care priorities into an intentional intervention? Make a commitment that you can adhere to in order to reach your goals.
4. If you are struggling to meet your goals, how can you take smaller steps to start?

Individualized Stress Management Template

Name- Mariel Hendricks

Care Area	Specific Goal/Objectives (SMART)**	Accountability Measure
Physical care	–Get at least 7 hours of sleep a night –Drink 2 Nalgene bottles of water per day –Attend 2 gym group sessions per week on Tuesday and Thursday –Walk my dogs 1 time on the weekend –Meal prep 5 meals a week	–Gym buddy –Sleep app –Accountability buddy
Psychological care	–Journal 3 times a week at bedtime –Breathing exercise each morning before I get out of bed	–Journal –Self-monitoring
Social care	–Call my brother every day –Call my parents once a week –Once a month mom's night out –Once a month date night with my significant other	–Calendar –Family and Friends
Professional/academic care	–Attend 1 in-person CE meeting a month through CIVMA –Attend 1 state conference and 1 national conference a year	–Calendar –Colleagues
Other areas of self-care (ex. hobbies)	–Do 3 Spartan races a year –Work on a puzzle instead of scrolling on my phone	–Accountability buddy –Screen time self monitoring

****SMART= specific, measurable, achievable, realistic, and time limited**

MentorVet

FIGURE 10.9 Mariel's Stress Management Plan.

5. Are there any resources you may need to meet your goals?
6. Be willing to put in the effort needed to make it a success. You may need to revise your initial self-care plan if you don't achieve initial success.
7. Acknowledge and accept. When you have achieved a goal, acknowledge that and celebrate!

SUPPORTING YOUR MENTEE'S SELF-CARE

Veterinarians often intertwine their professional and personal identities so closely that it can be challenging to see themselves beyond their careers. As a mentor, you can help your mentee explore who they are outside of veterinary medicine.

PERSONAL IDENTITY DEVELOPMENT

Ask about their hobbies, interests, and passions beyond their work, and encourage them to engage in activities that nurture their well-being. By encouraging a balanced approach to personal interests and their professional role, you can reinforce the importance of maintaining a strong sense of self beyond their role as a veterinarian.

You can also have them complete the stress management plan we discussed earlier in this chapter.

CULTIVATE INTROSPECTION

Self-reflection is a critical component of identity development, allowing individuals to understand their values, beliefs, and motivations. Encourage your mentee to engage in introspection through:

- Thoughtful, open-ended conversations that explore their perspectives, aspirations, and personal values.
- Journaling about their experiences in veterinary medicine, helping them process their emotions and thoughts.
- Examining their underlying assumptions and biases to promote self-awareness and growth.

By fostering introspection, mentees can gain deeper insight into their professional identity and how it aligns with their personal values.

CLARIFY CORE VALUES

Encouraging mentees to define their core values can help guide their professional and ethical decision-making. Utilize value-identification exercises to help them articulate what matters most to them, both personally and professionally.

When mentees have a strong grasp of their core values, they are better equipped to make aligned decisions, navigate ethical dilemmas, and understand sources of conflict in their professional lives. By supporting identity development, mentors empower veterinarians to cultivate a fulfilling and sustainable career while maintaining a well-rounded personal identity.

ENCOURAGE BOUNDARY SETTING

The best mentors encourage their mentees to set healthy boundaries in the workplace. Early in my career, I often struggled with this because I feared being judged or seen as less committed. But when my mentors encouraged me to take time for myself, I began to feel more confident in prioritizing my well-being. As a mentor, you have the opportunity to normalize these conversations and empower your mentees to care for themselves, too (Figure 10.10).

PROVIDE WELL-BEING RESOURCES

We should also provide our mentees with additional resources to support their mental health. There are a range of resources now available to individuals in the veterinary profession:

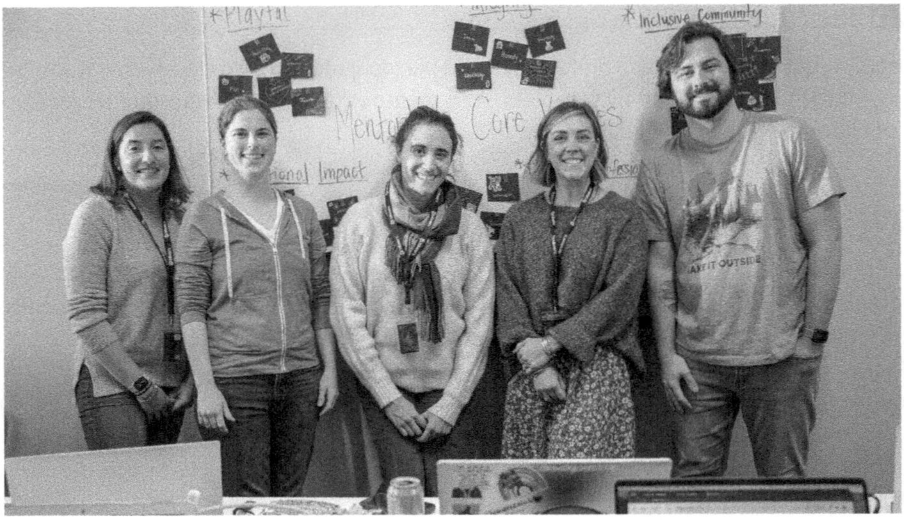

FIGURE 10.10 MentorVet team completing a core values exercise.

- Invest in an Employee Assistance Program (EAP) for your clinic, which can provide free short-term counseling for individuals in need of support.
- Share resources such as free peer support groups offered by Veterinary Hope Foundation and NOMV.
- Consider an embedded veterinary social worker in your practice or have a mental health professional come into the clinic regularly for team support.
- Refer your mentees to external mentorship programming for additional support.

The journey to sustainable well-being in veterinary medicine is challenging, but it doesn't have to be walked alone. Work alongside your mentees to establish self-care goals. Remember, taking care of yourself isn't selfish—it's foundational. Let your story, like mine, be one of resilience, growth, and compassion—for yourself and those you mentor.

CONCLUSION

Resilience and adaptability are not innate traits but skills that can be developed through intentional support, structured self-care practices and shifts in how veterinary professionals relate to perfectionism and change. The stressors of early-career practice—ethical dilemmas, self-doubt, team conflict, and the weight of responsibility—are predictable and manageable when met with the right tools.

Effective mentorship helps new graduates build emotional competence, create personal resources, maintain life balance, and develop well-being strategies that sustain long careers. This means fostering self-compassion over harsh self-judgment, helping mentees shift from "I should" to "I choose," and supporting the creation of concrete stress management plans that address physical, emotional, intellectual, occupational, and social well-being. When mentors model vulnerability, normalize imperfection, and provide access to mental health resources, they equip mentees to not only survive the transition to practice but also to build sustainable, fulfilling careers.

BIBLIOGRAPHY

American Psychological Association (2025). Resilience. https://www.apa.org/topics/resilience (accessed 31 March 2025).

Bartram, D.J., Yadegarfar, G., and Baldwin, D.S. (2009). A cross-sectional study of mental health and well-being and their associations in the UK veterinary profession. *Social Psychiatry and Psychiatric Epidemiology* 44 (12): 1075–1085.

Cake, M.A., McArthur, M.M., Matthew, S.M., and Mansfield, C.F. (2017). Finding the balance: uncovering resilience in the veterinary literature. *Journal of Veterinary Medical Education* 44 (1): 95–105. https://doi.org/10.3138/jvme.0116-025R.

Curran, T. and Hill, A.P. (2019). Perfectionism is increasing over time: a meta-analysis of birth cohort differences from 1989 to 2016. *Psychological Bulletin* 145 (4): 410–429.

Gardner, D.H. and Hini, D. (2006). Work-related stress in the veterinary profession in New Zealand. *New Zealand Veterinary Journal* 54 (3): 119–124.

Maslach, C. and Leiter, M. (2016). Understanding the burnout experience: recent research and its implications for psychiatry. *World Psychiatry* 15 (2): 103–111.

Merck Animal Health (2022). Veterinary mental health and wellbeing and how to improve them. https://www.merck-animal-health-usa.com/wp-content/uploads/sites/54/2022/02/2021-PSV-Veterinary-Wellbeing-Presentation_V2.pdf (accessed 31 March 2025).

Neff, K.D. (2011). *Self-Compassion: The Proven Power of Being Kind to Yourself.* New York: William Morrow.

Reinhard, A.R., 2021. Stress, Burnout, and Well-Being in New Veterinary Graduates: Evaluating a Pilot Online Professional Development Program Theses and Dissertations—Community & Leadership Development, 54. https://uknowledge.uky.edu/cld_etds/54 (accessed 31 March 2025).

Reinhard, A.R., Hains, K.D., Hains, B.J. and Strand, E.B., 2021. Are they ready? Trials, tribulations, and professional skills vital for new veterinary graduate success. Frontiers in Veterinary Science, 8, 785844. https://doi.org/10.3389/fvets.2021.785844

Tomasi, S.E., Fechter-Leggett, E.D., Edwards, N.T. et al. (2019). Suicide among veterinarians in the United States from 1979 through 2015. *Journal of the American Veterinary Medical Association* 254 (1): 104–112. https://doi.org/10.2460/javma.254.1.104.

Volk, J.O., Schimmack, U., Strand, E.B. et al. (2022). Executive summary of the Merck Animal Health Veterinarian Wellbeing Study III and Veterinary Support Staff Study. *Journal of the American Veterinary Medical Association* 260 (12): 1547–1553. https://doi.org/10.2460/javma.22.03.0134.

CHAPTER 11 Navigating Challenging Situations

INTRODUCTION

Dani Rabwin

Adverse medical outcomes and euthanasia represent two of the most emotionally and ethically complex aspects of veterinary practice. Both are inevitable realities that profoundly affect veterinarians, teams, and clients, yet they are rarely discussed in ways that prepare early-career practitioners for the weight of these experiences. How veterinarians respond to medical errors, disclose outcomes, and support one another can shape not only client trust but also professional identity and well-being.

The challenge for mentors is that these situations demand both technical competence and emotional wisdom—qualities that develop differently and at different paces. A mentee may be clinically skilled enough to perform a procedure but unprepared for the psychological aftermath of an unexpected outcome or understand the medical indications for euthanasia but struggle when client requests don't align with animal welfare considerations.

For this chapter, I brought together Dr. Lauren Forsythe and Dr. Barry Kipperman, whose combined expertise addresses these challenges from both systematic and philosophical perspectives. I chose Lauren because she is among the small group of veterinary professionals actively publishing on medical-error management and patient-safety systems. As a veterinary pharmacist and Diplomat of the International College of Veterinary Pharmacists, she brings a unique perspective from her work at major veterinary teaching hospitals where she has witnessed firsthand how errors occur, how they impact teams, and what systems' changes actually prevent future incidents.

I invited Barry because his unique combination of clinical experience and ethical scholarship offers mentors frameworks for navigating situations where there may be no clear "right" answer. As a diplomate in both internal medicine and animal welfare with a master's degree in ethics, he has devoted his career to understanding the moral complexities of veterinary practice, particularly around euthanasia decisions and moral stress.

Together, their perspectives illuminate how mentors can prepare the next generation of veterinarians to navigate errors and end-of-life decisions with honesty, resilience, and compassion.

ADVERSE MEDICAL OUTCOMES

Lauren Forsythe

In veterinary and human medicine, healthcare professionals all want to believe that we provide the best treatment possible for our patients, and in theory that is what we do. However, despite the best-laid plan, things can go wrong and errors do happen. The reality is that medical errors are an inevitable part of healthcare delivery. If humans are involved in providing care, errors will continue to occur, so we need to develop the capacity to handle them, learn from them, and prevent future errors to the best of our ability.

In human medicine, the initial push into studying the impact of medical errors came in the late 1990s and early 2000s with the report *To Err is Human* (Institute of Medicine [US] Committee on Quality of Health Care in America, 2000). While veterinary medicine has just begun to address this issue, we recognize there is a real need to study and learn more about medical errors and how to (and how not to) handle them. This section explores the foundational considerations of addressing and preventing medical errors as well as how to effectively use these foundations to enhance your mentor–mentee discussions even if there is still much to be learned in the regards to medical-error management.

THE UNDERLYING PROBLEM OF ADDRESSING MEDICAL ERRORS

When you realize a mistake has been made with a patient such as an incorrect medication that was dispensed and now the patient is experiencing serious side effects, do you get a sick feeling and start trying to figure out if it was you who made the mistake? I do. Think about our journey to become medical professionals. We undergo extensive training that emphasizes excellence at every step. We are rewarded for being good students, working hard, and getting the correct answers on exams. Throughout this process, getting an answer wrong is consistently framed as a negative. We also see the consequences when people around us make mistakes and the patient harm, disciplinary action, distrust, and/or loss of respect that results from an error. Whether happening to us directly or to someone working in our vicinity, these consequences send one very clear message: errors are unacceptable. Saying mistakes aren't tolerated leaves us with only one alternative: perfection. Clearly, perfection in healthcare delivery is not attainable. Where does that leave us? Let's look at human medicine examples to explore the complexities inherent in our work as health care providers.

HOW FREQUENT ARE MEDICAL ERRORS?

In human medicine, medical errors are the third leading cause of death in the United States with more than 200,000 patient deaths occurring annually due to preventable errors. However, errors can have negative consequences besides death. An estimated 400,000 hospitalized patients experience preventable harm each year (Rodziewicz et al., 2025). Preventable harm can be caused by any one of the numerous incidents under the umbrella term "medical errors." These errors include, but are not limited to, the following:

- Surgical errors
- Diagnostic errors
- Medication errors
- Equipment failures
- Patient falls
- Hospital-acquired infections

- Communication failures
- System failures

Of the error types listed above, the most commonly seen in veterinary medicine are “medication errors” and “communication” (Oxtoby et al., 2015). Regardless of error type, it is clear that those involved with the error experience high levels of emotional distress as well as significant impacts on all facets of their lives—both professional and personal. A tragic, but illustrative, case is that of Emily Jerry.

CASE EXAMPLE EMILY JERRY

(Emily Jerry’s Story 2014; Berger 2018)

Emily Jerry was a two-year-old girl with a yolk sac tumor the size of a grapefruit. After surgery and extensive chemotherapy treatment the tumor was gone—MRIs couldn’t even detect any residual scar tissue. She was in an Ohio hospital receiving one last round of chemotherapy to ensure the cancer was completely eliminated when her life ended from the saline bag used for her chemotherapy. She was supposed to receive her chemotherapy in a bag of normal saline and instead received a bag of hypertonic saline (23.4% NaCl) which caused swelling of her brain and her subsequent death. Several factors contributed to this error:

- The premade normal saline bags were on shortage, so saline was being compounded.
- The pharmacy was understaffed.
  - A single pharmacist was supervising seven pharmacy technicians, and pharmacy technicians were not required to be licensed in Ohio at this time.
  - The pharmacist had worked 16-hour shifts on both Friday and Saturday and was unexpectedly called in for a double shift on Sunday, the day the error occurred.

These contributing factors were not associated with any specific person, but the impact on the medical team was immense.

- The pharmacist:
  - Lost his job
  - Spent six months in state prison
  - Spent another six months in home confinement
  - Served three years of probation
  - Served four hundred hours of community service
  - Paid a 5000 fine
  - Permanently lost his license
- The pharmacy tech that made the compounding error lost her job
- The nurse that administered the saline quit
- The doctor treating Emily that day changed professions
- The hospital settled for $7 million

The Emily Jerry case shows how medical errors can create impacts far beyond the patient—creating the dynamic of the "second victim." This term refers to the healthcare professional(s) that made the error which resulted in patient harm and identifies the need to ensure they are supported as the consequences of the medical error unfold. However, this type of support network is difficult to implement in a culture that places blame on individuals—and not systems or processes—when errors occur. A more recent case occurred at Vanderbilt where a patient died after receiving vecuronium (a paralytic agent) instead of midazolam (a benzodiazepine). The nurse that obtained and administered the incorrect drug faced prison for the deadly error despite immediately coming forward to report the error (Lusk et al., 2022).

When healthcare professionals see their colleagues having criminal charges placed against them for medical errors, this sends the message to others that if they aren't perfect, then they better appear perfect. The result is hiding errors or close calls to avoid getting reprimanded. When this happens, we all lose because these errors or near misses cannot be analyzed to develop strategies that would prevent similar problems in the future.

To build a meaningful support network when medical errors occur, mentors need to be intentional about the culture established within their practice, as well as aware of the cultures in which mentees have learned and developed. Even if a practice has a very proactive culture around addressing medical errors in a productive way that focuses on processes, if a mentee comes from a culture of blame and hiding errors, it will take some time to rewire their default reactions. Luckily, reteaching and rewiring can begin before any errors occur. Open conversations about medical errors—from minor mistakes or near misses with no patient harm to errors leading to death—will help mentees recognize the ways they (and others) have handled these errors and any resulting consequences. Initiating these discussions before any errors actually occur establishes a relationship of trust and understanding, allowing mentors and mentees to address future errors with intention and compassion.

Table 11.1 compares data from two veterinary teaching hospital studies examining medical error rates, their frequency, and outcomes.

As Table 11.1 shows, the majority of errors included in these two studies did not cause patient harm. These near-miss errors are the type that lend themselves to covering up the error in blame-prone cultures, but in cultures that focus on system flaws these errors are valuable tools to prevent future patient harm. This is where you can have an impact as a mentor. Create a safe learning environment by regularly discussing near-miss events with your mentee. By openly sharing your own minor mistakes and encouraging your mentee to do the same, you establish that errors are universal learning opportunities rather than professional failures. These conversations about harmless errors build the foundation for addressing more serious incidents and reinforce a culture of continuous improvement rather than blame.

Table 11.1 Error Data Obtained from Two Veterinary Teaching Hospitals

	Teaching hospital study one (Wallis et al., 2019)	**Teaching hospital study two (Barazowski et al., 2025)**
Incident rate	0.5% (5 out of every 1000)	1.2% (12 out of every 1000 visits)
• Summary of harm	• 85% no harm events • 15% resulted in harm • 8% resulted in permanent harm or death	• 66% were medication errors • 43% of med errors reached the patient of which 8% caused harm

WHAT TO DO WHEN ERRORS OCCUR?

When an error occurs and results in patient harm, there are six steps that should be taken (Davidow, 2021):

1. Treat the patient first
2. Notify the client promptly
3. Support the veterinary staff involved
4. Investigate
5. Circle back to the client
6. Fix internal systems

By going through these steps with each error causing harm, you do right by the patient and the client, as well as support the staff. If your mentee is involved with the error or patient, it's likely that they could really benefit from some mentorship at this point.

You have an opportunity to guide your mentee through each step of this process. Even if they weren't directly involved with causing the error, but it's their patient, you can use it as an opportunity to mentor them through supporting the staff and leading the client communication and investigation process. In both scenarios, emotions have the potential to impact judgment and productive communication, so as the mentor you need to help your mentee address the error without allowing emotions to cloud their thought and decision-making process.

A challenging area with errors often involves notifying the client. It can be tempting to think that letting the client know about an error that occurred will decrease their trust in you as a doctor as well as in the practice. This is especially common in new graduates that are likely lacking confidence in themselves. However, errors that result in serious harm must be disclosed, and, in human healthcare, most patients say that they want to be informed of all mistakes even if no harm resulted. Not informing the client in a timely manner and then having the client find out later is much more likely to erode trust than admitting the error up front. Studies in human healthcare have shown that disclosing errors reduces the intent to sue, reduces the size of awards if a case goes to court, and discourages attorneys from taking these cases (Davidow, 2021).

When notifying a client about an error, the doctor should plan to provide the following information:

1. What the error was and the clinical implications?
2. Why the error happened and how recurrences will be prevented?
3. A sincere apology that conveys genuine empathy from the team.
4. Additional follow-up to provide closure once the incident has been investigated, and they can be given a clear explanation of what happened and plans to prevent future issues.

Ideally, when your mentee's patient experiences an error, you should discuss these key points and review their client communication plan before the contact occurs. However, errors might happen when you aren't available to coach your mentee through these points prior to them contacting the client. That's why I recommend practicing this process with minor errors and near misses or talking about past cases when you both have time. That way your mentee has practiced the process prior to an emotionally charged error.

Supporting the staff involved in errors includes supporting your mentee if they made the error as well as teaching your mentee how to support others when they make an error. As the doctor on a case, your mentee will be the person people look to for guidance, support, and reassurances when errors occur. Therefore, they need to be prepared to provide this support. Key factors to keep in mind include the following:

1. Address the situation without assigning blame
2. Asking "Are you okay?" is important for healing
3. Support, perspective, and technical and emotional learning help with moving on and becoming resilient

Sometimes supporting the people involved can be difficult especially when considering if the person that caused the error needs to be held responsible. To determine if there is a person-specific issue that needs to be addressed, ask the following four questions:

1. Did the staff member cause the harm deliberately?
    a. This is almost always no.
2. Was the staff member drunk, high, or otherwise impaired at work?
    a. If yes, refer the staff member to appropriate substance use resources.
3. Does the staff member have a history of mistakes that cannot be explained?
    a. If yes, this may indicate that the tasks they are expected to complete are above their skill set. Retraining or reassignment of tasks may be indicated here.
4. Could another person in the same situation have made the same mistake?
    a. This is almost always yes and serves as the litmus test for when there is a process problem that needs to be addressed.

ERROR EVALUATION

In Crossing the Quality Chasm (Institute of Medicine [US] Committee on Quality of Health Care in America, 2001), the authors state, "Trying harder will not work. Changing systems of care will. Poor designs set the workforce up to fail, regardless of how hard they try." This insight is crucial for mentorship because it shifts focus from individual blame to system improvement. **As a mentor, you can help your mentee understand that errors typically stem from process flaws, not personal failings—a perspective shift that builds both confidence and competence. This is why it's important to teach your mentee how to reflect on errors and evaluate what system changes will help prevent future issues.** By engaging in this Root Cause Analysis (RCA), your mentee must set aside the self-blame language that is likely going through their head and focus on the system issues that contributed to the error. While individuals can think through an RCA on their own, the best results come from a group working together to consider all angles of a problem. This is where you and your mentee can work together to identify others that can provide insights. You can support your mentee by taking the lead on getting the group together and lead the meeting to discuss the error. The benefit to your mentee isn't that they need to lead the process (although you can work towards that), but rather that they are included as a critical component in the discussion focused on system problems that contributed to the error. While these evaluations are essential when patient harm occurs, they should also be used for near-miss events, especially when a trend of similar near misses is noticed. By analyzing near-miss events, your mentee and others involved in the process are learning how to utilize RCA in a less emotionally charged situation as well as fixing system issues before they lead to patient harm.

There are several different ways to consider the root cause, but regardless of which method is used, the five rules of causation must be followed:

1. Clearly establish the cause-and-effect relationship.
2. Use specific and accurate descriptors for what occurred, rather than negative or vague words.
3. Identify that human errors must have a preceding cause.
4. Recognize that violations of procedure are not root causes but must themselves have a preceding cause.
5. Understand that failure to act is only causal when there is a duty to act.

Methods of considering the root cause include:

- The 5 Whys: State what happened, then ask "why" at least five times to get to the true cause.
- The Swiss Cheese Model: Consider each layer of cheese as a safeguard and each hole as a potential way that safeguard could fail. If all of the holes line up and the error reaches the patient, should there be additional safeguard layers or should changes be made to existing safeguards to close up some of the holes?
- Fishbone Analysis: Use preset categories to create a list of things that contributed to an error. Categories can vary based on what makes sense for an error type. For example, medication errors may have the categories of measures, people, process, materials, equipment, and environment.

Early on in your mentor—mentee relationship, set aside time to discuss these different methods for identifying the root cause and which ones resonate most with you versus which ones resonate most with your mentee. For me, the 5 Whys make the most sense and the Fishbone Analysis frustrates me because I get too focused on trying to decide exactly which category each thing should fall into. However, I've spoken to others that prefer the Fishbone Analysis because they feel they forget contributing factors with the less specific methods. There is no right answer, and often using multiple methods can give a more comprehensive picture. Knowing what you and your mentee each prefer means that you can both work from your areas of strength and decrease frustration associated with the RCA process (Figure 11.1).

ERROR PREVENTION FROM CULTURE CHANGE

If we don't talk about errors, then the same mistakes will continue to happen. However, to be able to talk openly about errors, we need to reframe the discussion from "who is to blame" to "what is to blame."

Culture has been shown to have a bigger impact on error prevention than equipment, technology, and facilities. To have a culture that effectively improves clinical outcomes, the mission and core values must reflect a commitment to quality and safety. However, simply having this in writing isn't enough. Leaders in the practice (and this includes mentors) must commit to asking people to speak up if they have concerns and when errors occur. When people do speak up, then you must listen to them and acknowledge the concerns to encourage future communication. Forward accountability is essential here, and it happens when you replace blame with curiosity.

Replacing blame with curiosity is a powerful way to communicate with your mentee about errors or near misses. When your mentee discusses a mistake they made, their internal dialogue is often dominated by self-blame, even if you express none yourself. To overcome this, use curiosity to redirect your mentee toward problem-solving.

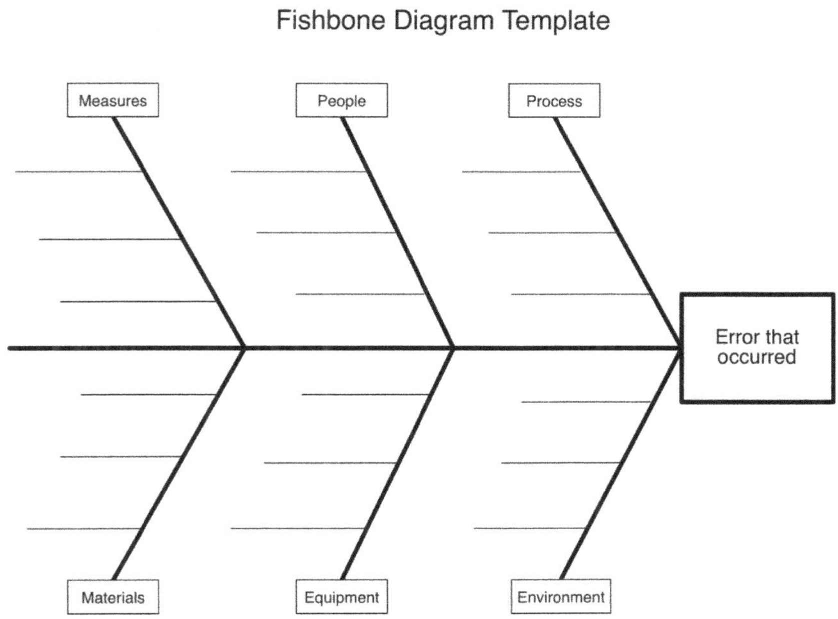

FIGURE 11.1 Fishbone diagram template showing six common categories that can be used.
Source: Lauren Forsythe

Begin by asking what external factors contributed to the mistake. If they respond with self-blame statements—"I wasn't paying attention" or "I should have looked something up"—probe deeper by asking why. For instance, if they were distracted, focus on identifying the source of that distraction and potential solutions, rather than accepting their assertion that they "just need to work harder to focus." Once external contributing factors are identified, collaborate on modifications. You likely either have made similar mistakes yourself or have already developed strategies to prevent them. Share these experiences during your brainstorming session. Work together to sort the external factors into three buckets:

1. Things your mentee can modify on their own → identify how they will modify these factors.
2. Things that could be modified from a practice standpoint → add these to the agenda for your next staff or doctor meeting.
3. Things that aren't feasible to modify → talk with your mentee about how awareness of these factors can help them know to be wary of the risk going forward.

Once the issues have been sorted into three categories then you can use the categories to help identify possible solutions. There may be more than one solution, or a contributing factor may fit into more than one bucket with different solutions depending on the bucket. An example discussion using the three buckets is provided.

EXAMPLE DISCUSSION WITH THREE BUCKETS

Setting the stage: You are meeting with your distressed mentee about an error that they made last week while you were on vacation. There were two young adult gray female cats in the clinic and both were named Bella. One cat was there for radiographs due to frequent vomiting and the other was there for a routine spay. Your mentee accidentally selected the wrong

Bella for the spay and didn't realize it until they had opened up the abdomen and saw that the patient was already spayed.

Your discussion: Your mentee is blaming themself for the mistake saying that they removed the cat and asked the technician to draw up the sedation without verifying the last name. You ask your mentee to identify what external factors contributed to the error and the following list is generated.

- Two gray Bellas in the hospital at the same time with similar age and health at first glance. Your mentee wasn't aware of the Bella getting radiographs because that case was another doctor's.
- A technician was off, and another had called in sick, so your mentee was helping get the patient ready for surgery since the technicians were overextended.
- There wasn't any name-alert indicator present on the cage, the patient, or the chart.
- Your mentee had a full day of surgeries scheduled, which was already stressful because they struggle to be thorough and efficient on surgery days.
- There was no double-check process in place for verifying the correct patient with their full name prior to starting a procedure.

Once you have the list, you sort each factor into a bucket and identify a plan to address it (Figure 11.2).

The end result: You have helped your mentee shift their focus from self-blame to the contributing external factors as well as identified immediate steps you and your mentee can take as well as items to discuss at an upcoming staff meeting.

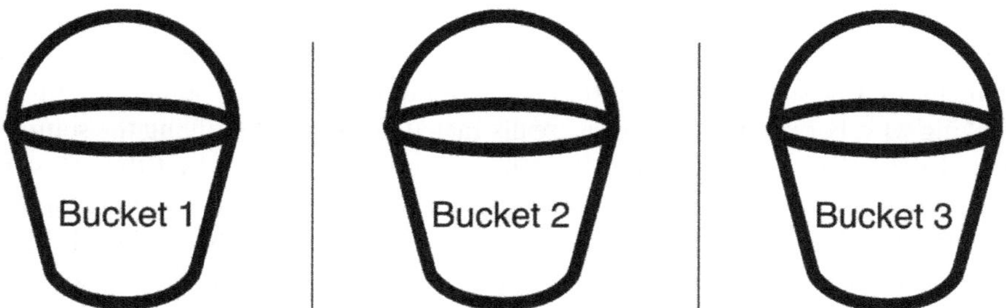

Mentee can address themselves	Can be addressed at practice level	Not able to be addressed
Mentee was helping get the patient ready for surgery ↓ Identify that having a technician do this provides a double check opportunity so if they need to bypass that, then identify a way to insert a double check elsewhere in the process.	No double check process prior to starting a procedure ↓ implement a surgical safety checklist led by the surgeon prior to starting each procedure.	Two similar looking cats named Bella ↓ Identify other ways discussed above to prevent problems.
Full day of surgeries ↓ Mentee works with you to identify procedures they are confident doing in the provided timeframe and ones that are still a struggle. Either decrease total number of surgeries per day or decrease number of more difficult procedures.	No name alert indicator ↓ Determine how to identify two patients that have the same (or very similar) first or last name such as using a bright cage card or name collar.	Short staffed ↓ If adjusting processes to compensate take a minute to consider what safeguards may be missed.

FIGURE 11.2 Examples of how the three buckets can be used to help your mentee address errors.
Source: Lauren Forsythe

MENTOR–MENTEE DISCUSSION TOPICS FOR DIFFERENT TIMEPOINTS

- Early On
  - Discuss previous experience with errors including culture surrounding errors in vet school/past practice and how your mentee has handled errors ranging from near misses to death.
    - To start this discussion, share your background with the culture surrounding medical errors. Do you have stories from vet school or early in practice that show a good or bad culture? Explain how the culture at this practice compares to your past experiences. Invite your mentee to share their past experiences and reflect on how they compare to the culture you have described. What do they think will be challenging when adapting to the current culture?
  - Discuss RCA and your mentee's experience with the different types.
    - To start this discussion, ask your mentee what they have done in the past to identify the cause of errors. Ask them what their knowledge of/experience with the different methods of doing an RCA is and which one they find most useful. Share your thoughts on which method you prefer. If your practice already has a process for evaluating the cause of errors, share that process with your mentee.
- After a Near Miss
  - Share near misses that you have made and ask your mentee to share any they have made. Brainstorm contributing factors, what prevented the error from reaching the patient, and steps that can be taken to prevent the same type of mistake in the future. Make this a regular touch point in your discussions.
    - To start this discussion, share a near miss you made since the last time you met with your mentee. Invite them to brainstorm ideas for prevention with you. Then ask your mentee what near misses they have had and help them brainstorm. Use RCA methods to help with brainstorming.
    - Note: Asking about your mentee's near misses as an open-ended question (i.e., "what near misses. . ." versus "have you had any near misses. . .") normalizes the fact that everyone makes mistakes vs. putting them on the spot to own up to their shortcomings.
  - Practice going through the process of notifying a client about an error that occurred. Use a near-miss situation for this practice discussion to help your mentee be prepared when an error reaches a patient.
    - To start this discussion, identify a near miss that you or your mentee brought up. Briefly outline what might have happened if it reached the patient. Then work with your mentee to identify how to communicate with the client using the points described in the section on responding to errors.
- During the Response to a Major Error
  - Assess how your mentee is handling the error emotionally.
    - To start this discussion, emphasize the stress of the situation and ask, "are you okay." Ask them what emotions they are fighting and if they are experiencing significant self-blame. Even if they didn't make the error themselves, they may still be distressed and blaming themselves. If your mentee didn't make the error, but it's their patient, ask them to reflect on what they know about the emotional state of the people involved with the error/patient. Provide guidance on checking in on these people.
  - Go through the client notification process with your mentee prior to them contacting the client. Let them practice explaining the facts in a client-friendly way based on the key points described in the section on responding to errors.

- To start this discussion, have your mentee explain what happened to you so that you are briefed on the situation. Ask questions to elicit the information that should be shared with the client. Then ask your mentee to go through the situation again, framing it in client-friendly language as if you are the client.

- After a Major Error
  - Talk with your mentee about the RCA process. Get their input on who should be involved.
    - To start this discussion, summarize the error that occurred and the eventual outcome, and check in on how your mentee is doing emotionally. Explain that now that the immediate issue has passed but the error is still fresh in our minds, we need to complete an RCA. Ask your mentee to identify individuals that they think have the experience or involvement to provide helpful perspectives regarding the process issues that may have contributed to the error. Set up a time for the RCA team to meet and explain to your mentee how the meeting will work.

Working with your mentee through medical errors can be challenging and emotional, especially if you still struggle to effectively manage your emotional resilience when you make mistakes. However, that doesn't mean you should avoid this topic. Instead, lean into the aspects you aren't comfortable with and share your struggles and use Table 11.2 to identify problematic thought patterns that you and/or your mentee may be struggling with and how to reframe those. Pushing past your comfort zone and being vulnerable can increase the value of the mentor–mentee relationship immensely.

Table 11.2 Problematic Thoughts and Strategies to Reframe

Problematic thought	Role this affects	Reframed version
I still get knocked off balance when I make a mistake that harms a patient. How can I be of benefit to my mentee when I can't even help myself?	Mentor	Handling errors in a productive manner is a lifelong learning process. By talking through my struggles with my mentee and asking them to identify when I'm falling into self-blame, we can both learn.
Who am I to provide advice on preventing errors when I make the same kind of mistakes?	Mentor	Having made the same type of mistake means that I know what my mentee is going through and we can brainstorm process improvements together to prevent future issues.
Our culture has been bad for so long there isn't anything we can do to address that, and errors are just going to keep happening.	Mentor and mentee	If our culture is problematic, then we should use the RCA process to identify what's contributing to that. Once we have ideas of the contributing factors, then we can sort them into the three buckets to determine what we can address.
I'm glad that mistake didn't reach the patient, and no one knows it was me who made it. I'll just keep it to myself, so people don't think less of me.	Mentor and mentee	I'm glad that mistake didn't reach the patient. I need to bring it up with my mentor/mentee/trusted colleague to discuss and identify what process improvements can be made to help prevent future instances that could reach the patient.
I really just need to double down and try harder, so I don't make stupid mistakes like this again.	Mentor and mentee	Trying harder won't work; to prevent future issues I need to address the root cause. I should brainstorm by myself and with others to identify the underlying problems, and if my lack of knowledge is a contributing factor, then I'll identify how to go about increasing my knowledge.
I make so many mistakes, maybe I wasn't cut out for being a vet.	Mentee	I'm human, so I will make mistakes, and, by reviewing the contributing factors, I can help improve systems to decrease my mistakes as well as help others avoid making mistakes.

Editor's Note: *Dr. Forsythe's framework for managing medical errors—replacing blame with curiosity, conducting RCA, and building cultures of learning—provides mentors with concrete tools for supporting mentees through unintended adverse outcomes. In this next section, Dr. Kipperman addresses the intentional decisions that carry equally complex ethical weight: euthanasia requests that may not align with animal welfare, clients whose financial limitations seemingly compromise care, and conflicts between professional obligations and practice pressures. While medical errors challenge us to learn from what went wrong, ethical dilemmas force us to grapple with fundamental questions about animal advocacy, client autonomy, and professional integrity.*

DEFINING EUTHANASIA AND ITS ETHICAL CLASSIFICATIONS

Barry Kipperman

Veterinary practice is unique in that clinicians are expected to intentionally end the lives of their patients. In a study of over 29,000 canine deaths in UK primary care practices, 89% occurred through euthanasia (Pegram et al., 2021). The term *euthanasia* derives from the Greek roots meaning "a good death" and, in human ethics, is typically reserved for circumstances of mercy killing, in which death is viewed as a respite from inevitable suffering that cannot be alleviated by reasonable means (Dyck, 1975).

The American Veterinary Medical Association (AVMA) Guidelines for the Euthanasia of Animals (2020) define euthanasia through two codependent requirements:

1. Method-Based: The use of humane techniques to induce the most rapid, painless, and distress-free death possible.
2. Intention-Based: The intent to induce death in a manner that is in accord with the animal's interests and/or because it is a matter of welfare.

The intention-based criterion is particularly important, as it distinguishes euthanasia from other acts that result in death but are not ethically justified. When euthanasia is justified using an "animal's best interest" paradigm, significant challenges may arise. Different stakeholders—including veterinarians, animal owners, colleagues, or multiple owners of the same animal—may hold differing views regarding an animal's quality of life, prognosis, and interests (Quain, 2021). Rollin (2011) characterized euthanasia as a double-edged sword: while it can relieve terminal suffering, it may also be used in circumstances that do not clearly serve the animal's interests.

Tannenbaum (1995) referred to euthanasia that does not align with an animal's best interests as *medically unnecessary euthanasia*. One commonly cited category is convenience euthanasia, which involves ending an animal's life due to changes in an owner's circumstances, such as insufficient time, capability (emotional or physical), or motivation to care for the animal (Batchelor and McKeegan, 2012; Rathwell-Deault et al., 2017). Although many clinicians would agree that euthanizing a healthy animal for trivial reasons is ethically indefensible, requests often arise in more ambiguous circumstances, such as euthanasia of an animal with manageable behavioral issues when the owner is unwilling to pursue mitigation strategies.

Another category is economic euthanasia, defined as euthanasia elected primarily due to the cost of veterinary care, or when minimal or no diagnostic testing or treatment is pursued for financial reasons, resulting in euthanasia as the eventual outcome (Kipperman, 2010). Economic constraints are a pervasive reality in veterinary practice and frequently place clinicians in ethically challenging positions, particularly when an animal's condition is treatable and the prognosis is favorable.

Quain (2021) proposed the term ethically indicated euthanasia to describe euthanasia performed in what are believed to be the animal's interests and not primarily motivated by convenience, financial limitations, or other reasons to which members of the veterinary team object. Euthanasia that does not meet this standard should be clearly classified in medical records as convenience, economic, or objectionable euthanasia. Using the term *euthanasia* without qualification in situations involving the intentional death of healthy animals or animals with treatable conditions risks obscuring its ethical meaning and may contribute to the normalization of medically unnecessary euthanasia.

While these definitions and classifications are grounded in ethical theory and professional guidelines, they often surface/apply in practice through mentorship conversations—particularly when early-career veterinarians encounter euthanasia requests that conflict with their values or professional identity. For mentors, fluency in this language is not about supplying answers or moral judgments, but about helping mentees accurately name the ethical dimensions of the situations they face.

Throughout this chapter, these foundational distinctions serve as a shared vocabulary for mentor–mentee dialogue. Subsequent sections focus on how mentors can support early-career veterinarians as they navigate ethically complex euthanasia decisions—by tolerating ambiguity, clarifying competing interests, and acting with integrity in environments where clinical, emotional, and organizational pressures often collide.

ETHICAL JUSTIFICATIONS FOR EUTHANASIA: WHEN ENDING LIFE IS WARRANTED

A pivotal decision veterinarians face is determining whether euthanasia is ethically appropriate or whether a patient's life remains worth living despite the presence of disease or disability. The concept of *a life worth living* is primarily an ethical consideration rather than a scientific one. Euthanasia should be considered when no reasonable alternatives exist to address significant and enduring suffering. Such suffering may be physical, psychological, or both, and not every manifestation of suffering warrants euthanasia.

The range of options available to address suffering may vary depending on factors such as access to resources, time, client capacity, and the veterinarian's autonomy within a practice setting. Consequently, euthanasia decisions rarely occur in a vacuum and are influenced by contextual constraints that shape what is practically achievable for a given patient and family.

Owners commonly cite perceived animal suffering as the primary reason for electing euthanasia (Marchitelli et al., 2020). Their assessment of suffering is therefore a central component of the decision-making process and must be considered alongside the veterinarian's clinical judgment. In some situations, veterinarians may believe euthanasia is warranted while owners disagree, potentially prolonging animal suffering. In others, owners may request euthanasia when veterinarians believe acceptable quality of life remains.

When consensus cannot be reached, outcomes may include continued suffering, premature death, or moral distress for the clinician. These situations are emotionally challenging and are particularly common during the early stages of a veterinarian's career, when confidence, experience, and professional autonomy are still developing.

Although euthanasia decisions are often framed as medical determinations, they are inherently value-laden and shaped by ethical judgment. For mentors, recognizing this complexity is essential—not to resolve these tensions for early-career veterinarians, but to help them articulate where disagreements arise and why they are difficult to navigate. Disagreement between owners and veterinarians does not necessarily indicate error or poor intent; rather, it reflects the competing obligations veterinarians must balance. Understanding when euthanasia may be ethically justified—and when it may not—provides mentors with a foundation for guiding mentees through requests for euthanasia that are emotionally charged, ethically ambiguous, or misaligned with the mentee's emerging professional identity.

REQUESTS FOR EUTHANASIA AND PROFESSIONAL DISCRETION

Veterinary practitioners frequently encounter requests for euthanasia that they perceive as ethically inappropriate. In a survey of North American veterinarians, 93% reported having received at least one euthanasia request they considered inappropriate (Moses et al., 2018). In another study, 45% of veterinarians agreed that euthanasia is sometimes used to resolve difficult cases even when it may not be in the animal's best interest and 42% reported having done so at least once during their career (Kipperman et al., 2018).

These findings underscore a central ethical tension in companion animal practice: euthanasia has the capacity to relieve suffering but can also be employed in circumstances that do not clearly serve the animal's interests. Veterinarians must balance obligations to the patient, the client, the veterinary team, their employer, and themselves—interests that frequently conflict.

When faced with euthanasia requests, veterinarians may choose to comply, attempt to dissuade the client, or decline the request. In a study of UK veterinarians, 71% reported wanting to refuse a euthanasia request but proceeded anyway (Yeates and Main, 2011). Similarly, US veterinarians have described feeling discouraged from exercising discretion to refuse euthanasia and experiencing pressure from employers or hospital administrators to comply with requests that conflict with their personal or professional values (Kipperman, 2017).

The rationale often offered—"*If I don't do it [euthanasia], someone else will*"—reflects an attempt to minimize personal responsibility for ethically troubling/dubious decisions. However, this reasoning diminishes professional integrity by normalizing the perception that veterinarians are willing to end patients' lives on demand. Avoiding conflict or retaining a client does not justify performing euthanasia that conflicts with one's ethical convictions, particularly given the moral stress that may follow.

When euthanasia is not ethically justified, veterinarians have a responsibility to propose reasonable alternatives that better serve the animal's interests. Nevertheless, declining a euthanasia request can be emotionally difficult, especially when owners are distressed or have already resolved to proceed. Ethical behavior in these situations requires courage and professional clarity.

MENTORSHIP IN PRACTICE: SUPPORTING MENTEES WHEN EUTHANASIA REQUESTS FEEL ETHICALLY WRONG

Requests for euthanasia that conflict with a veterinarian's values are among the most destabilizing experiences for early-career clinicians. Mentees often arrive at these moments seeking reassurance, certainty, or validation that there is a "right" answer. Mentors play a critical role not by supplying that answer, but by helping mentees clarify *how* to respond in a way that aligns with their developing professional identity.

Effective mentorship in these situations begins with normalizing ethical discomfort. Mentors can help mentees understand that feeling unsettled does not indicate weakness or inexperience; rather, it reflects engagement with the moral dimensions of practice. Asking questions such as, "*What feels hardest about this request?*" or "*Which interests are in conflict for you right now?*" can help mentees articulate their concerns without rushing toward resolution.

Mentors should also be attentive to power dynamics/imbalances. Early-career veterinarians may feel constrained by employer expectations, client pressure, or fear of negative consequences if they decline a euthanasia request. Rather than directing mentees toward compliance or refusal, mentors can explore available options, model language for difficult conversations, and help mentees anticipate the emotional and professional impact of different paths forward.

Ultimately, mentors support mentees not by eliminating ethical tension, but by helping them act deliberately, transparently, and with integrity in situations where no option is without cost.

TIMING OF EUTHANASIA AND ADVOCACY FOR THE PATIENT

Justifying *why* euthanasia may be appropriate is distinct from determining *when* it should occur. One of the most challenging aspects of euthanasia decision-making involves timing—particularly whether veterinarians should initiate discussions about euthanasia or wait for owners to do so. Veterinarians should feel empowered to raise the topic when delaying the conversation is likely to prolong animal suffering.

Because euthanasia may be indicated at any life stage, early discussion of end-of-life considerations is especially important for animals with congenital disease, chronic or progressive illness, or relatively short life expectancy. Avoiding conversations about death and dying may prevent owners from understanding disease trajectories and preparing for decisions that may arise later (Kipperman and Cooney, 2024). Owners consistently identify advance planning around euthanasia as a key component of a "good death" experience (Cooney and Kogan, 2022).

After euthanasia is discussed, owners may choose to take time to process the information and say goodbye. In some cases, owners propose timelines measured in weeks when the animal's condition suggests that euthanasia should be considered within days or even hours. These situations create ethical tension between advocating for the suffering patient and respecting the owner's emotional readiness to let go. Veterinarians must sometimes advocate for timely euthanasia even when doing so conflicts with owner preferences.

Conversely, owners may request euthanasia earlier than medically necessary, motivated by fear of witnessing decline or concern about potential crisis events. In these cases, veterinarians should provide clear information about expected disease progression, possible complications, and whether symptoms can be managed—temporarily or long term—to support informed decision-making and prevent premature euthanasia.

MENTORSHIP IN PRACTICE: COACHING CONVERSATIONS ABOUT TIMING

Mentors can help early-career veterinarians prepare for euthanasia discussions by emphasizing that conversations about timing often improve with rehearsal. Role-playing difficult dialogues—particularly those involving delayed or premature euthanasia requests—allows mentees to practice language that is compassionate, clear, and grounded in patient advocacy.

Rather than scripting exact responses, mentors can help mentees identify core messages they wish to convey, such as concern for the animal's comfort, transparency about likely disease progression, and respect for the owner's emotional process. Practicing these conversations in advance can reduce anxiety, improve confidence, and help mentees remain present and thoughtful when emotions are high.

Importantly, mentors can reinforce that advocating for appropriate timing is not a failure of empathy, but an expression of professional responsibility.

EMOTIONAL AND MORAL CONSEQUENCES OF EUTHANASIA

Performing euthanasia can evoke both positive and negative emotional experiences for veterinary professionals. While euthanasia may be perceived as a compassionate act that relieves suffering, it is also associated with significant emotional burden. Negative consequences include burnout, compassion fatigue, and reduced career satisfaction (Scotney et al., 2015). Individuals who perform euthanasia may experience perpetration-induced traumatic stress, a form of post-traumatic stress disorder (PTSD) characterized by distress following participation in acts that violate deeply held moral beliefs (Bennett and Rohlf, 2005).

Veterinary professionals may also experience secondary traumatic stress, particularly veterinary technicians and support staff who witness the physical and emotional distress of patients and owners during euthanasia procedures (Hanrahan et al., 2018). Because euthanasia-related stress affects the entire veterinary team, attention to its emotional consequences should extend beyond those who directly perform the procedure.

A substantial source of distress associated with euthanasia arises from moral conflict. Moral distress has been defined as the psychological distress that results from engaging in or being unable to prevent actions that conflict with one's moral or ethical beliefs (Crane et al., 2013). Moral stress more broadly encompasses distress arising from persistent value conflicts or constraints within the workplace (Fawcett and Mullan, 2018). Rollin (1987) first articulated the concept of moral stress in veterinary medicine, particularly in relation to killing animals for reasons deemed ethically objectionable.

I still have remorseful feelings regarding patients I euthanized where, in hindsight, I wish I had acted differently. These experiences remain emotionally salient and continue to shape how I approach ethical decision-making in practice.

Despite these challenges, euthanasia may also be associated with compassion satisfaction—the sense of fulfillment derived from helping others and alleviating suffering (Cooney and Kipperman, 2023). Medically indicated euthanasia is often described as the final act of love an owner can provide for their animal companion. Quain (2021) has referred to this as "the gift" of ending suffering, and many veterinarians report receiving more expressions of gratitude from owners following euthanasia than for any other clinical service.

MENTORSHIP IN PRACTICE: RECOGNIZING AND RESPONDING TO MORAL STRESS

Mentors are often among the first to notice signs of moral stress in early-career veterinarians, even when mentees themselves minimize or normalize their distress. Mentees may describe feeling "fine" while recounting experiences that reveal unresolved ethical conflict, emotional numbing, or persistent self-doubt. Mentors can help by naming moral stress explicitly and reinforcing that distress following euthanasia—particularly when it feels ethically fraught—is a predictable response, not a personal failing.

Effective mentorship involves creating space for reflection without judgment or urgency to "move on." Asking open-ended questions such as, *"Which part of that experience is still sitting with you?"* or *"What do you wish had been different?"* allows mentees to process ethical residue rather than suppress it. **Mentors can also model self-compassion by acknowledging their own difficult experiences and emphasizing that professional integrity includes attending to one's emotional well-being.**

By helping mentees recognize moral stress early and respond to it deliberately, mentors play a critical role in supporting long-term professional sustainability.

The AVMA offers useful euthanasia decision-making guidelines (Figure 11.3).

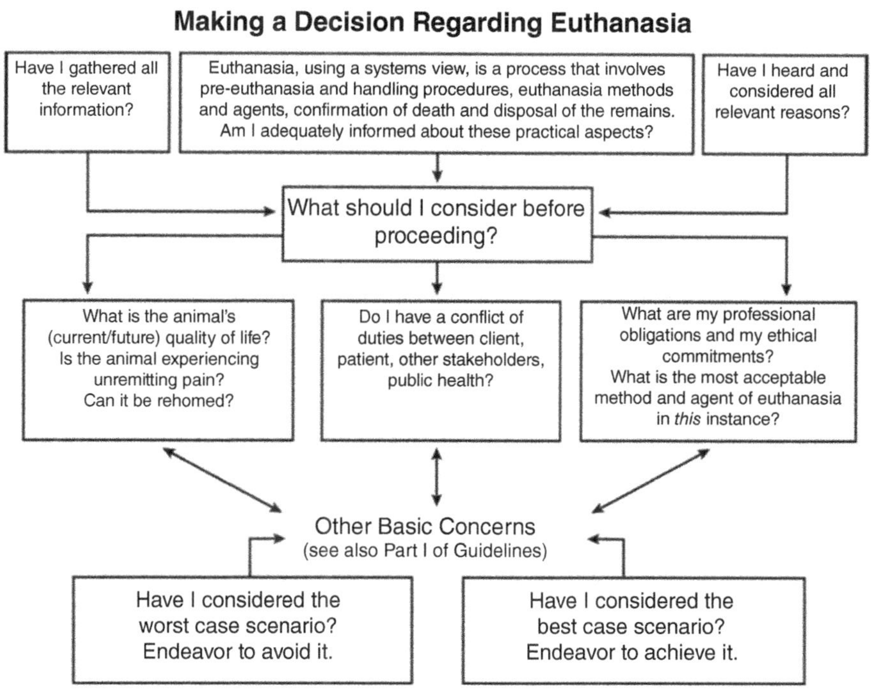

Figure 1—Veterinarians may appeal to this decision tree as a way to decide whether euthanasia is warranted when the proper course of action is not clear.

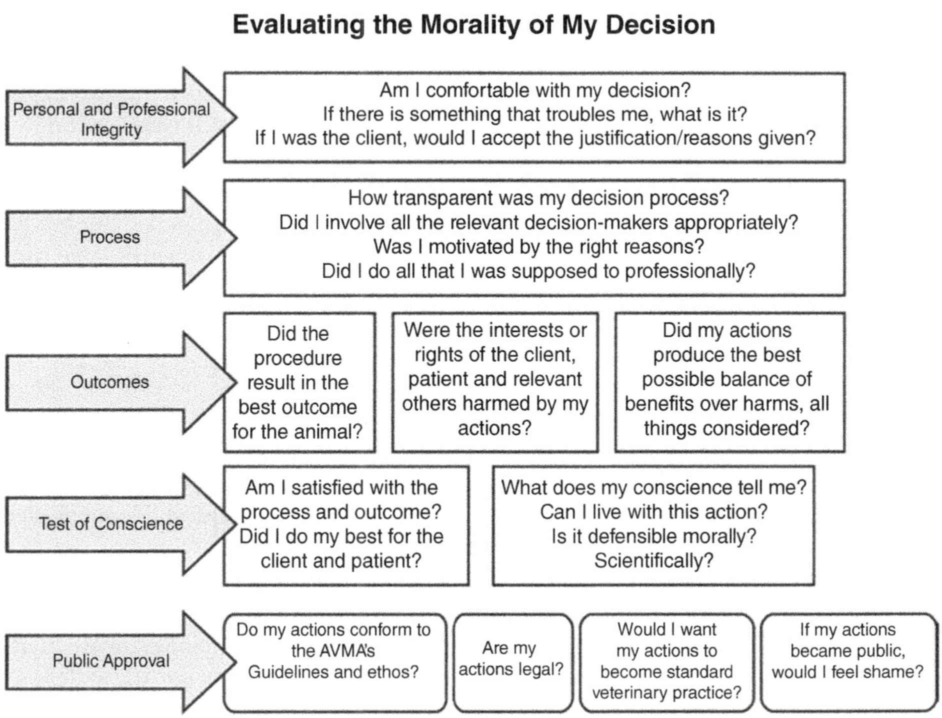

Figure 2—When attempting to make the best decision possible in a thorough and balanced way, veterinar-ians may find this decision matrix helpful. It can assist in assessing the morality of euthanasia in particular cases, especially if they are less straightforward

FIGURE 11.3 AVMA guidelines for decision-making associated with euthanasia. *Source:* With permission of AVMA (2020).

NAVIGATING ETHICAL DILEMMAS: DECISION-MAKING AND SUPPORT

Barry Kipperman

Ethical dilemmas arise when competing interests of perceived equal moral weight conflict, and there is no clear rule to determine the "right" course of action (Morgan and McDonald, 2007). In many circumstances, the ethically appropriate response may be apparent but difficult to enact because of anticipated negative consequences, such as conflict with clients, employers, or colleagues.

Veterinary professionals routinely encounter ethical dilemmas in practice, including those involving euthanasia decisions, financial limitations, futile treatment, conflicts between animal welfare and client preferences, and professional obligations within hierarchical workplace structures (Table 11.2). Despite the prevalence of these challenges, veterinarians often rely on intuition or personal value systems rather than structured ethical frameworks to guide decision-making (Kipperman et al., 2018).

Decision-making frameworks are not intended to produce definitive answers, but to support systematic consideration of relevant interests, potential consequences, and ethical principles. Such approaches are designed to guide reflection on pertinent ethical concerns and facilitate ethical problem-solving (Grimm et al., 2018).

Veterinary practitioners consistently report that sharing experiences with colleagues is one of the most helpful ways to navigate ethical dilemmas (Richards et al., 2020; Quain et al., 2021). Professionals often feel more comfortable discussing ethically or emotionally challenging cases with peers who understand the realities of clinical practice, particularly given the difficulty of sharing traumatic experiences with those outside the profession (Blum, 2018).

When ethical concerns are openly recognized and discussed in supportive environments, an ethical culture can begin to develop within the practice (Kong, 2015). Structured forums such as ethics rounds or facilitated discussion groups have been associated with improved identification of ethical dilemmas and reductions in moral stress (Quain et al., 2022; Ashall, 2023). Ideally, these discussions are led by individuals with both clinical experience and ethics training and include exploration of possible responses to real cases encountered by participants.

However, ethical discussion forums are not without limitations. Revisiting distressing cases may evoke negative emotions, and lack of perceived autonomy within a practice can inhibit open conversation. Practical barriers—including limited time and insufficient organizational support—remain significant obstacles to implementation (Ashall, 2023).

MENTORSHIP IN PRACTICE: HELPING MENTEES NAVIGATE ETHICAL AMBIGUITY

Mentors play a critical role in helping early-career veterinarians move from seeking certainty to tolerating ethical ambiguity. Many mentees enter practice accustomed to environments where problems have correct answers and success is defined by resolution. Ethical dilemmas challenge this mindset, as no option may fully satisfy all interests or values.

Rather than using ethical frameworks as checklists or decision trees, mentors can introduce them as conversation tools—ways to slow down thinking, clarify competing priorities, and make implicit values explicit. Walking through a framework together allows mentees to articulate their reasoning, recognize constraints, and understand that ethical clarity does not always lead to emotional comfort (Figure 11.4).

Mentors also serve as containers for uncertainty. By acknowledging that discomfort, doubt, and lingering questions are normal responses to ethical conflict, mentors help mentees build resilience and professional maturity. Encouraging reflection—rather than premature

Decision Tree

This Decision Tree has been devised in order to give guidance to vets when faced with euthanasia as a management option for an animal under their care.

It may be useful to consider the following scenarios when using the Decision Tree:

- Owned but unwanted healthy animal.
- Owned terminally ill, suffering animal; owner wants euthanasia.
- Owned terminally ill, suffering animal; owner refuses euthanasia.
- Owned terminally ill, mildly suffering animal; owner refuses euthanasia; owner very attached.
- Owned terminally ill, mildly suffering animal; owner not available.
- Owned animal with illness with minor effect on quality of life—for example, mild heart failure; owner wants euthanasia.
- Owned healthy animal with incontinence/ minor behavioural problem—owner requests euthanasia.
- Unowned wild animal with major injuries.
- Unowned wild non-indigenous species (for example, grey squirrel).
- Injured wild non-indigenous/pest species.

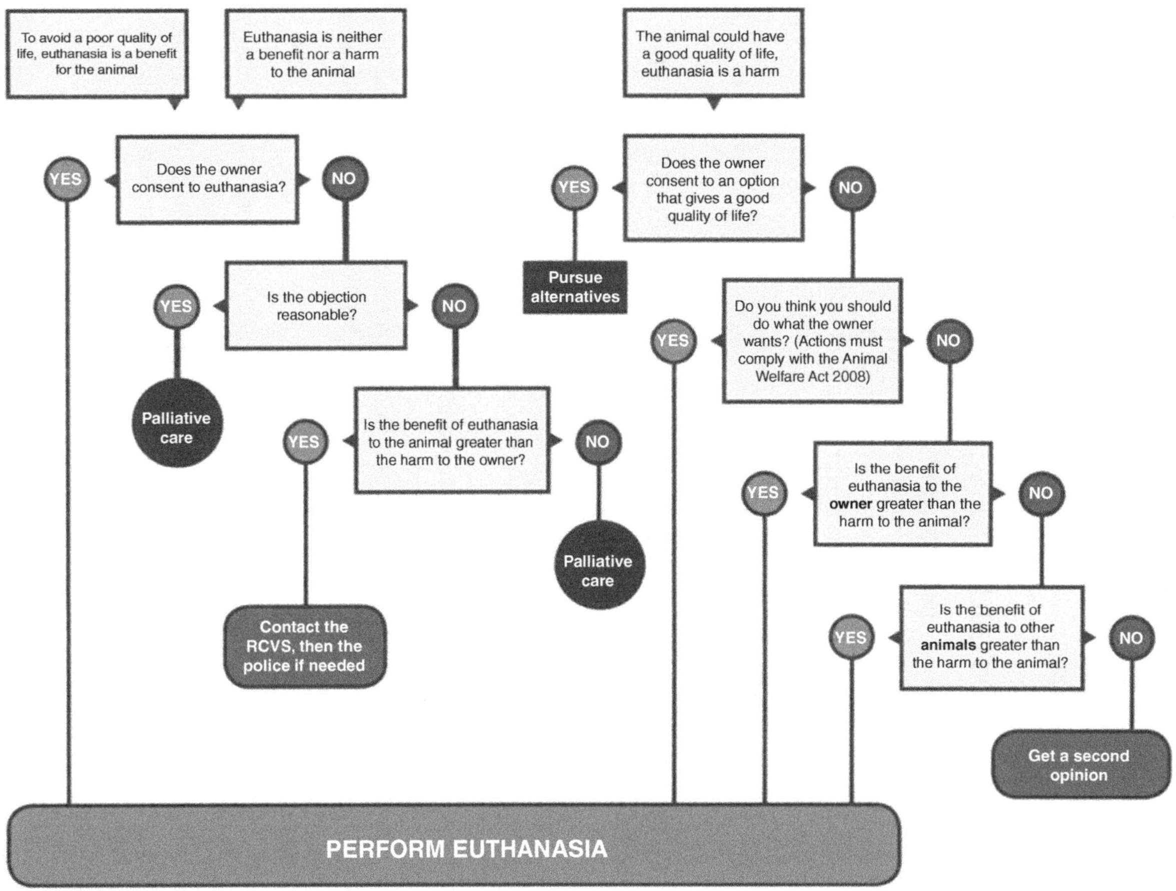

FIGURE 11.4 BVA euthanasia decision tree.

closure—supports identity formation and reduces the pressure to justify decisions solely by outcomes.

Effective mentorship does not aim to eliminate ethical tension. Instead, it helps mentees develop the capacity to remain thoughtful, grounded, and aligned with their values in situations where ambiguity is unavoidable.

CASE-BASED APPLICATION FOR MENTORS

Ethically complex euthanasia decisions are an inevitable part of veterinary practice. While ethical frameworks and professional guidelines provide structure, mentors often encounter these issues most vividly through the real cases their mentees bring forward. The following case examples illustrate common euthanasia-related dilemmas that arise early in veterinary careers. These cases are not intended to model "correct" decisions, but to support thoughtful discussion, reflection, and mentorship.

CASE EXAMPLE 11.1: REQUEST FOR EUTHANASIA OF A FELINE PATIENT WITH SUSPECTED DIABETES MELLITUS

Mrs. A, a new client, presents her 12-year-old cat, Debra, for euthanasia. Mrs. A reports that Debra drinks water constantly, eats voraciously, and is losing weight. She explains that she believes Debra has diabetes mellitus and states that she "can't bear to watch her waste away." No diagnostic testing has been performed.

On physical examination, Debra is alert, thin, ambulatory, and able to jump onto a chair in the exam room. Your mentee does not perceive that Debra is currently suffering. Mrs. A is clear that she has no interest in pursuing diagnostic testing or long-term treatment and requests euthanasia at this visit. There is no hospital policy addressing the refusal of euthanasia requests.

Ethical Considerations

Relevant interests in this case include the patient, the client, the veterinarian, the veterinary team, the practice, the mentor, and the profession. Debra's clinical signs raise concern for diabetes mellitus, hyperthyroidism, chronic kidney disease, or a combination of conditions—many of which are treatable and compatible with an acceptable quality of life. Mrs. A appears distressed and motivated by concern for Debra's future suffering but is unwilling or unable to pursue treatment.

Possible responses include:

- Proceeding with euthanasia at the client's request
- Declining euthanasia and outlining parameters for when euthanasia may be ethically appropriate
- Encouraging diagnostic testing or treatment
- Suggesting referral or rehoming options

This case illustrates the ambiguity inherent in euthanasia requests involving animals who are not clearly suffering but may face chronic illness. While some view euthanasia in such cases as a form of convenience euthanasia, others argue that veterinarians cannot fully know the circumstances driving a client's decision. The AVMA Guidelines for the Euthanasia of Animals (2020) encourage discussion and consideration of alternatives when an animal is believed to have a life worth living.

Proceeding with euthanasia not only may relieve the client's distress but may also result in moral stress for the veterinarian and create tension within the veterinary team. Declining the request may protect the animal's interests but risk damaging the client relationship or place the mentee in conflict with employer expectations. Mentors can help mentees explore these competing considerations without rushing toward resolution.

MENTOR REFLECTION PROMPTS: CASE 11.1

- What aspects of this request might feel most destabilizing/troubling for an early-career veterinarian?
- How might a mentee's discomfort differ if the pressure is coming primarily from the client versus from an employer or practice culture?
- What language could a mentor help a mentee practice if they choose to decline or defer euthanasia?
- How can mentors support mentees when the ethically preferable option may carry professional or emotional risk?

CASE EXAMPLE 11.2: ECONOMIC LIMITATIONS TO LIFE-SAVING SURGERY

You are a new graduate working with a mentor when you examine Molly, a six-month-old dog presenting for three days of vomiting, progressive lethargy, and declining appetite. You recommend bloodwork and abdominal radiographs, providing an estimate of $500, which the owners accept.

Radiographs reveal segmental dilation of the small intestine consistent with intestinal obstruction, most likely due to a foreign body. You explain that surgery is required and that, without intervention, Molly's condition will worsen and likely result in death. The estimated cost for surgery and postoperative care is $5000.

Molly's owners respond that if surgery cannot be performed for less than $1000, they will elect euthanasia. You offer financing options available through hospital policy, but their application is declined. The hospital has no formal financial assistance policy.

Ethical Considerations

Relevant interests include the patient, the client, the veterinarian, the mentor, the veterinary team, the practice owner, and the profession. Molly has an excellent prognosis with surgical intervention and is otherwise young and healthy. Her owners appear emotionally invested but financially constrained.

Potential responses include:

- Proceeding with euthanasia at the owners' request
- Seeking external funding or charitable support
- Having the hospital subsidize care, with or without transfer of ownership
- Referring Molly to a lower-cost facility

Each option carries ethical and practical implications. Euthanasia may relieve suffering but conflicts with the veterinarian's role as patient advocate when a readily available, life-saving treatment exists. Subsidizing care may improve team morale and save Molly's life but raises concerns about sustainability, fairness, and precedent. Referral may preserve the animal's life but introduce tension regarding perceived differences in cost or quality of care.

For early-career veterinarians, these situations are particularly challenging. Mentees may feel torn between advocating for the patient, respecting client autonomy, and navigating employer expectations. Mentors play a critical role in helping mentees process the ethical weight of these decisions and the emotional residue that may remain regardless of outcome.

MENTOR REFLECTION PROMPTS: CASE 11.2

- Where does moral stress arise most strongly in this case, and how might it persist even after a decision is made?
- How can mentors help mentees avoid personalizing client financial limitations as professional failure?
- What support might a mentee need if the outcome conflicts with their sense of patient advocacy?
- How can mentors help mentees reflect on this experience in a way that supports long-term professional resilience?

TABLES AND DECISION-MAKING TOOLS

The following tables are intended to support structured discussion and reflection when navigating ethically complex cases. Mentors may find these tools most useful when introduced after emotional processing has begun, rather than as prescriptive checklists.

Table 11.3 summarizes the interests that may influence veterinarians' clinical and ethical decision-making

Table 11.4 summarizes common types of ethical dilemmas encountered in veterinary practice.

Table 11.5 presents a framework for addressing ethical dilemmas by systematically identifying interests, consequences, and ethical principles.

Table 11.6 provides the Veterinary Ethics Tool (VET) to facilitate ethical deliberation in clinical practice.

Table 11.3 Veterinarian Interests

Animal
Client
Veterinarian
Practice owner/employer
Financial compensation
Public health
Referring veterinarian
Research/publications/teaching

Source: Kipperman (2022)/with permission of John Wiley & Sons.

Table 11.4 Types of Ethical Dilemmas in Veterinary Practice

Financial limitations compromise patient care (Kondrup et al., 2016; Kipperman et al., 2018; Quain et al., 2021)
Futile intervention: Client wishes to continue treatment despite poor animal quality of life and prognosis (Batchelor and McKeegan, 2012; Moses et al., 2018)
Euthanasia based on economic factors or for client convenience (Batchelor and McKeegan, 2012; Rathwell-Deault et al., 2017; Kipperman et al., 2018)
Balancing interests of animal against interests of client (Tannenbaum, 1995; Rollin, 2006a; Kipperman et al., 2018; Quain et al., 2021)
Whether to confront or report a colleague providing incompetent or substandard care (Rollin, 2006a; Crane et al., 2015)
Whether to report suspected animal abuse (Kogan et al., 2017; Joo et al., 2020)
Being asked to do something that feels like the wrong thing to do (Moses et al., 2018; Lehnus et al., 2019)
Being asked to do things that are outside of your skill set for financial or other reasons (Moses et al., 2018)
Disclosing bad news or medical errors (Kogan et al., 2018)
Whether to offer referral when this may provide a better outcome (Rollin, 2006b)
Whether to perform cosmetic or convenience surgeries (Mills et al., 2016)

Source: Data from Fawcett (2020).

Table 11.5 Framework for Addressing Ethical Dilemmas

1. Who are the relevant interests?
   What are the strengths of each interest?
   How do these interests conflict?
2. What are the available choices and their potential consequences for each interest?
3. What ethical theory best addresses this specific situation? (Kipperman and Rollin, 2022)
4. Are there any relevant laws or codes of conduct to consider?
5. Choose a course of action or inaction.
   Have I advocated for my patient/s to the best of my ability?

Source: Kipperman (2022)/with permission of John Wiley & Sons.

Ethical dilemmas surrounding euthanasia rarely resolve easily. Mentors are not tasked with eliminating uncertainty or protecting mentees from discomfort. Instead, mentors support early-career veterinarians by helping them think critically, reflect honestly, and act in alignment with their values—even when outcomes are imperfect. Through guided discussion, shared experience, and thoughtful use of ethical tools, mentors help transform ethically challenging moments into opportunities for professional growth and resilience.

Table 11.6 Veterinary Ethics Tool (VET) to Facilitate Decision-Making in Clinical Veterinary Medicine

	Relationship	Questions to facilitate ethical deliberation	No	I don't know	Possibly	Definitely
Animal-centered factors (justificatory reasons)	Clinician–patient (clinical responsibility)	A. Do you perceive the proposed treatment to be in the best interests of the patient?	X	—	✓	✓
		A1. Will the proposed treatment improve the patient's health?	X	—	✓	✓
		A2. Will the proposed treatment improve the patient's quality of life: (a) immediately	X	—	✓	✓
		(b) long term	X	—	✓	✓
		B. Is the proposed treatment option the one with the least potential to cause harm and suffering while still achieving the intended clinical goal?	—	—	✓	✓
		C. Have measures been taken to minimize the potential for harm and suffering?	—	—	✓	✓
		D. Do the expected benefits outweigh the potential harm and suffering inflicted on the animal or are they at least in balance?	X	—	✓	✓
Secondary factors (explanatory reasons)	Clinician–profession (professional responsibility	E. Does the primary clinician/team have experience in carrying out the proposed treatment and/or is it a well-documented recognized treatment?	—	—	✓	✓
		F. Is this case an example of good ethical decision-making for students/ trainees/colleagues?	—	—	✓	✓
		G. Would you feel comfortable justifying the proposed treatment to professional colleagues?	—	—	✓	✓
	Client–patient	H. Would proceeding with the proposed treatment have a positive impact on the owner-animal relationship?	—	—	✓	✓
		I. Would proceeding with the proposed treatment have a positive impact on the client's quality of life and/or financial benefits (e.g. the proposed treatment will allow breeding from a valuable animal)?	—	—	✓	✓
	Clinician–client	J. Is the proposed treatment financially viable for the client?	X	—	✓	✓
		K. Is the client capable of providing a suitable home environment and/or administrating medication during the recovery period?	X	—	✓	✓
Priority check	Professional responsibility	L. Are the secondary factors E–K (explanatory reasons) more influential in your clinical decision than the animal-centered factors A–D (justificatory reasons)?	✓	—	X	X
X	Consider alternative treatment options.					
—	Reconsider procedure and the clinician's responsibility.					
✓	Valid reasons for clinical procedure.					

Source: Data from Grimm et al. (2018).

CONCLUSION

Medical errors and euthanasia decisions represent inevitable realities of veterinary practice that demand both technical competence and emotional resilience. Errors occur in even the best systems, and the path forward lies not in assigning blame but in building cultures of curiosity, conducting RCA, and implementing process improvements that prevent future harm. Transparent disclosure to clients, support for affected team members, and systematic investigation create environments where learning replaces fear.

Euthanasia decisions carry equally complex weight, particularly when client requests conflict with animal welfare or when economic limitations compromise care. Mentors must prepare new graduates to navigate these dilemmas by fostering patient advocacy, providing frameworks for ethical analysis, and creating safe spaces for team discussion. When practices establish clear policies around euthanasia declination and financial assistance, they reduce the moral burden on individual clinicians while supporting more consistent, ethically defensible decisions that honor both professional integrity and compassionate care.

BIBLIOGRAPHY

American Veterinary Medical Association (2020). Guidelines for the euthanasia of animals. https://www.avma.org/sites/default/files/2020-02/Guidelines-on-Euthanasia-2020.pdf (accessed 24 January 2025).

Ashall, V. (2023). Reducing moral stress in veterinary teams? Evaluating the use of ethical discussion groups in charity veterinary hospitals. *Animals* 13 (10): 1662.

Barazowski, J.A., Forsythe, L.R., and Gochenauer, A.E. (2025). Assessment and categorization of medication errors in a veterinary teaching hospital. *Journal of the American Pharmacists Association* 102: 362.

Batchelor, C.E.M. and McKeegan, D.E.F. (2012). Survey of the frequency and perceived stressfulness of ethical dilemmas encountered in UK veterinary practice. *Veterinary Record* 170: 19.

Bennett, P. and Rohlf, V. (2005). Perpetration-induced traumatic stress in persons who euthanize nonhuman animals in surgeries, animal shelters, and laboratories. *Society & Animals* 13: 201–220.

Karen Berger (2018). Eric Cropp discusses medical error that sent him to prison [WWW Document]. https://www.pharmacytimes.com/view/getting-to-know-the-caring-eric-cropp (accessed 5 February 2025).

Blum, N.R. (2018). Professional development groups help physicians; why not veterinarians? *Journal of the American Veterinary Medical Association* 253 (6): 704–708.

Cooney, K. and Kipperman, B. (2023). Ethical and practical considerations associated with companion animal euthanasia. *Animals* 13: 430. https://doi.org/10.3390/ani13030430.

Cooney, K. and Kogan, L. (2022). How pet owners define a 'good death': new study reveals some surprising facts. *DVM360 Magazine* 53: 12.

Crane, M.F., Bayl-Smith, P., and Cartmill, J. (2013). A recommendation for expanding the definition of moral distress experienced in the workplace. *Australian & New Zealand Journal of Organisational Psychology* 6: e1. https://doi.org/10.1017/orp.2013.1.

Crane, M.F., Phillips, J.K., and Karin, E. (2015). Trait perfectionism strengthens the negative effects of moral stressors occurring in veterinary practice. *Australian Veterinary Journal* 93: 354–360.

Davidow, B. (2021). Communicating patient quality and safety in your hospital. *Veterinary Clinics of North America: Small Animal Practice* 51: 1111–1123.

Dyck, A. (1975). Beneficent euthanasia and benemortasia: alternative views of mercy. In: *Beneficent Euthanasia* (ed. M. Kohl), 117–129. Buffalo, NY: Prometheus Books.

Emily Jerry's Story (2014). Patient Safety Movement Foundation [WWW Document]. https://psmf.org/story/emily-jerry/ (accessed 5 February 2025).

Fawcett, A. (2020). Moral distress in veterinarians: why ethical challenges impact wellbeing. *VetFest 2020 Proceedings* https://vetfest.ava.com.au.

Fawcett, A. and Mullan, S. (2018). Managing moral distress in practice. *In Practice* 40: 34–36.

Grimm, H., Bergadano, A., Musk, G.C. et al. (2018). Drawing the line in clinical treatment of companion animals: recommendations from an ethics working party. *Veterinary Record* 182 (23): 664.

Hanrahan, C., Sabo, B.M., and Robb, P. (2018). Secondary traumatic stress and veterinarians: human–animal bonds as psychosocial determinants of health. *Traumatology* 24: 73–82.

Institute of Medicine (US) Committee on Quality of Health Care in America (2000). *To Err Is Human*. Washington, DC: National Academies Press.

Institute of Medicine (US) Committee on Quality of Health Care in America (2001). *Crossing the Quality Chasm*. Washington, DC: National Academies Press.

Joo, S., Jung, Y., and Chun, M.S. (2020). An analysis of veterinary practitioners' intention to intervene in animal abuse cases in South Korea. *Animals* 10 (5): 802.

Kipperman, B. (2010). Economic euthanasia: a disease in need of prevention. https://www.hsvma.org/economic_euthanasia_disease_in_need_of_prevention#.Y1mdNC-B30o (accessed 19 January 2025).

Kipperman, B. (2017). Ethical dilemmas encountered by small animal veterinarians: characterization, responses, consequences and beliefs regarding euthanasia. MSc thesis. University of Edinburgh, UK.

Kipperman, B. (2022). Veterinary advocacies and ethical dilemmas. In: *Ethics in Veterinary Practice* (ed. B. Kipperman and B.E. Rollin). Hoboken, NJ: Wiley-Blackwell.

Kipperman, B. and Cooney, K. (2024). Euthanasia. In: *Decision Making in Veterinary Practice*. Hoboken, NJ: Wiley-Blackwell.

Kipperman, B. and Rollin, B.E. (2022). Introduction to veterinary ethics. In: *Ethics in Veterinary Practice* (ed. B. Kipperman and B.E. Rollin). Hoboken, NJ: Wiley-Blackwell.

Kipperman, B.S., Kass, P.H., and Rishniw, M. (2017). Factors that influence small animal veterinarians' opinions and actions regarding cost of care and effects of economic limitations on patient care and outcome and professional career satisfaction and burnout. *Journal of the American Veterinary Medical Association* 250 (7): 785–794.

Kipperman, B., Morris, P., and Rollin, B. (2018). Ethical dilemmas encountered by small animal veterinarians: characterisation, responses, consequences and beliefs regarding euthanasia. *Veterinary Record* 182: 548. https://doi.org/10.1136/vr.104619.

Kondrup, S.V., Anhoj, K.P., Rodsgaard-Rosenbeck, C. et al. (2016). Veterinarian's dilemma: a study of how Danish small animal practitioners handle financially limited clients. *Veterinary Record* 179: 596.

Kogan, L.R., Schoenfeld-Tacher, R.M., Hellyer, P.W. et al. (2017). Survey of attitudes toward and experiences with animal abuse encounters in a convenience sample of US veterinarians. *Journal of the American Veterinary Medical Association* 250 (6): 688–696.

Kong, W.M. (2015). What is good medical ethics? A clinician's perspective. *Journal of Medical Ethics* 41: 79–82.

Lehnus, K.S., Fordyce, P.S., and McMillan, M.W. (2019). Ethical dilemmas in clinical practice: a perspective on the results of an electronic survey of veterinary anaesthetists. *Veterinary Anaesthesia and Analgesia* 46 (3): 260–275.

Lusk, C., DeForest, E., Segarra, G. et al. (2022). *British Journal of Anaesthesia* 129: e61–e62.

Marchitelli, B., Shearer, T., and Cook, N. (2020). Factors contributing to the decision to euthanize: diagnosis, clinical signs, and triggers. *Veterinary Clinics of North America: Small Animal Practice* 50 (3): 573–589.

Mills, K.E., von Keyserlingk, M.A., and Niel, L. (2016). A review of medically unnecessary surgeries in dogs and cats. *Journal of the American Veterinary Medical Association* 248 (2): 162–171.

Morgan, C.A. and McDonald, D. (2007). Ethical dilemmas in veterinary medicine. *Veterinary Clinics of North America: Small Animal Practice* 37: 165–179.

Moses, L., Malowney, M.J., and Boyd, J.W. (2018). Ethical conflict and moral distress in veterinary practice: a survey of North American veterinarians. *Journal of Veterinary Internal Medicine* 32 (6): 2115–2122.

Oxtoby, C., Ferguson, E., White, K., and Mossop, L. (2015). *Veterinary Record* 177: 438.

Pegram, C., Gray, C., Packer, R. et al. (2021). Proportion and risk factors for death by euthanasia in dogs in the UK. *Scientific Reports* 11: 1–12.

Quain, A. (2021). The gift: ethically indicated euthanasia in companion animal practice. *Veterinary Sciences* 8: 141. https://doi.org/10.3390/vetsci8080141.

Quain, A., Mullan, S., McGreevy, P.D. et al. (2021). Frequency, stressfulness and type of ethically challenging situations encountered by veterinary team members during the COVID-19 pandemic. *Frontiers in Veterinary Science* 8: 647108.

Quain, A., Mullan, S., and Ward, M.P. (2022). "There was a sense that our load had been lightened": evaluating outcomes of virtual ethics rounds for veterinary team members. *Frontiers in Veterinary Science* 9: 922049.

Rathwell-Deault, D., Godard, B., Frank, D. et al. (2017). Conceptualization of convenience euthanasia as an ethical dilemma for veterinarians in Quebec. *Canadian Veterinary Journal* 58: 255–260.

Richards, L., Coghlan, S., and Delany, C. (2020). "I had no idea that other people in the world thought differently to me": ethical challenges in small animal veterinary practice and implications for ethics support and education. *Journal of Veterinary Medical Education* 47: e20190013.

Rodziewicz, T.L., Houseman, B., Vaqar, S., and Hipskind, J.E. (2025). *Medical Error Reduction and Prevention*. Treasure Island, FL: StatPearls.

Rollin, B.E. (1987). Euthanasia and moral stress. *Loss, Grief & Care* 1: 115–126.

Rollin, B.E. (2006a). *An Introduction to Veterinary Medical Ethics*, 2e. Ames, Iowa: Blackwell Publishing.

Rollin, B.E. (2006b). The ethics of referral. *Canadian Veterinary Journal* 47 (7): 717.

Rollin, B.E. (2011). Euthanasia, moral stress and chronic illness in veterinary medicine. *Veterinary Clinics of North America: Small Animal Practice* 41: 651–659.

Scotney, R.L., McLaughlin, D., and Keates, H.L. (2015). A systematic review of the effects of euthanasia and occupational stress in personnel working with animals in shelters, clinics, and research. *Journal of the American Veterinary Medical Association* 247: 1121–1130.

Tannenbaum, J. (1995). *Veterinary Medical Ethics: Animal Welfare, Client Relations, Competition and Collegiality*, 2e. St. Louis: Mosby – Year Book.

Wallis, J., Fletcher, D., Bentley, A., and Ludders, J. (2019). *Frontiers in Veterinary Science* 6.

Yeates, J.W. and Main, D.C.J. (2011). Veterinary opinions on refusing euthanasia: justifications and philosophical frameworks. *Veterinary Record* 168: 263.

CHAPTER 12

Fostering Growth Through Feedback

INTRODUCTION

Dani Rabwin

Feedback represents an important yet challenging aspect of effective mentorship. The transition from veterinary school—where feedback flows through structured assessments, grades, and clinical evaluations—to practice often leaves new graduates uncertain about their progress and development. Without clear guidance on their performance, even talented veterinarians can struggle with confidence, repeat mistakes, and fail to reach their potential.

The challenge lies not in recognizing feedback's importance, but in delivering it effectively. Most mentors understand that new graduates need guidance, but many struggle with how to provide feedback that fosters growth and maintains trust. The fear of damaging relationships, uncertainty about timing and delivery, and lack of a structured approach often results in mentors either avoiding difficult conversations entirely or delivering feedback so poorly that it creates more problems than it solves.

Both giving and receiving feedback can feel uncomfortable and risky. Mentors worry about hurting feelings or damaging trust, while mentees may feel vulnerable and defensive when hearing about areas for improvement. These natural human reactions can turn what should be growth-oriented conversations into awkward or counterproductive exchanges that neither party wants to repeat.

The encouraging reality is that giving and receiving feedback effectively are learnable skills with proven frameworks and strategies. Rather than relying on intuition or hoping for the best, mentors can master specific models and approaches that transform feedback from an uncomfortable necessity into a powerful catalyst for professional development.

For this chapter, I chose Dr. Kelly Cooper, whose career embodies the balance between practical leadership and compassionate mentorship. After stepping into practice ownership just one year after graduation, Dr. Cooper went on to build a thriving mixed-animal practice before taking on leadership roles at Banfield Pet Hospital, where she coached doctors and led medical operations at district, regional, and national levels. Now the founder of Reality Vet Coaching & Consulting, she combines her experience in both independent and corporate settings to guide veterinary leaders in building strong teams and sustainable businesses. Her return to hands-on clinical practice keeps her deeply connected to the realities of everyday veterinary life, ensuring her insights into feedback are both evidence-based and eminently practical.

FEEDBACK AND MENTORSHIP

Kelly C. Cooper

WHEN FEEDBACK FALLS SHORT: LACY'S STORY

Lacy graduated from veterinary school only one year ago, yet she's already made the decision to move on from her first job as an associate veterinarian. If she stays with her current employer for just two more months, she won't be asked to pay back any of the $20,000 sign-on bonus she accepted when she was hired. Lacy is applying for a similar position across town at a general practice offering structured mentorship and more support staffing.

Lacy had been promised mentorship for her first year at her current position in a three-doctor general practice. She was paired with a more senior doctor as her mentor, who was encouraging and readily answered all her questions, but Lacy received little constructive feedback about her progress from her mentor or her manager. As a result, she was often unsure about how she was doing and uncertain if she was fulfilling the expectations of her role. She felt stuck, stagnant, and she lacked confidence. She really wants to work somewhere she feels her development will be well supported.

Unfortunately, Lacy's story is common among new graduates. Even in multi-doctor hospitals, novice veterinarians often lack structured guidance, and when mentorship is available, many mentors struggle with delivering quality, constructive feedback. This gap between what new graduates need and what they receive doesn't just represent a personal setback—it creates professional uncertainty that can undermine confidence, hinder development, and ultimately lead to career dissatisfaction.

THE FEEDBACK GAP: FROM ACADEMIA TO PRACTICE

In the evolving field of veterinary medicine, where competence and accuracy expectations are high, transitioning from student to practitioner is challenging. In veterinary school, structured feedback is built into the academic environment through test scores, grades, and guidance from professors during classroom learning and clinical rotations.

When new graduates enter practice, they leave this safe, predictable feedback structure and enter a new reality. Unless they have a dedicated and effective mentor, their only feedback comes through patient outcomes, client interactions, customer ratings, and formal reviews. This shift explains why most veterinary graduates prioritize strong mentorship when choosing their first employer.

The transition highlights two critical feedback responsibilities for employers and mentors: creating an environment where feedback flows intentionally with a focus on learning and ensuring mentors have skills to deliver growth-fostering feedback in a psychologically safe setting.

When experienced veterinarians mentor new graduates, they accept responsibility to share knowledge through teaching, coaching, and feedback. Their skills will directly impact their mentee's engagement, learning, and success. Thankfully, a mentor with positive intentions and a growth mindset can learn to give feedback, though mastery develops through practice.

My own early feedback attempts were rough. I once delivered criticism so bluntly to a new associate that she avoided me for weeks afterward, teaching me that how you communicate matters as much as what you communicate. This is why building a trusting relationship with your mentee creates such an important foundation—it covers your inevitable human flaws. Keep practicing this vital skill. Your mentees will value your efforts and with time, you'll develop mastery in this essential aspect of mentorship.

FEEDBACK AS ESSENTIAL NOURISHMENT

When learning new skills or starting a job, everyone wants to perform well. This requires feedback from those who have the experience and knowledge to provide guidance. Effective feedback answers critical questions about progress: "How am I doing? Where am I going? Am I meeting expectations? How can I do better?" "A McKinsey survey of 12,000 managers indicated they consider 'candid, insightful feedback' critical to career development" (Blanding, 2022).

Merriam-Webster defines feedback as "the transmission of evaluative or corrective information about an action, event, or process to the original or controlling source" (Definition of FEEDBACK, 2025). In professional settings, feedback provides a reflection on performance, behavior, or appearance with the specific goal of fostering improvement and development.

Think of a newly planted seed that needs soil, water, and sunlight to thrive. In a growth environment, feedback serves as these essential nutrients. Without them, development stagnates, growth stunts, and desired outcomes become unattainable.

"Gallup data show that 80% of employees who say they have received meaningful feedback in the past week are fully engaged" (Mclain and Nelson, 2022). As a mentor, your feedback should help your mentee develop skills, knowledge, and confidence in the most positive, affirming way possible. Through effective feedback, you'll facilitate their self-awareness, receptiveness to input, and commitment to continuous learning.

TABLE: THE FEEDBACK BALANCE SHEET

This table illustrates the stark contrast between the positive and negative impacts on both individuals and organizations when feedback is delivered effectively versus ineffectively.

Impact on the...	Effective feedback	Ineffective or lack of feedback
Individual	• Clarifies performance expectations • Reinforces positive behaviors • Fosters continuous improvement • Creates mentee self-awareness • Builds mentee confidence, competence, and motivation • Highlights mentee strengths • Enhances trust between mentor and mentee	• Perpetuates unclear expectations • Mentee repeats incorrect behaviors • Increases anxiety due to uncertainty • Decreases engagement and motivation • Reduces risk-taking by mentee • Allows for missed growth opportunities • Erodes trust between mentor and mentee
Organization	• Builds trust between the mentee, peers, and the organization • Improves overall performance and productivity • Creates a culture of continuous learning • Reduces errors and performance gaps • Promotes innovation • Increases employee retention • Develops a pipeline of future leaders	• Reduces communication across the team • Leads to inefficiency and poor performance • Increases medical errors and safety risks • Creates strained workplace relationships • Reduces employee engagement • Leads to higher turnover

HONEST FEEDBACK: A RARE GIFT

Billionaire investor Warren Buffet is famously quoted, "Honesty is a very expensive gift. Don't expect it from cheap people." Consider your last request for feedback—you likely received vague positivity like "you did great." People default to these pleasant but unhelpful responses because they want to be nice, lack clarity about what feedback you need, or haven't developed enough trust to risk offering constructive criticism.

This is how leaders end up with blind spots. Without effective feedback, they believe they're doing well, unaware of their faults. When you don't receive needed feedback, those hidden gaps impact your effectiveness and reputation. Left unnoticed, they become more challenging to address.

A recent Gallup poll found that only 26% of employees strongly believe feedback helps them work better. Another survey found 72% rated "managers providing critical feedback" as important for career development, yet only 5% believe managers provide such feedback (Blanding, 2022).

This is why honest feedback is truly a gift—it's hard to obtain. I've worked in situations where I never received constructive feedback, and it was frustrating. Being told "everything is great" is unhelpful, especially when I knew I could do better but didn't know what was missing.

Like most people, I don't love hearing about my flaws but realize not knowing is worse for my growth than the short-term discomfort of hearing I'm not perfect. One benefit of working in a corporate environment was the professional development I received. After years of coaching and feedback sessions, I've learned to identify and lean into strengths while acknowledging and managing my weaknesses.

As a mentor, your feedback is a precious gift to your mentee's development. They cannot grow optimally with vague platitudes. They need specific feedback. Seek feedback for yourself too—it builds trust while modeling the growth mindset essential in this profession. Temporary discomfort always beats long-term consequences of issues left unaddressed.

Warren Buffet—"Honesty is a very expensive gift. Don't expect it from cheap people."

CREATING A CULTURE OF OPEN EXCHANGE

In thriving organizations, effective feedback flows continuously between colleagues—vertically between leadership levels and horizontally across peer groups. The most successful teams actively promote and engage in a culture where feedback is expected and normalized (Blanding, 2022). This culture rarely develops naturally. Creating such a culture requires intention, structure, and consistent reinforcement.

Less effective cultures restrict feedback to one-way communication, offer virtually none, or focus exclusively on criticism. These environments typically lead to disengagement and frustration. If you are mentoring where a feedback culture is absent, you can still create your own culture with your mentee and team. As a doctor, mentor, or manager, you shape culture through relationships and have significant influence over your mentee's experience. I strongly encourage building your own culture of feedback, regardless of your broader organizational context.

RECOGNIZING FEEDBACK CHALLENGES

Despite the clear benefits of a healthy feedback culture, many struggle with feedback exchanges. Mentors hesitate to deliver honest feedback, while recipients often resist receiving it. These mirror-image challenges create barriers to growth, leaving individuals uncertain about their performance and development needs.

Let's explore the key factors that make both giving and receiving feedback difficult:

1. Fear of relationship damage vs. threat to self-esteem:
   - Givers prioritize harmony over honesty, worrying that constructive feedback might label them as difficult or damage relationships. Past experiences where feedback created tension reinforce this avoidance.
   - Receivers perceive feedback—especially criticism—as threatening to their self-image and confidence. The fear of feeling inadequate leads many to avoid feedback situations altogether, limiting growth opportunities.
2. Skill deficiency vs. inner criticism:
   - Givers lack confidence in their ability to provide feedback effectively. Without frameworks for structuring observations, many struggle to distinguish between subjective judgments and objective assessments.
   - Receivers often wrestle with imposter syndrome or perfectionism, avoiding feedback for fear of being "exposed" or seeing any critique as failure rather than opportunity. Both mindsets protect these deep-seated insecurities.
3. Fear of consequences vs. protective instinct:
   - Givers worry that honest feedback could lead to negative professional consequences, especially when addressing those in positions of influence. This concern is heightened in organizations where psychological safety is limited.
   - Receivers develop protective instincts after previous encounters with harsh feedback, becoming reluctant to seek input even in new situations with different people.
4. Empathy vs. vulnerability:
   - Givers hesitate to deliver feedback that might hurt someone's confidence or emotional well-being, sometimes withholding important observations that could ultimately benefit growth.
   - Receivers find asking for feedback requires vulnerability—something particularly challenging for veterinary professionals accustomed to demonstrating competence and certainty.
5. Cultural norms affecting both sides:
   - Both giving and receiving direct feedback may be viewed as inappropriate in certain cultural contexts—spanning ethnic backgrounds, family upbringings, organizational environments, and professional industries.
   - In competitive environments, seeking feedback may be seen as weakness while giving it may violate unspoken rules about maintaining professional distance.

For mentors, understanding these barriers from both perspectives is crucial. Many veterinary professionals are overachievers plagued by perfectionism, making feedback exchanges particularly challenging. This emphasizes the importance of establishing trust and practicing various feedback methods. Through seeking feedback yourself and modeling openness to growth, you'll discover what works best for your mentee while building a culture where feedback becomes a valued tool rather than a dreaded experience.

As you develop your mentoring skills, reflect on your comfort level with delivering both positive and constructive feedback. If you notice hesitation when feedback is needed, explore the reasons behind your reluctance. Seek perspective from trusted colleagues and deliberately practice the techniques presented here to build your confidence.

BREAKING THROUGH DEFENSIVE BARRIERS

"What do I do when the feedback I give isn't heard or the receiver becomes defensive?" This is one of the most common questions I hear after my feedback presentations. When your mentee feels threatened, their natural response will be to defend themselves—a reaction rooted in fear of criticism or failure.

Dictionary.com defines defensiveness as "excessive concern with guarding against the real or imagined threat of criticism, injury to one's ego, exposure of one's shortcomings" (DEFENSIVENESS, 2023). Defensiveness creates a significant barrier to effective feedback because once someone enters this state, they stop receiving your input. Defensiveness typically manifests as:

- **Explanations**—when the receiver quickly explains away their decisions, they've stopped listening to your feedback.
- **Deflection**—"Other people do this too" shifts responsibility away from themselves onto others instead of taking ownership.
- **Emotional reaction**—appearing as anger, frustration, sadness, or shutting down completely. If your mentee loses composure after uncomfortable feedback, you've lost the opportunity for constructive dialogue until they regain their composure. Wait for a calmer moment, then seek to understand what triggered the reaction while maintaining a neutral stance.

These reactions may indicate your mentee isn't open to coaching—at least in that moment. If defensiveness becomes a pattern, you may have a mentee who resists coaching altogether. Someone truly open to growth will remain curious and listen actively to your input.

When timing and setting are appropriate, your mentee needs feedback about how they receive feedback. Their inappropriate responses will undermine your efforts and diminish your ability to mentor effectively. For a recent graduate who depends on guidance to develop professionally, this resistance can indicate broader performance concerns.

CREATING PSYCHOLOGICAL SAFETY FOR FEEDBACK

To minimize defensiveness and create an environment where feedback can be received, incorporate these proven communication techniques:

- **Be empathetic**: Every individual is unique and carries different capabilities and challenges. Put yourself in their shoes.
- **Focus on observed behaviors** rather than making assumptions about intentions or character.
- **Be curious instead of judgmental**: Seek to understand the mentee's perspective by asking open-ended questions.
- **Use "I" statements**: The word "you" can feel accusatory. Start sentences with "I." For example, Say "I noticed you arrived after the agreed upon time" instead of "You were late this morning."
- **Avoid "why" questions**: Like "you" statements, "why" can create defensiveness. Try more inviting alternatives: "Could you help me understand what affected your arrival time today?" instead of "Why were you late?"

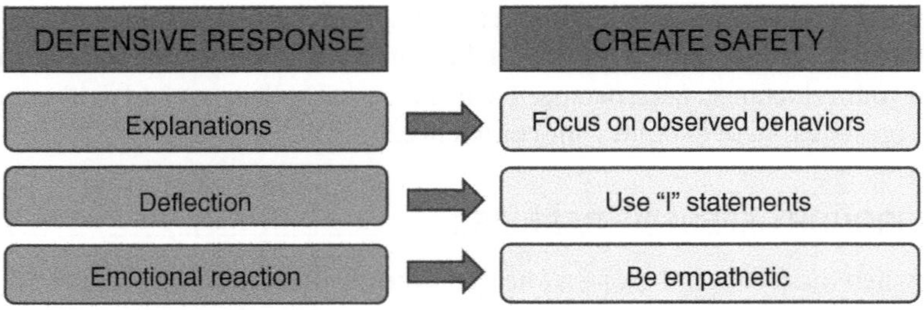

FIGURE 12.1 Create safety to reduce defensiveness. *Source:*

Recognizing defensiveness is a critical skill that can transform your mentoring relationship from one of resistance to one of growth. By approaching with empathy, focusing on behaviors rather than character, and shifting your language to be more inviting, you create the psychological safety needed for meaningful feedback exchanges. Remember that your ultimate goal isn't just delivering feedback—it's ensuring that feedback becomes the gift it's meant to be: one that's actually received and appreciated.

Figure 12.1 maps specific defensive responses to communication techniques that help create psychological safety and reduce defensiveness. By strategically applying these approaches—focusing on observed behaviors rather than intentions, using "I" statements to reduce accusatory language, and responding with empathy to emotional reactions—mentors can transform defensive barriers into productive learning conversations.

Understanding the psychological foundations of feedback—why it matters, what makes it challenging, and how to create psychological safety—provides the groundwork for effective mentorship. But knowing why feedback is important isn't enough; mentors need practical tools and structured approaches to deliver feedback that truly drives growth. **The difference between a mentor who understands feedback conceptually and one who can implement it effectively lies in mastering specific methods and models that transform good intentions into meaningful conversations.** Let's explore the practical frameworks that will help you deliver feedback with confidence and consistency.

FEEDBACK IN ACTION: METHODS AND MODELS

BLINDSIDED BY A TRUSTED MANAGER

When I was in my second year of field leadership as a medical director, overseeing 14 hospitals and 35 doctors, I had my first annual performance review with my manager, whom I had worked with for about nine months.. He had traveled with me in my market three times, and I had been on numerous group calls,two in-person team development meetings, and monthly one-on-ones with him. Along the way, he had provided encouraging and positive feedback, and constructive suggestions to improve my impact. My market had just come off of a stellar year for growth and we had top results in the region for client experience, patient safety, and employee engagement. I thought my review would be equally stellar, expecting an "exceeds expectations" rating.

I was quite surprised and disappointed when my manager presented a short laundry list of my shortcomings to me as we sat in a busy Starbucks. The list included several soft skills he had never mentioned to me before. He also shared that it was rare for such a new leader to receive an "exceeds" rating, so my rating was a "meets expectations." He then tried to soften the blow, by telling me how great a rating that was.

In hindsight, I admit I was overconfident, but I was blindsided and disappointed to say the least. My team had worked hard for our achievements, and we were head and shoulders above our peers. In that moment, I stopped trusting my manager, knowing he could have provided timely feedback and when it was relevant along the way. I did not feel he had my best interests at heart and saw that he was conflict avoidant. It also caused me to question my ability and shook my confidence, stirring up the voices of impostor syndrome inside my head.

Because of my experience, I vowed to never blindside my own people. I committed to giving them the feedback they deserved along the way, so they could develop awareness and have the opportunity to improve and develop with support. I would not let my discomfort with constructive feedback be the barrier to their success. That experience also taught me that I could not assume that my managers would provide the feedback I needed to grow, and it was up to me to proactively ask for it and keep asking for it.

Since then, I've discovered that many veterinarians do not receive the candid feedback they need for growth. They continue believing everything is fine until they're blindsided by a manager who finally voices concerns that could have been addressed earlier. This feedback vacuum creates unnecessary anxiety, erodes trust, and stunts professional development. As a mentor, you have the power to break this harmful cycle by providing the consistent, thoughtful feedback your mentee deserves—feedback that helps them recognize both their strengths and areas for improvement before small issues become significant problems.

Having explored the importance of feedback and the psychological factors affecting its exchange in the previous sections, let's turn our attention to the practical aspects of feedback delivery. In the next section, we'll examine specific methods and structures for providing feedback that resonates with your mentee and drives professional growth. My experience of being blindsided during that performance review highlights why implementing these methods consistently is crucial—not only for the mentee's development but also for maintaining trust in the mentoring relationship. By mastering these feedback techniques, you'll ensure your mentees receive the guidance they need when they need it most.

THE 5:1 PRINCIPLE: BALANCING POSITIVE AND CONSTRUCTIVE INPUT

Delivering effective feedback requires understanding the fundamental types and maintaining the right balance between them. When mentors grasp this balance, they transform feedback from a potentially stressful interaction into a powerful catalyst for growth and development. Let's examine how to create this crucial equilibrium in your mentoring relationships.

Feedback comes in two essential forms: positive and constructive. Positive feedback recognizes strengths, expected behaviors, and appreciation for the individual. It motivates, builds confidence, and reinforces desired behaviors through praise, recognition, compliments, and rewards.

Constructive feedback addresses gaps in knowledge, skill, behaviors, outcomes, or results. I prefer the term "constructive" over "negative" because it emphasizes learning and growth opportunities rather than simply pointing out flaws. People respond more openly to constructive feedback rather than negative feedback because it focuses on development rather than criticism.

Stephen Covey's popular business book, "The 7 Habits of Highly Effective People," introduces the "emotional bank account" metaphor to describe relationship quality and the trust built between people. Covey notes, "In relationships, the little things are the big things. . . We make deposits through kindness, honesty, keeping promises, and being courteous. We make withdrawals by being unkind, disrespectful, overreacting, ignoring, being harsh, or rude" (Covey, 2004).

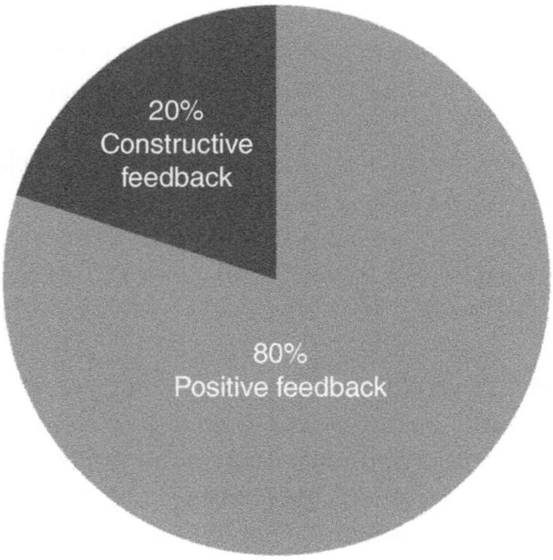

FIGURE 12.2 The ideal positive to constructive feedback ratio. *Source:* Image created by Dr Kelly Cooper.

When you provide positive feedback and recognition, you make emotional bank account deposits. Conversely, constructive feedback, even when delivered skillfully with positive intentions, can feel like a withdrawal to the receiver. Balance these carefully to maintain a healthy relationship (Figure 12.2).

What is the best ratio of positive to constructive feedback? A 2004 study by Losada and Heaphy revealed that the highest performing teams have a ratio of 5.6 positive interactions to every 1 negative interaction (Zenger and Folman, 2013). According to marriage expert John Gottman "That 'magic ratio' is 5 to 1. This means that for every negative interaction during conflict, a stable and happy marriage has five (or more) positive interactions" (Benson, 2017). And while a mentoring relationship is not a marriage, it is an important and close working relationship.

As a mentor, this concept highlights the importance of delivering feedback in a balanced fashion. Positive feedback drives motivation and engagement. "A Gallup survey found that 67% of employees whose managers focused on their strengths were fully engaged in their work, as compared to only 31% of employees whose managers focused on their weaknesses" (Porath, 2016).

While giving positive feedback only on wins and strengths would be preferable, the new graduate's learning curve also makes frequent constructive feedback necessary. Be focused and intentional about providing plenty of recognition and praise to maintain the balance and keep your mentee motivated.

To achieve the right emotional bank account balance:

- Be mindful of your feedback ratio (aiming for that 5:1 positive-to-constructive ratio).
- Make regular "deposits" through specific, meaningful positive feedback.
- Carefully frame necessary constructive feedback to minimize unnecessary "withdrawals."
- Recognize when an "account" needs replenishment.

STRUCTURED VS. SPONTANEOUS: THE TWO CHANNELS OF FEEDBACK

Understanding the balance between positive and constructive feedback is essential, but equally important is knowing when and how to deliver each type. Mentors can provide feedback through two complementary channels: formal and informal.

Formal feedback follows a structured, scheduled format, often with written documentation. It carries greater weight than informal feedback and typically involves advance planning and regular scheduling. The mentee, mentor, and line manager (if different from the mentor) usually participate together. Use formal feedback to discuss behavioral or performance trends or to address behaviors that don't meet expectations. When documentation is part of the process, share it with the receiver and add the documents to their employment record.

Examples of formal feedback can include:

- Monthly one-on-ones
- Quarterly, semiannual, or annual performance reviews
- Development planning and follow-up meetings
- Performance improvement plans and corrective action discussions

Informal feedback occurs more frequently and happens more spontaneously and with minimal planning. It lacks the formal structure but offers immediate impact when timing delivery soon after the observed behavior. While you might keep personal notes from these conversations for future reference, these notes stay private rather than entering into official records.

The more consistently you provide informal feedback, the clearer your mentee's understanding of their performance becomes. This clarity prevents surprises during formal, documented feedback sessions like performance reviews. As a mentor who may not be your mentee's direct manager, you'll likely focus primarily on informal feedback while providing performance observations to the manager for more formal evaluations.

THE ELEMENTS OF EFFECTIVE FEEDBACK

As previously discussed, feedback can be given effectively, ineffectively, or not at all, which is also considered ineffective. What is meant by the term effective feedback? Effective feedback is feedback provided in the most productive way possible so that the receiver obtains the most value from the experience. It is provided with positive intention and planning. The ability to give effective feedback is a critical management skill to be learned, practiced, and improved over time. Effective feedback is characterized by several key qualities:

- Respectful and Supportive:
  Deliver feedback using emotional and situational intelligence (see Chapter 7 for more details), using respect and empathy, and considering the graduate's perspective and potential emotional state. Don't just point out what went wrong—that's negative feedback—but help them explore alternatives and opportunities for learning.
- Collaborative:
  Effective feedback is often a collaborative, two-way discussion between the mentor and the mentee, one that focuses on the mentee's own reflections, observations, and learnings, where the mentor serves as a facilitator for the mentee's learning by asking open-ended questions and allowing the mentee to lead.

- Well-Timed:
  Feedback is most effective when given promptly. This ensures that the context and memory of the event are fresh in the mentor's and mentee's minds. By doing so, the mentor can "connect the dots" between the event and the feedback and allows for accurate reflection and adjustment if needed.
  This doesn't mean feedback should always be given in the moment. Be aware of the potential impact of the timing, considering the mentee's ability to receive the feedback in that moment and delaying for a more appropriate time.
- Well-Placed:
  Location matters, especially when the feedback is constructive. In most situations, positive feedback, such as recognition, can be given publicly and privately, although knowing the mentee's preference is helpful in making this decision, as some people do not appreciate public recognition. As a rule, give constructive feedback privately, especially when corrective, to avoid embarrassing the receiver or the feedback being diluted by distraction.
- Specific:
  Feedback with specific details has greater impact than generalizations. When you refer to a date, time, situation, or people involved, the mentee will be able to clearly connect the feedback to the event. As an example, instead of saying "you did a nice job today," you could say "I noticed you delegating to the technicians when working up the dog-attack patient this morning. You were clear and concise in what you needed from them. Nice work." See the difference?
- Actionable:
  Actionable feedback includes clear steps for improvement instead of vague suggestions that can leave the mentee unsure of how to proceed. Offer specific actions. As an example, instead of saying "try to be more welcoming when you enter the exam room," you could say "here are some ways to be more welcoming when you enter the exam room: make eye contact with the client, shake their hand, introduce yourself and welcome them by name." This feedback highlights specific, repeatable behaviors.

Mastering the elements of effective feedback—being respectful, collaborative, well-timed, appropriately placed, specific, and actionable—transforms your mentorship from simply transferring information to genuinely empowering growth. These characteristics aren't just nice-to-have features but essential elements that determine whether your feedback will be embraced or rejected. By consistently applying these elements with intention and care, you'll create a feedback environment where your mentee can truly flourish, building both competence and confidence that will serve them throughout their veterinary career.

FEEDBACK FRAMEWORKS

Now that you understand what makes feedback effective, let's explore the structured approaches that can help you deliver it consistently. You can choose from many different models to provide feedback to your mentee. Using a consistent feedback model helps you provide clarity, ensuring your feedback is most effective. Whichever models you end up using—and I recommend a combination of Situation-Behavior-Impact (SBI) and the Coach Approach—apply them consistently to develop your skill and create a culture of feedback.

THE SBI AND STAR FRAMEWORKS: CREATING CLEAR CONNECTIONS

The SBI and STAR models offer clear frameworks that simplify feedback delivery, whether positive or constructive. By connecting specific events to behaviors and outcomes, these structures create powerful mental links that enhance learning. While these models might feel formulaic initially,

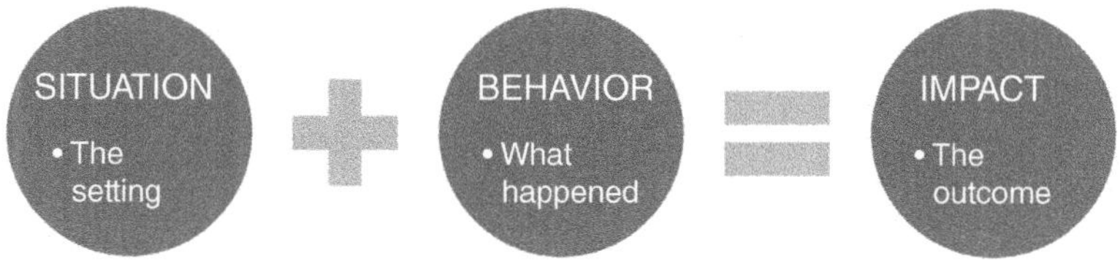

FIGURE 12.3 The SBI feedback model. *Source:* Image created by Dr Kelly Cooper.

with practice they become second nature, allowing your feedback to flow naturally and authentically (Figure 12.3).

- SBI Model (Situation-Behavior-Impact):
  - Situation: Describe the specific situation, timing, or location, which allows the receiver to visualize when and where the event occurred.
  - Behavior: Next, describe the behavior that was observed, avoiding judgmental statements..
  - Impact: Last, describe the impact (or outcome) of the behavior.
  - Example: "When you were evaluating Max this morning (situation), you slowed down and thoroughly palpated his abdomen (behavior). As a result, you were able to detect an enlarged spleen (impact)."
- STAR Model (Situation-Task-Action-Result):
  - Situation: Similar to SBI, describe the specific situation, timing, or location.
  - Task: Describe the task or goal.
  - Action: Describe the action (or behavior) observed.
  - Result: Describe the result (outcome or impact) of the action.
  - Example: "Yesterday, in surgery (situation), when you were working on your surgical efficiency (task), I noticed you made a rather small incision (action). As a result, you had a difficult time locating the uterus, and the procedure took longer than your intended goal."

The SBI model's straightforward formula connects specific context to observed behavior and outcomes, creating clear, judgment-free feedback that enhances learning and becomes natural with practice (Figure 12.4).

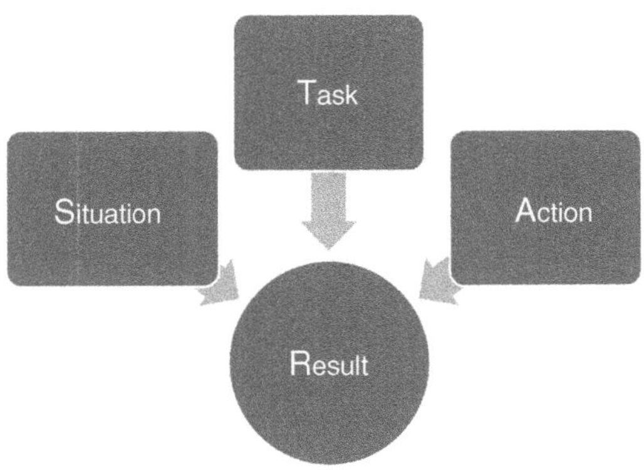

FIGURE 12.4 The STAR feedback model. *Source:* Image created by Dr Kelly Cooper.

WHY THE SANDWICH APPROACH FALLS FLAT

The feedback sandwich arises when someone uncomfortable with constructive criticism cushions it between two positive comments—like placing meat between slices of bread. For example, "You did a great job with client interactions today. I also noticed that you aren't completing your records by the end of the day, but the team enjoys working with you." This approach ultimately confuses recipients, who struggle to determine whether they're receiving praise or correction. Rather than clarifying important feedback, it dilutes the message and should be avoided in effective mentoring relationships.

EMPOWERMENT THROUGH INQUIRY: THE COACH APPROACH

The "coach approach" offers a more engaging feedback method that transforms the mentoring dynamic. Instead of simply giving the mentee their assessment and direction, the mentor asks powerful, open-ended questions that stimulate reflection and self-awareness. Through active listening and thoughtful follow-up questions, the mentor guides the mentee toward self-discovery, helping them identify their own strengths, improvement areas, and solutions. This approach feels less threatening than direct instruction and empowers mentees to take ownership of their development, teaching them the valuable skill of self-reflection while creating sustainable change through personal insight.

QUESTIONS THAT UNLOCK GROWTH

Powerful, open-ended questions form the foundation of the coach approach. Rather than imposing your perspective, these questions stimulate critical thinking, clinical reasoning, and self-awareness in your mentee. They create space for mentees to voice their own thoughts and feelings and ultimately develop solutions they truly own. In this dynamic, your role shifts from being the authority to being the facilitator—asking thoughtful questions and listening actively to help your mentee explore their own thinking process. The following examples demonstrate how coach-approach questions can transform your feedback conversations:

- How did that go? Which parts went well? What was the most challenging?
- Can you tell me more... (to elaborate the thought to a deeper level)
- How did you feel about that situation?
- What would you do again? What would you do differently?
- How do you want to move forward?
- What will you commit to?
- How can I help you with this? What support do you need from myself or others? (Figure 12.5)

This flowchart illustrates a simple yet powerful structure for engaging mentees in reflective, growth-oriented dialogue. By asking open-ended questions, mentors help mentees process their experiences, identify takeaways, and commit to meaningful next steps.

A successful coach approach hinges on active listening followed by thoughtful exploration of deeper meaning. I call this "pulling the thread"—keeping your questions connected as you carefully unravel what happened. You could also think of it as "peeling the onion," where each layer you remove reveals more insight until you reach the root cause. This investment in getting to

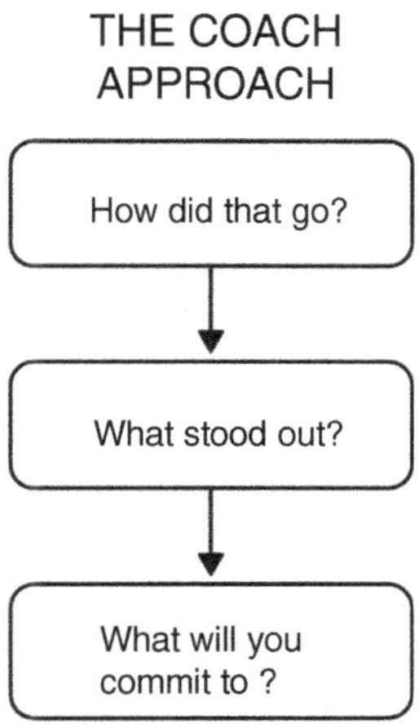

FIGURE 12.5 The coach approach to feedback. *Source:* Image created by Dr Kelly Cooper.

the core issue pays remarkable dividends: your mentee feels truly seen and understood, trust deepens between you, and the likelihood of addressing the real issue—not just its surface symptoms—increases significantly.

SIDEBAR

Sir John Whitmore—"Coaching for Performance"

"Coaching is unlocking people's potential to maximize their own performance. It is helping them to learn rather than teaching them. It is a way of relating to people that moves beyond models, tools and techniques and embraces a philosophy, an attitude, a belief in the potential of people" (Whitmore, 2017).

A COMPREHENSIVE FEEDBACK CYCLE: FROM DAILY INTERACTIONS TO FORMAL REVIEWS

With these feedback models as your foundation, the next step is creating a complete feedback system that combines formal and informal approaches. Many successful leaders have developed processes for combining formal and informal feedback that work well, engage their teams, and are easily applied to most mentorship or management situations where supervisors work closely with team members and can observe their behaviors. Here is an example:

- Create a foundation
  First you need the basis and standard from which you plan to provide feedback. This includes the expectations for your mentee in their role, which is usually defined in the job description and employee handbook. A skills checklist is also a valuable tool to align on the critical skills to be learned or performed.

  The next helpful tool is an agreed-upon development or learning plan that outlines the skills your mentee will focus on. Those skills should be defined in a specific or SMART goal format, so both of you are clear on the plan.

HOW TO WRITE A SMART GOAL

Specific: Clearly defined what needs to be accomplished
Measurable: Quantifiable to track progress
Achievable: Realistic and attainable
Relevant: Aligned with career development needs
Time-bound: Has a defined timeline for completion

- Feedback in the moment
  As you work together side-by-side on the clinical floor, seek opportunities to provide informal positive feedback in the moment that will motivate and encourage your mentee. When you see opportunities for constructive feedback, mentally note them or jot them down. Note the time, circumstance, and the behavior that you witnessed, as well as the impact. Decide how important it is for the mentee to hear this feedback and remember the goal of 5 deposits to 1 withdrawal. You must also decide how important it is to deliver the feedback immediately or to wait for a quieter, more effective time to do so.
- Daily huddles
  Have a plan to informally huddle at the end of each shift or day where you can debrief about how it went. This is your opportunity to discuss informal constructive feedback in private as well as takeaways, action items, and planning for the next day. Both the mentor and mentee should take informal personal notes for themselves for future reference. As time passes and your mentee grows so that less hands-on support is needed, daily huddles may turn into weekly huddles.
- Weekly check-ins
  These are 15 to 20 minutes, scheduled, and private check-ins, where recent events and learnings are discussed and plans for the coming week are discussed. Encouragement and recognition for progress is given as well as course correction where needed.
- Monthly one-on-ones
  These more formal meetings are used to assess progress, update training and development plans, provide and ask for feedback, and strengthen the relationship between the mentor and mentee. At these meetings, it's important to discuss any trends that affect overall success for future performance evaluations.
- Performance evaluations
  These are the formal meetings where progress is evaluated and documented against expectations. Managers are also involved if the mentor is not the manager. They can happen as part of the new graduate mentoring program, perhaps as a midway or final check-in. They also occur as routine annual or semiannual performance reviews. Ideally, if you've been executing the entire feedback strategy well, there will be zero feedback surprises for the mentee because you have created a culture of ongoing, collaborative feedback, and the mentee is well aware of their strengths, opportunities, and what's next. They could likely lead the discussion, facilitated by the mentor and/or manager. This is the ideal outcome for an effective feedback cycle (Figure 12.6).

While implementing this multilayered feedback system will significantly benefit your mentee, even the most thorough approach must evolve through ongoing refinement. This is where

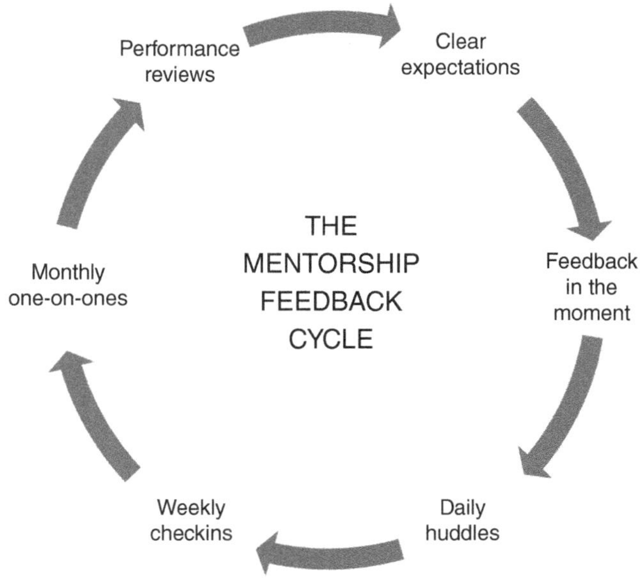

FIGURE 12.6 The mentorship feedback cycle. *Source:* Image created by Dr Kelly Cooper.

your own development as a mentor comes into play. Just as you've created a structure to help your mentee grow, you need similar input to enhance your mentoring abilities. The feedback cycle is never complete unless it flows in both directions.

THE MENTOR'S GROWTH JOURNEY

Let's talk about seeking effective feedback for yourself. While we've focused on how feedback helps your mentee grow, the same principles apply to you as a mentor. Even as an experienced veterinarian, you continue to develop—both in clinical skills and in mentorship abilities. When you step into mentoring, you're learning new communication and relationship skills that might feel awkward. Some aspects will come naturally, while others won't. You'll stumble occasionally, and yes, sometimes fail—but those moments are all a part of the learning process.

Remember, your mentee doesn't expect perfection. They want a collaborative mentor who recognizes their own need to grow. The most effective leaders have become so because they actively sought feedback and applied it, adapting their skills, knowledge, and behaviors to meet changing demands. While perfection isn't expected—we're all human, after all—a commitment to learning and growth is essential.

Where should you look for feedback? Start with your mentee. A healthy feedback culture flows in both directions—you not only give feedback to your mentee but also receive and act on their input. Keep in mind that, for a new graduate, providing feedback to somebody in authority, such as a mentor, can feel intimidating and risky, so build trust and psychological safety first. Your manager and daily teammates are also valuable feedback sources. Now that you understand effective feedback principles, seek out that honest, constructive input that will strengthen your mentoring and leadership abilities.

CONCLUSION

The mentor's ability to provide quality, effective feedback is one of the most critical skills in developing your mentee's competence and confidence. When feedback is given with skill, thought, and intention, it builds bridges of trust and creates a foundation for continuous growth and development. The feedback models and approaches we've explored—from SBI to the Coach Approach—are designed to make these conversations more approachable, actionable, and meaningful for both you and your mentee.

Remember that effective feedback is a two-way street. By not only providing feedback to your mentee but also seeking it for yourself, you model the growth mindset essential for success in veterinary medicine. Even as an experienced practitioner, your willingness to receive feedback demonstrates that learning is a lifelong journey. This reciprocal relationship builds trust and shows your mentee that nobody—not even their mentor—is perfect, but everyone can improve with honest reflection and open communication.

As you develop your feedback skills, be patient with yourself. Like any clinical skill, becoming proficient at delivering effective feedback takes practice and refinement. The awkwardness you may feel at first will gradually give way to more natural, fluid conversations that genuinely support your mentee's development. By creating a culture where feedback flows freely in both directions, you're not only helping your mentee navigate their transition from student to practitioner—you're also contributing to a healthier profession where continuous learning and improvement are valued above perfection. This is the true gift of feedback, and it's one worth giving.

BIBLIOGRAPHY

Benson, K. (2017). *The Magic Relationship Ratio, According to Science.* Gottman Institute https://www.gottman.com/blog/the-magic-relationship-ratio-according-science/ (accessed 28 March 2025).

Blanding, M. (2022). *Why People Crave Feedback—And Why We're Afraid to Give It.* Working Knowledge [WWW Document]. Harvard Business School. https://www.library.hbs.edu/working-knowledge/why-people-crave-feedback-and-why-were-afraid-to-give-it (accessed 16 February 2025).

Covey, S.R. (2004). *The 7 Habits of Highly Effective People.* New York: Free Press.

DEFENSIVENESS (2023). Definition & meaning. Dictionary.com [WWW Document]. https://www.dictionary.com/browse/defensiveness (accessed 28 March 2025).

Definition of FEEDBACK (2025). [WWW Document]. https://www.merriam-webster.com/dictionary/feedback (accessed 4 March 2025).

Mclain, D. and Nelson, B. (2022). How effective feedback fuels performance [WWW Document]. Gallup.com. https://www.gallup.com/workplace/357764/fast-feedback-fuels-performance.aspx (accessed 28 March 2025).

Porath, C. (2016). Give your team more-effective positive feedback [WWW Document]. Gallup.com. https://hbr.org/2016/10/give-your-team-more-effective-positive-feedback (accessed 28 March 2025)

Whitmore, J. (2017). *Coaching for Performance: The Principles and Practice of Coaching and Leadership*, 5e. London: Nicholas Brealey Publishing.

Zenger, J. and Folman, J. (2013). The ideal praise-to-criticism ratio [WWW Document]. HBR.org. https://hbr.org/2013/03/the-ideal-praise-to-criticism (accessed 16 February 2025).

Measuring Success

CHAPTER 13

INTRODUCTION

Dani Rabwin

Measuring mentorship success requires looking beyond good intentions and positive relationships to understand whether mentees are actually developing the skills and confidence they need to thrive. While some of the most meaningful aspects of professional growth—communication skills, clinical reasoning, and team collaboration—can be difficult to quantify, veterinary practices also generate valuable data that can reveal important patterns about a mentee's development and the effectiveness of mentorship approaches.

The challenge for mentors is learning how to use both quantitative metrics and qualitative observations to guide their mentees' growth. Financial indicators like monthly revenue, average client transactions, and patient visits per day offer objective insights into how clinical decisions, time management, and communication skills translate into practice impact. But these numbers tell only part of the story. Understanding whether a mentee is building confidence, improving their diagnostic reasoning, or becoming a more effective team member requires different kinds of observation and measurement.

Many mentors feel unprepared to discuss performance metrics with their mentees, whether financial or otherwise. They may lack confidence in interpreting practice data or worry that focusing on numbers will compromise their mentee's commitment to patient care. This uncertainty can leave new graduates operating without clear feedback about their progress, missing opportunities to see how their professional development contributes to both patient outcomes and practice success.

For this chapter, I chose Dr. Lindsey Hedges because her journey from new graduate to practice owner to Senior Director of Medical Learning at Mission Pet Health has given her a comprehensive understanding of how thoughtful measurement enhances rather than detracts from mentorship relationships. As someone who built her own practice while prioritizing leadership development, Lindsey understands that sustainable veterinary medicine requires both excellent patient care and sound business awareness.

Lindsey's current role developing mentorship programs at scale has shown her how to use data—both financial and operational—to tell stories about professional growth, helping mentees understand that performance metrics are simply tools for measuring progress and identifying opportunities for development, not judgments about their worth as veterinarians.

EVALUATING THE SUCCESS OF YOUR MENTORSHIP PROGRAM

Lindsey Hedges-Gieseking

Measuring mentee performance relies on a complex system of interdependence. Many veterinarians understand the basic concepts of doctor production and profits and losses, but few deeply understand the complex interworking of financial management in veterinary practice. Mentorship is a great opportunity to learn together through practical application. With goal setting, reflection, and analysis, you can track the impact that teamwork, quality medicine, and time management can have on month-to-month financials.

KNOW *YOUR* NUMBERS

When familiarizing your mentee with provider revenue reports, it's important that you give them context to what normal looks like in *your* hospital. As you prepare for your role as a mentor, review your practice financials by asking the following questions:

- What's the average monthly revenue per doctor in your practice? What is the range for the experienced doctors there?
- How long did it take each doctor to build their client base to achieve that revenue? What would you expect for a new graduate veterinarian?
- How many days does each doctor work, on average, per month? What is the average revenue per doctor day at your practice? What is the range?
- How many pets do your experienced doctors see on average per day?
- What is the average client transaction (ACT) for your entire hospital? For each doctor?
- What is the average % of revenue that comes from goods vs. services for each doctor? For services, what is the breakdown for laboratory, radiology, surgery, and dentistry?
- What financial goals have you set as a hospital for this year? How is the team involved in reaching those goals?

Every hospital and practice management system functions differently in how their numbers are calculated; work with your hospital leaders to understand how your reports are generated. If you have not had prior experience with interpreting provider revenue reports in the past, this is a great opportunity to learn. Ask your hospital leaders if they would be willing to sit down with you each month to review your performance and financial statements, ideally well before your mentee starts. Compare your financial performance to the same time period last year or last quarter to gain a deeper understanding of how your numbers change over time. Once your mentee starts, include them in these meetings, familiarizing them with the process and defining the key performance indicators (KPIs) in your reports, even before they have generated any revenue of their own.

When you define KPIs for your mentee, it's important to help them understand not just how the number is calculated but also why each number is important to day-to-day practice. Here are a few descriptions of common KPIs and their why's.

MONTHLY REVENUE

Why: Monthly Revenue gives us a high-level view of the income generated in the practice. There is not one single threshold that divides "good" and "bad" across the industry. Many doctors view monthly revenue only in relation to production percentages—whether for production bonus calculations or salary increases year over year. However, tracking monthly revenue also allows us to observe trends and ask more questions—why are we seeing the changes we are seeing? What should we do in response to these changes?

How: Monthly Revenue is the sum of all invoices paid that are assigned to a particular provider in your practice information management system (PIMS) from the 1st to the last day of the month. Commonly, this includes all services, prescriptions, and diagnostics performed during visits that include an exam fee. However, there can be huge variability clinic to clinic, depending on their policies. Over-the-counter sales, prescription refills, technician appointments, internet pharmacy, telemedicine visits, cremation, and prescription diet sales may be assigned only partially to a doctor, or the entire category may be assigned to a general hospital provider code.

Influenced by:

- Average client transaction
- Number of patient visits
- Service category mix
- Appointment availability
- Total appointment capacity
- Client compliance
- Hospital policies on allocation of charges to providers
- Active clients, new clients, and total number of doctors in the practice

Once you know how monthly revenue is calculated and how it is influenced, it's important to understand your hospital's benchmarks within that monthly revenue. Benchmarks allow you to look at different categories of revenue based on percentage of total revenue. To accurately calculate benchmarks, it is important to have standard categories within your PIMS. Most systems have standard categories that must be assigned to every item that can be invoiced; some allow even more detailed categories to be created. If your software has not been organized with a standardized coding system, the AAHA/VMG Chart of Accounts is considered the gold standard for veterinary practices and can be accessed at no charge on both organizations' websites (AAHA, 2019) (https://www.aaha.org/resources/chart-of-accounts/).

Using a standard chart of accounts also allows you to be sure you are comparing apples to apples when using national benchmark data for similar practices in similar demographic areas (AAHA and AVMA, 2020). Common revenue category benchmarks to track include:

- Professional services
- Pharmacy
    - Prescription medications
    - Prescription flea/tick parasite control
    - Prescription heartworm or combination HW/parasite control
    - Internet pharmacy revenue
- In-house laboratory
- Reference laboratory
- Imaging

- Surgery
- Dentistry
- Anesthesia
- Retail/over-the-counter sales
- Dietary sales

Depending on the way your provider reports are generated in your PIMS, the category breakdown may be listed as percentages or total dollar amounts. Use accounting software or Excel to convert all total dollar amounts to percentages of total revenue to monitor trends. These relative ratios are key when comparing data from different time periods or between different providers to normalize data for goal setting and decision-making (Felsted, 2021).

When you start discussing financials, start with an overview of the hospital averages in month one. Wait to share the new grad's performance metrics until there are at least two to three months of data to compare. If you share your own monthly revenue with your new grad as an example, be sure to tell them how long you expect it might take for them to reach those averages. Some new graduates come in with the unrealistic expectation that they must make production by month two or three, but they may not understand what "making production" even means. Do they earn different production amounts for goods versus services? How much monthly revenue do they have to generate to exceed their base salary? What factors are inside their control that influence their monthly revenue amount? What factors are outside their control? What are their financial goals, and how do those tie into your practice's financial goals? We will discuss this more in depth as we work through a monthly provider report example in PROGRESS, NOT PERFECTION below.

AVERAGE CLIENT TRANSACTION

Why: Tracking trends in ACT allows for an objective assessment of changes to the quality of medicine and client compliance.

How: ACT is calculated by the total amount of monthly revenue divided by the number of invoices for that doctor over a particular period of time. It is a measure of how much the average client spends during a hospital visit.

Influenced by:

- Quality of recommendations
  - Thorough diagnostics and treatment options
- Client education
- Client compliance
- Types of cases
- Invoices included
  - Refills, diets, and over-the-counter sales, if included, decrease ACT

Understanding the factors that influence ACT can help you objectively examine ACT differences between doctors in your practice. One by one, ask each doctor in your practice what factors they think contribute to their ACT. What is their biggest strength? What is their greatest opportunity? If your team is open to it, this can be a great source of peer learning during a doctors' meeting. Often one person's strength is another's opportunity; ACT gives us an objective measure that can directly influence behavior.

New graduate veterinarians typically start out with high average client transactions compared to the average in most practices. This often stems from their commitment to client education; they may have longer appointment times early on and spend that time discussing differentials, necessary diagnostics, and all possible treatment options when building a plan for each patient. They also have more new clients and new patients, resulting in fewer low invoice totals from rechecks or invoices "lost" to refills. Encouraging collaboration with the other doctors will help them learn different ways to hone their communication, maintain high-quality recommendations without overeducating, and how to better manage their time through delegation and teamwork. It may also help remind our experienced doctors about the value of thorough early recommendations through mutual mentorship.

These types of discussions are a great reminder that we don't have to compromise quality for efficiency as doctors gain experience. In the absence of these discussions, new graduate ACTs may decrease over time, even falling below hospital averages as clinical confidence and client education wane. Create a system of peer support, curiosity, and feedback from the start, and your entire team will benefit.

> *You do not rise to the level of your goals. You fall to the level of your systems.*
> *—James Clear, Atomic Habits (2018)*

AVERAGE PATIENT VISITS PER DAY

Why: Average Patient Visits (APV) per Day is a critical factor that can make or break monthly revenue, and it can be one of the most contentious topics within a practice. This number may vary greatly from doctor to doctor, depending on the amount of control they have over their own appointment schedule.

How: Simply put, APV per Day is the average number of patients seen per day per doctor. Depending on your practice management system, this number may be generated for you, or you may have to calculate it using raw data from the month. After pulling your numbers for a month, the equation is:

$$\frac{\text{Number of appointments seen}}{\text{Number of days worked}} = \text{Average patient visits per day}$$

Influenced by:

- Schedule management
  - Time per appointment
  - Appointment blocks
  - Drop off or work in protocols
- Doctor availability
  - Hours worked per day
  - Alignment with high-demand hours

- No-shows and cancellations
- Exam room availability
- Teamwork and workflow
    - Number of support staff per doctor

Just as muscle is generated in the gym, monthly revenue is generated in the appointment schedule. And, just as everyone can find a reason not to go to gym when they don't feel up to it, everyone in the practice can find a reason to block off the schedule. We have all had those days where you feel that the schedule is controlling you, and it is tempting to take back control by limiting availability to allow time to catch up. However, at the end of the day, every appointment seen improves the health of our patients and the health of our practice. That is not to say that we must work in every patient, stay late every night, or eliminate all non-receiving time from our schedules. Time for recovery must be included for long-term gain. There is no one routine that will work for every practice everywhere all the time. A healthy mindset, including celebrating a full schedule rather than dreading it, can undo some of our own schedule control issues and help our mentees get started on the right foot.

At the end of the day, the metrics that matter most are those that are hardest to measure. How is your mentee improving their communication skills? How is their confidence growing? How do they collaborate within the team? These qualitative metrics are just as important as the quantitative financial metrics. In the next section, we will explore how to use trend data to ask questions and set goals with your mentee.

GATHERING AND ANALYZING DATA

Dr. New Grad walks into their 4:00pm appointment with Mrs. Jones. Romeo, a 10-year-old MN DSH tuxedo cat has a 2-day history of inappetence. He has been vocalizing at home at night, vomiting digested food 4 times daily, and urinating outside of the litter box for the last 2 weeks. On exam, he has multiple resorptive lesions present, mostly on lower premolars and molars. He's down from 11 lbs to 7 lbs since his last visit 1 year ago. A thyroid slip is present and his kidneys are small upon palpation. He has a grade II systolic heart murmur. And. . . by the way. . . Romeo needs a nail trim.

A new graduate may view their revenue reports much like they would view Romeo: so many abnormals that they don't know what to analyze first or how to prioritize interventions. They may try the "do everything" approach and try to get every single number to increase toward their hospitals "normal." When, inevitably, there's a complication in the process, they will label themselves a failure and decide that these more complicated problems should be referred.

Just as we teach our mentees to develop a standardized approach in the exam room, we can teach a standardized approach to analyzing revenue data.

NOSE-TO-TAIL EVALUATION

If we focused on only the resorptive lesions in Romeo, we might schedule dental surgery without considering any other concurrent issues. Similarly, if we only focus on monthly revenue, we might miss other trends in the data.

In veterinary school, I was taught to perform a nose-to-tail exam, using the same thorough process every time while developing my clinical reasoning. When evaluating provider revenue reports, analyzing the data one line at a time, from left to right, top to bottom, can help you develop the perspective needed for better financial reasoning.

Dr. New grad	June	July	August	Hospital average
Monthly revenue	$19,567	$38,645	$52,468	$76,123
ACT	$284	$269	$260	$256
APV per day	5	9	13	18
Doctor days per month	14	16	16	17
Professional services	65%	60%	50%	34%
Pharmacy	21%	25%	22%	23%
Laboratory	12%	15%	20%	21%
Imaging	2%	0%	4%	50%
Surgery	0%	0%	3%	10%
Dentistry	0%	0%	1%	7%

FIGURE 13.1 Revenue report.

If you aren't sure how to start, here is template and example (Figure 13.1):

1. Look at three months of provider data and compare it to overall hospital averages for the same period.
2. Highlight or circle the values you want to come back to investigate further as you go.
3. Assess Monthly Revenue first, ACT second, and APV third
4. Assess trends in revenue categories.
5. View the entire report to see how many areas I've highlighted before asking more questions.

This is the process that works for me and reports that are available to me—work with your mentee to develop a process that works for your hospital reporting.

PROGRESS, NOT PERFECTION

When comparing these key performance indicators, it can be daunting for a new graduate to constantly compare themselves against the average for the practice. While it's important to understand those averages as a goal that your new graduate is working toward, it's also important that you stress that we're looking for progress, not perfection.

Let's compare this month's numbers to last month's numbers. What's changed? Why do you think it's changed?

Increases or decreases are not good nor bad, but there's often an explanation. That explanation is the key to tracking progress over time. Let's look at an example:

Dr. New grad	June	July	August
Monthly revenue	$21,487	$43,825	$72,148
ACT	$295	$215	$185
APV per day	5	11	19

Looking at these numbers, you may assume you know what's going on. It is human nature to use our own experience to define causation. However, if we don't ask questions, our assumptions might hold our mentee back from progress or reinforce a fixed, right vs. wrong mindset. Here are two potential scenarios that require different approaches for the same data:

Question	Scenario 1	Scenario 2
What is my mentee's body language as I show them their Provider Report?	They stare past the numbers. Shoulders are hunched, they cross their arms, and I notice dark circles beneath their eyes.	They smile and take a snapshot to send to their mom before turning toward me to discuss the data.
How many days did you work last month?	*20. I helped cover Dr. Smith's sick days and worked the last 2 weekends in a row.*	*20! I came in an extra day to scrub in on that splenectomy and ended up seeing a few drop-off appointments and then I worked an extra weekend day to give Dr. Smith time off for her son's birthday.*
What's changed over the last three months with your numbers? Why do you think it's changed?	*My ACT is tanking, I don't have the time to research the right diagnostics, so I treat the pet's symptoms and ask clients to schedule a recheck exam. When I call them to talk about possible diagnostics, they either say the pet is better and cancel, or they say they will call back and schedule the recheck and they don't.*	*I made production this month! I have been saying yes to every work in, and sometimes I am running behind, but I feel like I'm getting faster in my appointments overall. I am so excited to make an extra payment on my student loans already. This is such a great feeling.*
What else? What would you like to change for next month?	*My revenue is up, which is great, but I don't think this is sustainable. I know I've been picking up more work ins, but I think it is negatively affecting client communication and I feel like I'm delaying patient care. I want to find ways to rest and recharge, even on hard days. And I want to do more diagnostics on sick patients again, like I did when I started.*	*My ACT is down, but I think that is because I have been scheduling a lot of recheck exams. My clients have been great about scheduling before they leave the room, and when they come back, it is often only an exam fee, so the invoice is much lower.*
Goals set:	• Take a walk around the neighborhood during lunch. • Take naps this weekend and fully unplug from work. • Stop delaying diagnostics—choose a minimum database for common sick cases and practice delivering the recommendation in our next mentorship meeting.	• Consider using telemedicine for rechecks to free up spaces on the scheduler. • Discuss which rechecks can be seen by Credentialed Technicians as tech appointments during our next mentorship meeting.

There's a bigger picture here and a story that the numbers tell, but we can't tell that story until we ask more questions. Through guided self-reflection, we can give an overwhelmed mentee the courage to rest, reset, and try again. We can avoid shaming a new grad who is eager to grow, and who may potentially explore innovative ways to make more space in the schedule. Through the power of mentorship, we can teach the next generation of veterinarians to value progress, not perfection, when measuring performance.

REFINING AND SCALING YOUR MENTORSHIP PROGRAM

When you fall in love with mentorship, it can be tempting to say yes to every opportunity to mentor that comes your way. Once you see one mentee grow and succeed, it's natural to want more. And if one mentee has a great mentorship experience, they tend to spread the word to colleagues and friends. While this can be great for scheduling student externships, summer break work, and recruiting future veterinarians, overcommitting to mentorship may pull a mentor away from other responsibilities and could create tension within the hospital team.

The key to scaling your mentorship program is to set the expectation from the start that mentorship is a team sport. All new team members have something to learn from everyone in the hospital. It shouldn't be the mentor's responsibility to teach their mentee everything—instead, they can be a guide, meeting their mentee where they are and helping them find resources and connect with the team members who can support them along their learning journey.

Refining and scaling a mentorship program is not about figuring out a formula that works for every individual mentee that comes to your hospital. Refining and scaling a mentorship program *is* about learning how to support diverse individuals with different skill sets and uniting them with the common purpose and vision of your hospital team.

A great mentorship program creates a waterfall of great mentorship. One great mentor becomes a head mentor, who trains a new mentor, who supports a new mentee. Eventually that mentee becomes a mentor in training, and the cycle continues (Figure 13.2).

How Early Is Too Early?

If we want our mentees to become mentors. . . how early is too early? Early-career veterinarians can be phenomenal mentors, but they may hesitate to volunteer for the role because of their perceived lack of experience. As a head mentor, prepare feedback for the early-career veterinarian to help build their confidence in their competence for the role. Here are a few questions to consider:

- Do they have a growth mindset? When mistakes are made, do they examine what they can learn from those mistakes vs. judging things as right vs. wrong?
- Do you feel that this veterinarian is a team player? Can they delegate effectively? Do they ask for input from their technicians or assistants?

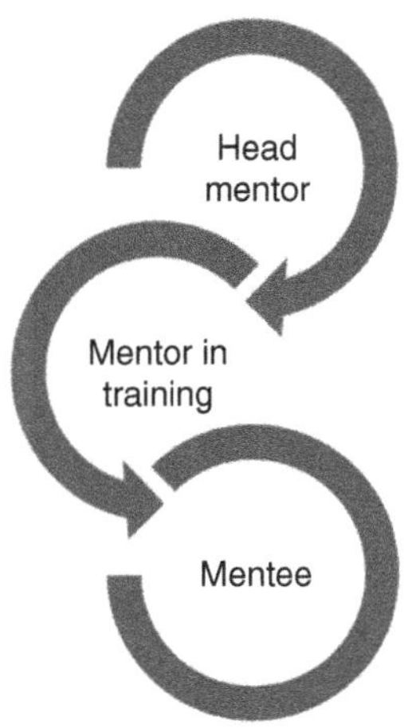

FIGURE 13.2 Cycle of Mentorship: Experienced mentors support new mentors as they support mentees.

- Do they create psychological safety within the team? Are team members willing to speak up about mistakes when working with this doctor?
- Have they reached the average KPIs for your hospital? Are they still undergoing their own growth? Where are their opportunities for development?
- Are they open to feedback? Have they successfully delivered feedback to other individuals within the team?

These questions are not meant to qualify or disqualify an individual from being a mentor. In an ideal world, every person can be a mentor and a mentee. Answering these questions can instead help you focus your support and set realistic expectations for your mentor in training as they prepare for their mentee. Often, knowing they have another mentor in their corner if they get stuck is all the courage they need to say yes.

Refining Your Program

As you grow and strengthen your mentorship program, focusing on feedback and continuous improvement will keep you on track to serve your mentees and meet your hospital's goals. Before developing systems to track overall program trends, determine which program metrics are most important for your hospital's goals. Why do you want to invest in mentorship? What is your ideal outcome of a successful mentorship program? Here are a few common hospital goals to consider:

- Improved retention rates
    - Track turnover; analyze exit interview data for areas of opportunity
- Improved team member engagement
    - Develop engagement surveys; track overall participation
- Higher employee satisfaction
    - Measure employee Net Promoter Score; develop satisfaction surveys for targeted aspects of the program or hospital

Scalability

Once you have multiple mentors trained within your practice, work together to consider outreach opportunities for mentorship throughout your local community. Invite high school students in for break work, or plan a "future doctor" program for the public schools in your area. Attend career fairs and networking events at veterinary schools to offer break work and externships. Once students see the learning environment you've created, word will spread. Seek feedback from break work students and externs in order to rapidly improve your mentorship program standards. At the same time, you will develop leadership skills in your associates, preparing them for future leadership roles in the hospital or in the veterinary community at large.

Scalability requires teamwork. By building a culture where mentorship is shared, supported, and aligned with your hospital's purpose, you create a sustainable path for long-term growth. Start now by identifying potential mentors in training, supporting them with feedback and guidance, and inviting your entire team into the mentorship conversation. The more you invest in your team's growth and development, the stronger your mentorship culture—and your hospital—will become.

CONCLUSION

Mentorship cultures are not built by chance; they're built with intention. Through understanding benchmarks, tracking KPIs, and fostering open discussions around trends, mentors can guide new graduates toward confidence and competence. It is possible to achieve the goals of both your mentee and your hospital, so long as we learn to value progress, not perfection, when measuring performance. The same holds true for building a strong, scalable mentorship program. Success requires balancing financial performance with professional development, data collection with continuous improvement, and team growth and retention with program expansion. The more you invest in mentorship, the stronger your team's culture and hospital will become.

BIBLIOGRAPHY

AAHA & AVMA (2020). *Financial Standardization in Veterinary Practices: Why It Matters and How to Do It.* Schaumburg, IL/Washington, DC: AAHA & AVMA https://www.avma.org/sites/default/files/2020-03/aaha-avma_financialstandardization.pdf March (accessed 8 April 2025).

American Animal Hospital Association (2019). *Chart of Accounts.* AAHA https://www.aaha.org/resources/chart-of-accounts/ 24 April (accessed 8 April 2025).

Clear, J. (2018). *Atomic Habits: an easy and proven way to build good habits and break bad ones.* London: Random House Business.

Felsted, K.E. (2021). Check the vitals of your practice financials: effective ways to use data and benchmarks. *AAHA Trends Magazine* (1 May). https://www.aaha.org/trends-magazine/publications/check-the-vitals-of-your-practice-financials/ (accessed 8 April 2025).

CHAPTER 14 The Mentoring Continuum

Dani Rabwin

INTRODUCTION

Veterinary mentorship is most often discussed in terms of initiation: whether a program exists, how mentors are assigned, and what resources are made available at the outset of a relationship. Considerably less attention is paid to what happens after mentorship begins. Mentorship relationships do not remain static over time, nor should they. As mentees gain experience, confidence, and professional identity, the type and intensity of support they require changes. When mentorship structures and expectations fail to adapt accordingly, misalignment can develop even in relationships that were initially effective.

The preceding chapters of this book advance a clear argument about what effective veterinary mentorship requires. Mentorship must be flexible, responsive to individual needs, attentive to nonclinical dimensions of practice, and grounded in trust, communication, and psychological safety. These principles apply across a wide range of mentorship models, from formal programs to informal, relationship-based support. Agreement on these foundations, however, has not resolved the practical challenges of sustaining mentorship over time, particularly as practice environments become more complex and constrained.

Mentorship relationships also exist within a longer professional arc than is often acknowledged. Supporting early-career veterinarians is necessary, but insufficient on its own. The profession depends on continued mentorship capacity, which requires attention to how relationships evolve, how roles shift, and how responsibility for mentorship is gradually distributed. When mentorship is treated as a fixed role held by a small group of experienced clinicians, it becomes increasingly fragile. When it is understood as a continuum that includes receiving mentorship, adapting within it, and eventually contributing to it, responsibility for sustaining the profession is shared more broadly.

My own mentorship relationship with Buff did not conclude when I no longer needed daily guidance. It changed. Early in my career, the questions I brought to him were primarily clinical and immediate. Over time, those questions became less about decision-making and more about judgment, context, and professional sustainability. The relationship remained valuable precisely because it evolved in response to changing needs rather than remaining fixed in its original form.

Even when mentorship is widely understood to require individualization, evaluation frameworks often prioritize outcomes that are more easily standardized and measured. This chapter examines how mentorship relationships change over time, how transitions and conclusions can be handled intentionally, and how mentees can be prepared to participate in mentorship themselves. It also surfaces unresolved tensions in contemporary veterinary mentorship, including the challenge of scaling mentorship in increasingly corporatized environments and the limitations of evaluating mentorship success primarily through financial or productivity-based metrics. These tensions are not resolved here. They are named deliberately because avoiding them limits the profession's ability to sustain mentorship in practice.

THE EVOLUTION OF MENTORING RELATIONSHIPS

Mentoring relationships are inherently variable. They differ in structure, formality, intensity, and scope depending on individual needs, practice environments, and professional context. Even within a single relationship, the type of support that is helpful at one point in time may become less appropriate as experience accumulates and responsibilities change. Recognizing this variability is essential to understanding why mentorship requires recalibration rather than static expectations (Elce, 2019).

As veterinarians gain experience, autonomy often develops unevenly across different areas of practice. Clinical decision-making may progress more quickly than communication, leadership, boundary setting, or emotional processing. A mentee may manage a full caseload confidently while still struggling with uncertainty, client conflict, or the emotional weight of adverse outcomes. In these cases, **reduced need for clinical guidance does not equate to reduced need for mentorship; it reflects a shift in what mentorship is supporting.**

WHAT SIGNALS A SHIFT IN MENTORSHIP NEEDS?

- Fewer "what should I do?" questions; more "what would you do?"
- Greater independence, with uncertainty still present
- Emerging clinical style that differs from the mentor's
- Less need for scheduled check-ins
- Continued value in knowing support is available
- Early interest in supporting others

Misalignment arises when mentorship expectations fail to adapt to these changing needs. Mentors may continue providing support in ways that no longer match the mentee's developmental priorities, while mentees may hesitate to articulate evolving needs out of concern for appearing ungrateful or insufficiently independent. In other cases, mentorship may recede prematurely under the assumption that fewer questions signal readiness for full independence. These dynamics more often reflect the absence of shared language around transition than deficiencies in commitment or skill.

Differences in clinical approach, communication style, or professional priorities often emerge as mentorship relationships evolve. This is rarely a problem to be corrected; more often, it reflects the development of professional identity. Veterinary medicine is not practiced by formula alone. It involves judgment, values, and personal style shaped by experience. When mentorship is flexible, these differences can become a source of learning and confidence. When mentorship is rigid, divergence may be misinterpreted as resistance or disengagement, creating strain that has little to do with competence or commitment.

Adapting mentorship over time requires attention, communication, and flexibility—resources that are not always supported within contemporary practice environments. Without mechanisms to support evolution, mentorship relationships may persist in forms that no longer serve their original purpose or dissolve without clarity or closure. Understanding mentorship as dynamic rather than fixed provides the foundation for examining how relationships conclude and how mentorship capacity is sustained over time.

WHEN MENTORING RELATIONSHIPS SHOULD END

Mentoring relationships are often assumed to be open-ended, with duration implicitly treated as a marker of success. In practice, mentoring relationships may appropriately conclude for a range of reasons, many of which reflect healthy development rather than failure. Ending a relationship does not negate its value; it often reflects a change in needs, roles, or context that makes the original structure less relevant.

Some mentoring relationships reach a natural conclusion as mentees gain confidence, competence, and professional autonomy. Defined goals may be met, developmental priorities may shift, or the relationship may evolve into a collegial dynamic that no longer requires a formal mentor–mentee framework. In these cases, formal mentorship may conclude while informal connection, consultation, or professional respect continues. Naming this transition explicitly helps reinforce that the relationship succeeded in its intended purpose.

Other relationships end because circumstances change. Relocation, specialty training, changes in practice setting, or shifts in professional role may require different forms of support. Mentors may also experience changes in availability, capacity, or expertise that limit their ability to continue in a primary mentorship role. These transitions reflect the contextual nature of mentorship rather than shortcomings of the relationship itself.

In some cases, relationships should end because they are no longer effective or appropriate. Persistent misalignment in expectations, communication, or values can limit the relationship's usefulness despite good intentions. Breaches of trust, boundary concerns, or ongoing disengagement may compromise psychological safety and professional development. Continuing a mentoring relationship under these conditions can create obligation without benefit, a concern echoed by Elce (2019), who describes how unresolved boundary issues or misaligned expectations can undermine mentoring outcomes.

In rarer but important cases, mentoring relationships should end because they are actively harmful. Patterns of dismissiveness, intimidation, coercion, retaliation, or repeated boundary violations undermine psychological safety and can impede learning, confidence, and professional identity formation. In these situations, the goal is not repair or recalibration, but protection. Ending the relationship promptly and clearly is an appropriate and necessary response, and responsibility for that decision does not rest solely with the mentee.

Difficulty ending mentorship relationships often stems from the absence of shared norms around closure. Without clear expectations for how mentorship relationships conclude, relationships may persist beyond their usefulness or end abruptly without discussion, leaving uncertainty or residual tension. Professional closure requires direct, respectful communication that acknowledges what the relationship provided, clarifies why it is no longer required, and emphasizes continuity of professional respect. Ending a mentoring relationship does not imply the end of mentorship altogether; rather, it allows space for support that is better aligned with current needs.

MENTOR TIP

Ending a mentorship relationship is not a failure when it reflects developmental progress or contextual change.

PREPARING MENTEES TO BECOME MENTORS

The sustainability of mentorship in veterinary medicine depends on whether mentees are prepared to participate in mentorship over time. This does not imply that all veterinarians should become formal mentors. Rather, it reflects the reality that mentorship capacity must be intentionally renewed if it is to remain viable within the profession (Yanke et al., 2023).

One of the most enduring strengths of effective mentorship is its capacity to extend beyond a single relationship. Many veterinarians who benefit from meaningful mentorship eventually find themselves offering support to others—not as a formal role, but as a natural extension of their own growth. This movement from receiving guidance to offering it helps sustain mentorship across teams and over time, reinforcing that professional development is not a solitary process.

The transition from mentee to mentor often begins informally. As confidence and judgment develop, early-career veterinarians start answering questions, sharing perspectives, and normalizing uncertainty for colleagues who are newer still. These peer and near-peer relationships do not replace experienced mentorship, but they play a meaningful role in reducing isolation, encouraging help-seeking, and strengthening team culture. Recognizing this form of mentorship as legitimate and valuable supports the broader mentoring continuum without placing all responsibility on a small number of senior clinicians.

Mentorship requires skills that extend beyond clinical expertise. Emotional intelligence, communication, feedback, boundary-setting, and the ability to support learning without fostering dependence are central to effective mentorship. Mentorship requires skills that extend beyond clinical expertise, and effective mentoring depends not only on what mentors provide but also on how mentees actively engage through reflection, goal setting, feedback-seeking, and ownership of their learning (Hodgson et al., 2022). Preparing mentees for mentorship therefore involves making these skills visible and explicit within the relationship, rather than assuming they will develop on their own over time.

Mentors can support this transition by involving mentees in developmentally appropriate mentoring activities, such as co-mentoring newer colleagues, supporting peer learning, or briefly talking through mentoring moments that come up naturally during day-to-day work. Explicit conversations about interest and readiness are essential. Not all excellent clinicians wish to mentor, and treating mentorship as an expectation rather than an option risks undermining both mentors and mentees.

MENTOR TIP

Mentoring others is not the next step for every veterinarian, and treating it as an expectation rather than an option risks undermining both mentors and mentees.

THE HARD QUESTIONS WE NEED TO ASK

The preceding chapters describe what effective mentorship requires at the level of individual relationships. The questions that remain are not primarily about intent, effort, or awareness. They are about whether current systems allow mentorship to function in the ways we now understand to be necessary. The tensions outlined below are not resolved here. They are named deliberately, with the intention of prompting reflection and conversation—within practices, among colleagues, and across the profession—about what mentorship is being asked to accomplish and whether current structures allow it to do so honestly.

THE COMPENSATION QUESTION

Mentorship requires time, attention, and cognitive labor. In many practice environments, this work is layered onto clinical roles without protected time or compensation, often framed as a professional expectation rather than as a distinct contribution. This approach relies heavily on the goodwill and personal capacity of individual mentors, while simultaneously operating within systems that prioritize productivity and efficiency.

Historically, mentorship was often tied to long-term professional incentives, such as partnership, ownership, or sustained collaboration. As practice structures have changed, particularly with increased corporatization, those incentives have become less consistent or less accessible. Mentors may be expected to provide substantial developmental support to early-career veterinarians while meeting unchanged production targets and performance benchmarks.

Elce (2019) notes that mentorship sustainability is compromised when mentoring responsibilities are not recognized structurally. The question, then, is not whether mentorship has value, but how that value is acknowledged within contemporary practice models. If mentorship is essential to recruitment, retention, and professional development, relying on uncompensated labor raises concerns about equity, burnout, and long-term viability.

THE SCALING QUESTION

As veterinary organizations grow, mentorship programs are increasingly expected to function at scale. Scaling introduces constraints that favor consistency, efficiency, and predictability. Program design often emphasizes standardized timelines, uniform milestones, and replicable structures that can be implemented across multiple sites or teams.

At the same time, effective mentorship is widely understood to require responsiveness to individual needs, learning styles, and contexts. These two realities exist in tension. Even when organizations acknowledge the importance of individualized mentorship, the mechanisms used to deliver mentorship at scale may limit flexibility in practice.

The challenge is not that scaling is inherently incompatible with mentorship, but that scale changes what is possible. When mentorship is embedded within systems designed for uniformity, there is a risk that relational nuance, developmental pacing, and fit between mentor and mentee are subordinated to programmatic consistency. This raises questions about what mentorship becomes when it must function within rigid structures and which outcomes are prioritized as a result.

THE MEASUREMENT QUESTION

Mentorship programs are frequently evaluated using metrics that are operationally convenient and easily quantified, such as speed to independent scheduling, production targets, and revenue benchmarks, often assessed at defined intervals such as six or twelve months. These measures align with broader business priorities in modern practice environments, but they provide insight primarily into operational readiness and capture only a narrow portion of professional development.

Less consistently measured are outcomes such as confidence in decision making, tolerance of uncertainty, psychological safety, sense of belonging within a team, and long-term professional sustainability. These dimensions are frequently cited by early-career veterinarians as central to their experience of mentorship, yet they are more difficult to assess and therefore less likely to be incorporated into formal evaluation frameworks (Yanke et al., 2023).

When mentorship success is defined primarily through financial or productivity-based indicators, programs may inadvertently prioritize rapid output over developmental readiness. This raises the question of whether current evaluation practices align with what mentorship is intended to support, and how success might be differently understood if nonclinical outcomes were taken seriously as markers of progress (Table 14.1).

Table 14.1 What Mentorship Programs Commonly Measure vs. What Often Goes Unmeasured

Commonly measured indicators	Often unmeasured or inconsistently measured outcomes
Time to independent scheduling	Confidence in clinical decision-making
Production or revenue benchmarks	Tolerance of uncertainty and complexity
Completion of program milestones	Psychological safety within the team
Retention at 6–12 months	Sense of belonging within the practice
Reduction in supervision needs	Long-term sustainability and wellbeing

THE PERFECTIONISM QUESTION

Veterinary education appropriately emphasizes precision, thoroughness, and high performance. Admission processes, grading systems, and clinical training reinforce expectations that errors should be minimized and competence demonstrated consistently under evaluation. These traits are adaptive in educational settings and play an important role in selecting and training capable clinicians.

In clinical practice, however, the same traits can become maladaptive in environments defined by uncertainty, time pressure, and incomplete information. New graduates may equate competence with error-free performance, experience disproportionate distress when outcomes fall short of ideal standards, or hesitate to ask for help or admit uncertainty, even when support is available and clinical reasoning is sound. In team-based practice environments, this can limit collaboration and slow growth.

This creates a difficult tension. Admissions committees and training programs must rely on what can be evaluated reliably, and performance under assessment remains one of the most defensible tools available. Yet the traits that are easiest to measure are not always the ones that best support help-seeking, teamwork, or long-term well-being in practice.

Cake et al. (2017), writing within the broader veterinary well-being literature, describe resilience as a dynamic process shaped by both individual capacities and professional context. Their analysis highlights how performance concerns, perfectionism, and organizational culture contribute to distress, raising questions about how standards of competence and success are defined and reinforced within the profession. Within mentorship relationships, this creates a tension between supporting growth and challenging deeply internalized norms—without framing those norms, or the distress they produce, as personal deficiency.

THE ACCESS QUESTION

Veterinary training environments expose learners to a wide range of potential mentors. Students interact with multiple clinicians, faculty members, residents, technicians, and peers across rotations and disciplines. Mentorship in this context is often diffuse, episodic, and distributed, even when relationships are informal.

Early-career practice environments frequently offer a much narrower mentorship landscape. In some settings, mentorship expectations are placed on a single doctor, technician, or supervisor, regardless of fit, capacity, or scope of expertise. This represents a significant contraction in mentorship access at the same time that expectations for independence, productivity, and professional confidence increase.

The issue raised here is structural rather than individual. If effective mentorship is relational and often distributed across multiple people, what does it mean to expect similar outcomes in environments where far fewer mentoring relationships are available? How mentorship is expected to function and what it can reasonably accomplish must be considered in light of these access constraints. Naming this gap is necessary before meaningful conversations about mentorship expectations, evaluation, and sustainability can occur.

CONCLUSION

The chapters in this book describe what effective mentorship requires at the level of individual relationships: trust, communication, psychological safety, feedback, adaptability, and attention to the full scope of professional development. Those elements are not theoretical. They are well supported by evidence and echoed consistently by early-career veterinarians themselves. The challenge the profession now faces is not a lack of clarity about what mentorship should be, but how that understanding is carried forward over time, across roles, and within systems that were not designed with mentorship as a central function.

Mentoring relationships evolve. They shift in intensity, focus, and form as experience grows and responsibilities change. Some conclude naturally, others require recalibration, and some must end because they no longer serve their intended purpose. Recognizing these transitions as part of a continuum rather than as failures allows mentorship to remain responsive rather than rigid. It also creates space for mentees to move from receiving support to contributing to it, in ways that reflect their interests, capacity, and context.

The tensions surfaced in this chapter—around compensation, scale, measurement, perfectionism, access, and expectations—do not have simple resolutions. They point instead to the limits of relying on individual effort to sustain mentorship in environments that reward efficiency, uniformity, and easily measured outcomes. Naming these tensions is not an indictment of existing programs or mentors. It is an acknowledgment that mentorship, as it is currently practiced and evaluated, is often asked to carry more than it reasonably can.

Every veterinarian is shaped by mentorship, whether formally acknowledged or not. The impact of mentorship extends beyond the medicine practiced to the confidence developed, the risks tolerated, and the sense of belonging sustained over time. The profession's legacy is not defined solely by clinical outcomes, but by the veterinarians who remain engaged, capable, and supported throughout their careers.

The veterinarian being mentored today will influence someone else tomorrow—through guidance, example, or absence. Whether that influence strengthens the profession depends on how mentorship is understood, supported, and allowed to evolve. Recognizing mentorship as a continuum places responsibility not only on individual mentors but also on the systems and structures that determine what mentorship is permitted to become.

BIBLIOGRAPHY

Cake, M.A., McArthur, M.M., Matthew, S.M., and Mansfield, C.F. (2017). *Finding the balance: uncovering resilience in the veterinary literature. Journal of Veterinary Medical Education* 44 (1): 95–104.

Elce, Y.A. (2019). *Mentorship in veterinary medicine: building capacity and retention. Journal of Veterinary Medical Education* 46 (5): 1099–1107.

Hodgson, J.L., Freeman, S.R., and Darling, A.L. (2022). Developing mentee skills: supporting effective mentoring relationships in veterinary medicine. *Journal of Veterinary Medical Education* 49 (4): 420–430. https://doi.org/10.3138/jvme-2021-0048.

Yanke, A.B., Weigand, K.A., and Hofmeister, E.H. (2023). *Addressing the needs and challenges of mentorship in veterinary medicine. Journal of Veterinary Medical Education* 50 (1): 83–90.

Structuring Effective In-Clinic Mentorship Programs

APPENDIX

Kate Boatright

Editor's Note: *This appendix expands upon concepts introduced in Chapter 2 ("The Mentor–Mentee Relationship") by Dr. Kate Boatright. It provides a practical framework and ready-to-use tools for developing in-clinic mentorship programs within veterinary practices. Clinics can adapt these templates and schedules to meet their own needs or pair them with the broader mentorship strategies discussed throughout this book.*

Most in-clinic mentoring focuses on supporting early-career veterinarians in the transition from student to doctor. These programs provide technical skills training and support professional skills development. The most effective programs also support mental health and well-being.

While early-career veterinarians are the primary target of mentoring programs, similar programs can be developed to support all roles on the team and support more experienced veterinary professionals through career and life transitions. The remainder of this section will focus on developing an in-clinic mentoring program for early-career veterinarians, but many of the core concepts can be applied to any position on the team and career stage.

STEP ONE: EVALUATE YOUR MOTIVATION FOR MENTORSHIP

Before jumping in to design a mentorship program, the leadership team of the clinic should carefully consider why they want to add a mentorship program. Developing a program will take time and delivering a program will also require time and monetary commitments. Before committing these resources, consider if your primary goal of mentorship is recruitment, retention, or both.

Mentorship is a powerful recruitment tool, particularly if you are looking to hire an early-career veterinarian. From 2020 to 2025, mentorship has been the most important factor for most new graduate veterinarians in selecting a first job (American Veterinary Medical Association, 2025). Many new graduates report accepting jobs with lower salaries in exchange for a formalized mentorship experience. Developing a mentorship program to help support recruitment is a reasonable goal, as long as you truly evaluate whether your clinic is the right environment for a new graduate veterinarian (see Box A.1).

Following through on the promise of a mentorship program with a well-executed delivery can help improve retention of new veterinarians. One of the most common reasons new graduates leave their first job is a lack of mentorship (Jelinski et al., 2009; Gates et al., 2020). It is important to realize that "lack of mentorship" can mean two different things: a true absence of mentorship or mentorship that did not meet the new graduate's expectations and goals of mentorship. Thus, clinics who hope to retain their new graduate hires should set specific expectations for what the mentorship program will include and follow through on delivery.

BOX A.1 DETERMINING IF YOUR CLINIC IS READY TO ADD A NEW GRADUATE VETERINARIAN TO THE TEAM

If you're considering adding a mentorship program to improve recruitment of a new graduate veterinarian, consider the following question: *How quickly do we need a veterinarian to be a fully productive member of the team?*

If the answer is *immediately*, then this is **not** the right time to hire an early career veterinarian. New graduate veterinarians need time and support to become fully productive members of the team. Not only will they initially be less efficient, productive, and confident compared to your experienced veterinarians, they will need the support of those veterinarians. This can decrease productivity and increase stress levels of your current veterinarians. So, if your clinic is looking for a new associate to hit the ground running with little to no adjustment period, then you should be looking for a more experienced colleague to add to the team.

If the answer is *within 6 to 12 months*, then it's reasonable to move forward with a mentorship program. Each new graduate veterinarian will develop at their own pace. While there's no set timeline for when an individual will be operating at full capacity, most new graduates will be able to handle a standard schedule and be producing enough to cover their salary within a year of graduation.

Adding a mentorship program to your hospital can also be a retention tool for existing employees who may want to learn new skills. For instance, if one veterinarian is skilled at ultrasound, they could mentor another associate who is interested in learning this skill. This can expand the availability of this service to clients and help to improve job satisfaction for both veterinarians. This type of mentorship program may be a good way to start introducing mentorship to your clinic before adding an entirely new hire.

STEP TWO: IDENTIFY AVAILABLE RESOURCES AND POTENTIAL GAPS

Before beginning a mentorship program, veterinary hospitals must determine what resources they have available to support the program and what resources they may need. At a minimum, you must have a primary mentor, experienced and engaged team members, and available time. Additional resources to consider include reference materials, continuing education platforms, and external mentorship support.

PRIMARY MENTOR

Having an engaged mentor is essential to the success of the mentorship program. This individual should be an experienced veterinarian who has an interest in providing mentorship and available time to do it. This may mean that other clinic duties may need to be decreased in the short term to allow time for mentoring. See "The Mentor-Mentee Relationship" in Chapter 2 for a more in-depth discussion of selecting an in-clinic mentor.

One of the biggest mistakes a veterinary clinic can make when it comes to developing a mentorship program is assuming someone will pick up the mentor role once the mentee arrives. If the practice owner or medical director is not planning to be the primary mentor, which is very reasonable given their managerial responsibilities, then have a team discussion to determine which—if any—of your associate veterinarians are interested and willing to take on the mentor role. If you do not have anyone interested in becoming a mentor, then the feasibility of a mentorship program needs to be reevaluated.

EXPERIENCED AND ENGAGED TEAM

The veterinary team plays a large role in creating a clinic environment that is supportive and provides opportunities for learning and growth. Even with the best primary mentor, an unsupportive team can detract from the overall mentorship experience and decrease job satisfaction for the mentee. This does not mean that every team member has to be actively engaged in teaching the mentee, but it does mean that the team should have reasonable expectations for the mentee's performance. Setting appropriate expectations among team members is a critical responsibility of clinic management and the primary mentor.

An early-career veterinarian should not be expected to be as efficient, quick, or confident as an experienced veterinarian. They may take longer to arrive at a diagnosis, need to look up more information, or ask questions of their mentor or other veterinarians more often. This does not mean that the mentee lacks knowledge or is a poor veterinarian. Most often, this is due to the mentee's lack of confidence in their skills and knowledge base. Team members should never judge the mentee's performance by comparing them to the experienced veterinarians they are used to working with.

Credentialed veterinary technicians and other experienced team members can provide exceptional support for early-career veterinary professionals. In some cases, they may work more closely with the mentee during the day than the primary mentor. Establishing a practice culture that encourages these team members to engage in mentorship by providing feedback, sharing their experiences, and making respectful suggestions based on their observations will help promote continued learning and development.

The mentee should be scheduled to work with experienced team members as much as possible. These individuals are familiar with the clientele, workflow, inventory, and clinic policies to work with the mentee. It is detrimental to the mentee and the team to pair a new graduate veterinarian with a newly hired or inexperienced team member. This can magnify inefficiency and increase the risk for mistakes.

TIME

Mentorship requires time, and it is important to ensure that your clinic has enough available time to provide a positive mentorship experience. Here are areas of the clinic schedule to evaluate before adding a mentorship program:

- Does your clinic schedule allow for a short-term decrease in appointment availability or will this create overwork for other veterinarians or significantly limit the ability of your clients to access care?
    - Many mentees benefit from having extended appointment lengths initially, which means they are seeing fewer patients.
    - In the initial stages of mentoring, the primary mentor may need to see fewer appointments to compensate for the time spent working with the mentee.
- Is there time open in the schedule that can be blocked for mentor meetings and formal feedback sessions?
    - While some mentors and mentees are willing to spend time outside of their scheduled clinic day for these meetings, it should never be an expectation that meetings will happen outside of normal clinic hours.

LEARNING RESOURCES

Mentees should be provided with resources that will support self-directed learning and encourage their independence in managing cases. These resources may include drug references, textbooks, online platforms, and access to specialty consultations. Some mentees and mentors may find it helpful to keep a wish list of resources that can support the mentee's continued development and consider using continuing education funds to purchase essential resources.

In some cases, sending the mentee to an intensive, external training program, like an ultrasound course, spay/neuter clinic, dentistry training program, or other wet lab, can provide concentrated training in a certain skill area. However, to capitalize on the mentee's training, be sure there are cases scheduled where the mentee can utilize their skills after returning home.

STEP THREE: DETERMINE GENERAL STRUCTURE

It is important to have a general idea of the structure of the program before it begins. This includes the total length of the program, appointment structure, mentor meeting schedule, and feedback plan. Knowing these details will help to set appropriate expectations between the mentor and mentee and should be included in the mentorship agreement. While it is important to have a framework planned, the ideal program should be flexible enough to adapt to the specific needs of an individual mentee as the mentorship progresses.

PROGRAM LENGTH

Formal mentorship programs vary in length. Often, these programs are offered as 6- or 12-month commitments in the clinic. For early-career veterinarians who are entering a second job or coming out of an internship, an accelerated timeline of three months may be sufficient.

Even though the formal mentorship program may end at a defined time, this does not mean that the mentoring relationship ends or that the mentee no longer has support. Some clinics may offer the option to extend the formal program or discuss how to move to a more informal approach after the conclusion of the initial program.

STRUCTURE OF APPOINTMENTS

In-clinic mentorship programs often offer the mentee a progressive plan for seeing appointments and performing procedures. These plans start with longer, less complex appointments and procedures. Over time, the appointment length is shortened while the complexity is increased (see Table A.1). Similar progressions can be developed for surgical (see Figure A.1) and dental (see Figure A.2) procedures.

The following questions should be considered when planning the schedule: (Boatright, 2023).

- How long will the mentee's initial appointments be?
- What is the ideal timeline for moving the mentee to standard appointment lengths?
- Will the mentee be initially restricted to specific appointment types and how will that change over time?
- Can drop-off appointments be utilized to increase case complexity without time pressure?
- How often will the mentee have time for surgical or dental procedures?
- When is the soonest the mentee could be expected to work as the only doctor in the building? Will that affect the length or type of appointments scheduled?
- If the mentee is feeling overwhelmed or rushed, is there an opportunity to slow down the planned progression?
- If the mentee is feeling bored or unchallenged, is there an opportunity to speed up the planned progression?

Table A.1 Sample Mentorship Schedule

Appointment stage	Length of stage	Goals of this stage
Coworking	1 to 4 weeks	• Mentor and mentee share the mentor's normal schedule (both appointments and procedures). • This is not meant to be time for the mentee to simply shadow. The mentee should be encouraged to actively take the lead on cases, but because there is a shared schedule, the mentor is uninterrupted in being able to provide support. • This time is ideal to allow the mentee to meet regular clients and patients, learn workflow, inventory, and computer systems.
Preventive care only	2 to 4 weeks	• Mentee begins to see solo preventive care appointments on extended appointment time (recommended double the length of standard appointments). • Mentor sees normal schedule with availability to support mentee as needed. In the initial week of this (and any stage), it may be helpful for the mentor to have 1–2 appointments blocked per shift to compensate for time spent assisting the mentee.
Mild medical concerns	3–4 weeks	• Mentee continues to see preventive care appointments but add in minor illness and injuries, such as itchy pets, check ears, check eyes, and acute lameness. • Some clinics will focus on adding appointments in a certain discipline each week (i.e. week 1 adds dermatology, week 2 adds ophthalmology, etc.) • If your clinic schedule can accommodate variable appointment lengths, consider starting to transition the mentee to shorter preventive care appointments during this phase. During the transition time, provide occasional blocked appointments as a buffer.
Complex medical concerns	3–4 weeks	• In this stage, add in management of chronic diseases, vomiting and diarrhea, weight loss, and ADR cases. • If your clinic schedule can accommodate variable appointment lengths, consider starting (or continuing) to transition the mentee to shorter preventive care appointments during this phase. It may be difficult to separate "mild" sick cases from "complex" ones for scheduling purposes, but recheck appointments could be offered in a standard appointment length.
Emergency appointments	3–4 weeks	• If your clinic sees emergencies, these are typically the last level of appointment that is added for a mentee. • Be sure that the mentee has experienced support staff and direct access to a mentor veterinarian for these cases as they can be more stressful.
Growing independence	Final 25–50% of the mentorship program	• During this time, the mentee should be on a standard schedule. • Regular mentoring meetings are still occurring, but the frequency may be slowing down.

Source: Adapted by Kate Boatright, VMD from the Veterinary Mentorship Manual (Boatright, 2023).

Stage 1:

Shadowing and Co-working Time

- This is an excellent time to discuss suture type and size choices for common procedures. Even though the mentee will have learned about different sutures during school, they may not have had the opportunity to use the suture material your clinic stocks.
- Start by splitting spays and neuters with the mentor doing half of the surgery and the mentee performing the other half. Be sure to give the mentee opportunities to both
- Once the mentee is comfortable with the procedure, allow them to perform at least one fully supervised surgery before being in the surgery room without a mentor.

Stage 2:

Routine Elective (spay, neuter) Procedures as Primary Surgeon

- Recommend starting with neuters then adding spays.
- Start with cat spays then add dogs in.
- For dog spays and neuters, consider an age or weight cap initially. Remember that even some experienced vets aren't comfortable performing the old, fat dog spay!

Stage 3:

Non-routine Elective (lumpectomy, cystotomy, enucleation, amputation, etc.)

- A mentor should scrub in or be immediately available any time a new procedure is performed by the mentee in case of questions.

Stage 4:

Emergency (exploratory laparotomy, pyometra, C-section, GDV, etc.)

- Since emergency surgeries may occur infrequently depending on your type of practice, give mentees the opportunity to assist on these procedures if the appointment schedule allows.

FIGURE A.1 Surgical procedure progression. *Source:* Reproduced from the Veterinary Mentorship Manual (Boatright, 2023) with permission from Dr. Kate Boatright.

Stage 1:

Shadowing and Co-working Time

- Review dental radiographs together and discuss decision-making around extractions
- Allow mentee to perform dental nerve blocks, flaps, and various extractions under direct supervision.

Stage 2:

Dental Cleaning/Comprehensive Oral Health Assessment and Treatment (COHAT) without anticipated extractions

- Of course there is always the potential for a surprise extraction after the sedated oral examination and radiographs are performed.
- A mentor should be available for support in the event unanticipated extractions are needed.

Stage 3:

Dental Cleaning/COHAT with few, simple anticipated extractions such as incisors and small premolars.

Stage 4:

Dental Cleaning/COHAT with extensive or more complicated anticipated extractions such as canine teeth, carnassial teeth, and lower molars.

Stage 5:

Planned full mouth extractions

FIGURE A.2 Dental procedure progression. *Source:* Reproduced from the Veterinary Mentorship Manual (Boatright, 2023) with permission from Dr. Kate Boatright.

FLEXIBILITY

While having a planned progression of appointment length and complexity is needed to fully structure your mentorship program, maintaining flexibility is of the utmost importance. Each mentee will progress at a different pace. This will be affected by their innate confidence, previous clinical experience, communication skills, and clinical training during school.

Some mentees may be ready for shorter appointments or more complex cases faster than planned. This is the easiest modification to make, as you can start to add additional appointments to the schedule. Drop-off appointments are also an excellent way to add more complexity without a time crunch.

Other mentees may feel unprepared to move to the next stage of their mentorship plan. The mentor and mentee should carefully discuss why these feelings are arising and what is needed to support the mentee. In some cases, it may simply be a lack of confidence or fear, which the mentor can help the mentee to work through—either during one-on-one mentoring time or by providing external resources for support. In others, the mentee truly may not be ready to see more appointments.

Slowing down the schedule is often more difficult due to the fact most clinics are scheduling appointments several weeks into the future. If this occurs, block any unfilled appointments during the transition period back to a slower schedule, discuss with other doctors if they are able to take on any additional cases (this should not be an expectation), and consider moving sick appointments to drop-off appointments to lighten the pace of appointments. Because it is easier to speed up the planned schedule than to slow down, it is likely better to plan for each of the scheduled stages to be on the longer side. The mentor and mentee should assess how the schedule feels from both appointment length and complexity at their weekly mentor meetings and adjust as needed.

MENTOR MEETINGS AND CASE DISCUSSIONS

These meetings are a key component of formalized mentorship programs. They provide a one-on-one opportunity for the mentor and mentee to discuss cases, successes, concerns, goals, and other topics that may not fit into the normal clinic day. These meetings can also incorporate time for formal feedback, evaluation of the mentoring relationship, and periodic review of the mentorship plan. Ultimately, having regular meetings also helps to deepen the relationship between mentor and mentee, build trust, and provide time for check-ins on mental health, well-being, and other concerns.

Mentors and mentees should determine how they want to handle case discussions. Some mentors can still operate efficiently and stay on track with frequent interruptions and prefer the mentee comes to discuss cases and questions throughout the day as they occur. Other mentors prefer to have designated time for case discussions to minimize interruptions during the day. This strategy can help to encourage mentees to triage their questions as urgent (need addressed before the patient leaves the building) and nonurgent (can be answered later by a follow-up call or email to the client after the appointment).

For mentors who prefer designated case review time, it is best to schedule multiple short sessions throughout the week, often for 15 minutes or less. They can be scheduled at the beginning of the day, over the lunch hour, or at the end of the day.

Regardless of how cases are handled, longer mentor meetings should still be scheduled regularly. In the initial stages of the mentoring program, weekly meetings are ideal. Some clinics argue that this takes away too much time from appointments to block 30 to 60 minutes every week for mentor meetings, but the value of these meetings generally outweighs the lost appointment time (see Box A.2).

BOX A.2 CAN WE *REALLY* AFFORD TO HAVE WEEKLY MENTOR MEETINGS?

Use this worksheet to calculate how much revenue you are losing during weekly mentor meetings and compare it to the cost of turnover if the mentee leaves because you didn't follow through or offer weekly meetings.

Calculate the financial cost of a meeting:

A. Mentor's average client transaction (____) X number of missed appointments (___) = Lost revenue from mentor not seeing appointments (_____)
B. Mentee's average client transaction (____) X number of missed appointments (___) = Lost revenue from mentor not seeing appointments (_____)
C. Total lost revenue from a single mentor meeting: Add A and B = __________
D. Total from C (_____) X number of meetings in a 6-month period (____) = Total lost revenue over 6 months (_______)

Now, remember that the cost of turnover is usually estimated at 50–75% of the position's annual salary:

E. Mentee's Salary (________) X 0.75 = Cost of replacement (____________)

Which amount would you rather be looking at: D or E?
Benefits to having weekly mentor meetings:

- Mentee feels more supported and has exceptional mentorship experience, leading them to stay with the clinic after the first year.
- Mentee likely to become a more productive member of the team due to that support, leading to higher long-term revenue.
- More consistency in patient care due to decreased turnover.

Risks of not having weekly mentor meetings:

- Mentee feels unsupported, has a poor mentorship experience, and decides not to renew their contract after the first year.
- Turnover will result in higher workload for remaining veterinarians, utilizing resources for another job search, decreased appointment availability, and interruptions to patient care.

BOX A.3 SAMPLE MENTOR MEETING AGENDA*

1. Check-in
    a. Opportunity for mentee and mentor to share how they feel things are going with work in the clinic, provide updates on personal life, and celebrate successes since the last meeting.
    b. Determine if there are any concerns that need to be prioritized during this meeting (i.e. a particularly difficult case, client interaction, or interaction with team member or a performance concern).

2. Case review
   a. Invite the mentee to bring cases they would like to discuss in more detail as well as their nonurgent case questions to this time.
   b. Consider doing a random chart audit of cases the mentee has seen recently.
   c. The mentor could also present an interesting or complicated case they saw recently.
3. Feedback
   a. This is not intended to be a formalized feedback session at every mentor meeting, though periodically the meetings could be lengthened to include these sessions as opposed to scheduling them separately *(see "Feedback Plan" section below for more details).*
   b. Including some feedback during each mentor meeting can help to decrease the stress of receiving feedback as it becomes routine. Be sure to provide positive feedback as well as opportunities for growth.
   c. This is also a time to evaluate how the mentorship is going and discuss any requested adjustments to the mentorship plan or schedule.
4. Goal assessment
   a. Discuss progress made on current goals and if adjustments are needed.
   b. Celebrate successes!
5. Discussion topic
   a. Consider saving time for a deep dive into a specific topic, which may include a medical condition, surgical procedure, communication skill, leadership skill, personal well-being, mental health, or other topic of interest to the mentee.
   b. Choosing these topics in advance can allow the mentee to engage in self-directed learning before the meeting and allow for a more productive discussion.
6. Looking forward
   a. Outline action steps for responding to any feedback discussed or identified in relation to ongoing goals (these may be for mentee, mentor, or both).
   b. List any resources that are needed to continue to work toward goals (i.e., an introduction to a colleague, new textbook, continuing education course, equipment, etc.).
   c. Choose discussion topic for next meeting.
   d. Confirm next mentor meeting is scheduled.

**This agenda is adapted from Dr. Kate Boatright's Online Mentoring Resources, available at* www.writetheboat.com/mentorship.

As the mentee gains confidence, meetings may be needed less frequently, but these meetings often still have value and allow for intensive discussion of more complex topics over time. The efficiency of these meetings can be improved by having a set agenda so that mentee and mentor know how to prepare for the meeting ahead of time and have a shared expectation of what will be covered (see Box A.3).

A planned frequency of mentor meetings should be included in the mentorship agreement and can be reevaluated over time. To ensure these meetings happen with minimal to no interruption, consider the following scheduling tips:

- Put mentor meetings on the clinic schedule. Do not allow any appointments or procedures during this time.

- Scheduling meetings at the beginning of a shift or right after a lunch break can prevent the meeting getting shortened or canceled because the mentor or mentee are running late in appointments.
- Consider holding meetings outside of the clinic (i.e., go for a walk to meet at a local park or coffee shop) to minimize interruption.

FEEDBACK PLAN

Regular feedback is a critical part of professional and personal development. While delivery of feedback should not be confined to formal feedback sessions or mentoring meetings, setting regular time points for feedback provides opportunities to move away from a "no news is good news" system. For more information on delivering feedback, see Chapter 12.

When determining how feedback will be structured, consider the following questions:

- How often will feedback be provided?
  - In an ideal world, feedback would be delivered multiple times per week, if not daily (Mclain and Nelson, 2022). While this may not always be feasible, it should certainly be delivered more regularly than an annual performance review. At a minimum, in the early stages of mentorship, formal feedback should be scheduled monthly.
  - Consider if this formalized feedback can be built into your regular mentor meetings instead of having a separate time allotted for it. You might consider lengthening some mentor meetings to accommodate this.
- Who is responsible for collecting and delivering feedback?
  - This is most commonly going to be the primary mentor, clinic management, or a combination. Be sure to define who is responsible so that feedback is delivered in a timely manner.
  - Sometimes, if a particular concern arises with a team member, this team member may be encouraged to deliver the feedback directly or be present for the meeting to avoid triangulation.
- How will feedback be delivered?
  - There are many models that can be used to deliver feedback. The preferred style of feedback will be determined by the situation that needs to be addressed and the individual preferences of both the person delivering and receiving the feedback.
- What opportunities are there for 360° feedback?
  - The mentee should be encouraged to provide their own feedback on the mentorship program and their experience with the mentor and the team on a regular basis.

STEP FOUR: THINKING BEYOND THE CLINIC

Most in-clinic mentorship programs rely on formal, in-person, local, and traditional models of mentorship (See "The Mentor-Mentee Relationship" in Chapter 2). These models can be highly effective when delivered well, but veterinary clinics should consider opportunities to augment their in-clinic mentorship by exploring other mentorship models.

One strong opportunity to augment in-clinic mentorship is to enroll the mentee in a formalized online mentorship program. These programs are particularly helpful for supporting the development of communication and leadership skills and supporting mental health and well-being.

Data from one national mentorship program found participants to have improved conflict resolution skills with both clients and team members following completion of the program compared to individuals of similar experience levels who did not participate (Reinhard, 2025). These programs often have a combination of self-directed learning through online modules, live online classes, group mentorship meetings, and peer mentorship support.

Another option to enhance in-clinic mentorship is to encourage the mentee to seek out mentors in their areas of interest, such as exotic companion animal medicine, rehabilitation medicine, or hospice care. This can be particularly helpful if no one in the clinic or local area has that area of expertise and may end up adding a new revenue stream to the clinic. Mentors may be able to use their own networks to make introductions to possible mentors. The clinic can encourage the mentee to engage in external mentoring relationships, which often will be through a distance model.

BIBLIOGRAPHY

American Veterinary Medical Association (2025). Chart of the month: what drives new grads' job choices? [WWW Document]. https://www.avma.org/blog/chart-month-what-drives-new-grads-job-choices (accessed 23 April 2025).

Boatright, K. (2023). Veterinary mentorship manual (PDF download). www.writetheboat.com/mentorship.

Gates, M., McLachlan, I., Butler, S., and Weston, J. (2020). Experiences of recent veterinary graduates in their first employment position and their preferences for new graduate support programmes. *New Zealand Veterinary Journal* 68: 214–224. https://doi.org/10.1080/00480169.2020.1740112.

Jelinski, M.D., Campbell, J.R., MacGregor, M.W., and Watts, J.M. (2009). Factors associated with veterinarians' career path choices in the early postgraduate period. *Canadian Veterinary Journal* 50: 943–948.

Mclain, D. and Nelson, B. (2022). How effective feedback fuels performance [WWW Document]. Gallup.com. https://www.gallup.com/workplace/357764/fast-feedback-fuels-performance.aspx (accessed 25 April 2025).

Reinhard, A. (2025). Fostering confidence and skills: the success of MentorVet leap in nurturing new talent at VCA [WWW Document]. MentorVet.Net. https://www.mentorvet.net/press/mentorvet-vca-fostering-confidence (accessed 23 April 2025).

Index

D

E

T

U

V

W

X